KETOGENIC DIET COOKBOOK FOR BEGINNERS

~ 700 ~

Easy to make and delicious low-carb, high fat recipes, **#2020 edition**. Includes a 21 day diet meal plan, nutritional facts and grocery shopping tips

STELLA RAY MARTIN

© Copyright 2019 by Stella Queen - All rights reserved.

The content contained within this book may not be reproduced, duplicated or transmitted without direct written permission from the author or the publisher.

Under no circumstances will any blame or legal responsibility be held against the publisher, or author, for any damages, reparation, or monetary loss due to the information contained within this book. Either directly or indirectly.

Legal Notice:

This book is copyright protected. This book is only for personal use. You cannot amend, distribute, sell, use, quote or paraphrase any part, or the content within this book, without the consent of the author or publisher.

Disclaimer Notice:

Please note the information contained within this document is for educational and entertainment purposes only. All effort has been executed to present accurate, up to date, and reliable, complete information. No warranties of any kind are declared or implied. Readers acknowledge that the author is not engaging in the rendering of legal, financial, medical or professional advice. The content within this book has been derived from various sources. Please consult a licensed professional before attempting any techniques outlined in this book.

By reading this document, the reader agrees that under no circumstances is the author responsible for any losses, direct or indirect, which are incurred as a result of the use of information contained within this document, including, but not limited to, — errors, omissions, or inaccuracies.

Table of Contents

INTRODUCTION 1
BREAKFAST 2
   01. Breakfast Granola 2
   02. Green Smoothie 2
   03. Muffins Breakfast 2
   04. Special Burrito 2
   05. Coconut and Almonds Granola 3
   06. Red Breakfast Smoothie 3
   07. Tomato and Eggs Breakfast 3
   08. Plantain Pancakes 4
   09. Strawberry and Kiwi Breakfast Smoothie 4
   10. Turkey Breakfast Sandwich 4
   11. Sweet Potato Breakfast 4
   12. Pork Skillet 5
   13. Squash Blossom Frittata 5
   14. Maple Nut Porridge 6
   15. Breakfast Waffles 6
   16. Nuts Porridge 6
   17. Eggplant French Toast 6
   18. Blueberry Smoothie 7
   19. Spinach Frittata 7
   20. Beef Burrito 7
   21. Eggs and Artichokes 8
   22. Italian Scrambled Eggs 8
   23. Egg and Ham Muffins 8
   24. Kale Frittata 9
   25. Shallots Muffins 9
   26. Turkey Frittata 9
   27. Veggie and Egg Mix 10
   28. Shallot and Egg Pancakes 10
   29. Pork and Turkey Mix 10
   30. Turkey Burger 11
   31. Turkey Balls 11
   32. Egg Cups 11
   33. Blackberry Muffins 12
   34. Pumpkin and Berry Muffins 12
   35. Zucchini Muffins 12
   36. Avocado Muffins 13
   37. Spinach Omelet 13
   38. Pesto Omelet 13
   39. Strawberry Sandwich 14
   40. Irish Brown Bread 14
   41. Fresh Fruit Crunch 14
   42. Apple and Quinoa Breakfast Bake 15
   43. Banana and Pear Breakfast Salad 15
   44. Apple Cinnamon Crisp 15
   45. Peanut butter & blueberry Parfait 15
   46. Quinoa Quiche 16
   47. Sweet Rosemary Oats 16
   48. Quinoa Breakfast Bars 16
   49. Granola Breakfast Pops 16
   50. Cinnamon Breakfast Quinoa 17
   51. Cinnamon Walnut Breakfast Parfait 17
   52. Breakfast Taco 17
   53. Egg Spinach Breakfast Muffins 18
   54. Whole Grain Toast with Fruited Ricotta Spread 18
   55. Cherries Oatmeal 18
   56. Strawberry Chia Breakfast Pudding 18
   57. Banana Nutty Oats 19
   58. Breakfast Apple and Raisin Oatmeal 19
   59. Fast Punch 19
   60. Chocolate Covered Banana Quinoa 19
   61. Egg Parsley Omelet 20
MAINS 21
   62. Lime Chicken Soup 21
   63. Spinach Soup 21
   64. Hot Turkey Meatballs 21
   65. Cauliflower Soup 22
   66. Tarragon Cod with Olives 22
   67. Kale Soup 22
   68. Salmon with Balsamic Fennel 22
   69. Carrot Soup 23
   70. Leeks Cream Soup 23
   71. Turkey and Artichokes 23
   72. Smoked Salmon Salad 24
   73. Shrimp with Zucchini 24
   74. Turmeric Broccoli and Leeks Stew 24
   75. Salmon and Green Beans 25
   76. Chicken Stew 25
   77. Spiced Turkey Stew 25
   78. Beans and Salmon Pan 26
   79. Turmeric Cauliflower and Cod Stew 26
   80. Chicken Chili 26
   81. Green Beans Soup 27
   82. Mashed Garlic Turnips 27
   83. Lasagna Spaghetti Squash 27
   84. Blue Cheese Chicken Wedges 27
   85. 'Oh so good' Salad 28
   86. 'I Love Bacon' 28
   87. Lemon Dill Trout 28
   88. 'No Potato' Shepherd's Pie 29
   89. Easy Slider 29
   90. Dijon Halibut Steak 29
   91. Cast-Iron Cheesy Chicken 29
   92. Cauliflower Rice Chicken Curry 29
   93. Bacon Chops 30
   94. Chicken in a Blanket 30
   95. Stuffed Chicken Rolls 30
   96. Duck Fat Ribeye 31
   97. Easy Zoodles & Turkey Balls 31
   98. Sausage Balls 31
   99. Bacon Scallops 31
   100. Buffalo Chicken Salad 31
   101. Meatballs 32
   102. Fat Bombs 32
   103. Cabbage & Beef Casserole 32
   104. Roast Beef Lettuce Wraps 32
   105. Turkey Avocado Rolls 33

106. Nearly Pizza 33
107. Taco Stuffed Peppers 33
108. Beef Tenderloin & Peppercorn Crust 34
109. Bratwursts 34
110. Bacon-Wrapped Hot Dog 34
111. Herb Shredded Beef 34
112. Herbed Butter Rib Eye Steak 34

SIDES 36

113. Grilled Artichokes 36
114. Mashed Yams 36
115. Balsamic Roasted Beets 36
116. Kale Mix 36
117. Pumpkin Fries 37
118. Pumpkin and Bok Choy 37
119. Pumpkin Mash 37
120. Pumpkin Salad 38
121. Turnips and Sauce 38
122. Lemon Fennel 38
123. Plantain Fries 38
124. Roasted Broccoli 39
125. Kumquat Side Salad 39
126. Baked Brussels Sprouts 39
127. Squash and Sweet Potato Mix 39
128. Tapioca Root Fries 40
129. Cauliflower and Turnips 40
130. Roasted Broccoli 40
131. Roasted Cauliflower 40
132. Garlic Plantain Mash 41
133. Sage Kohlrabi 41
134. Spaghetti Squash Mix 41
135. Coconut Butternut Squash 42
136. Cinnamon Butternut Squash 42
137. Stir Fried Veggies 42
138. Flavored Carrots 42
139. Quinoa and Spinach Mix 43
140. Minty Asparagus 43
141. Chard Mix 43
142. Cabbage and Tomatoes 43
143. Carrots Salad 44
144. Sweet Potatoes and Raisins Mix 44
145. Turmeric Okra 44
146. Creamy Green Beans 44
147. Radish and Cabbage Salad 45
148. Baked Beets Mix 45
149. Roasted Sprouts and Carrots 45
150. Coconut Corn and Tomatoes 45
151. Squash Mix 46
152. Cinnamon Carrots Mix 46
153. Brown Rice Salad 46
154. Curry Green Beans 46
155. Onion and Avocado Salad 47
156. Chili Green Beans and Radish 47
157. Broccoli and Peas 47
158. Bok Choy Mix 47
159. Garlic Kale and Bok Choy 48
160. Endives and Watercress Salad 48
161. Zucchini and Kale Mix 48
162. Chili Corn and Zucchinis 49
163. Spinach and Radish Salad 49
164. Low-Carb Pizza Crust 49
165. Bacon-Wrapped Onion Rings 49
166. Smoked BBQ Toasted Almonds 50
167. Roasted Eggplant 50
168. Low-Carb Pita Chips 50
169. Keto Flatbread 50
170. Buffalo Cauliflower 51
171. Brussels Sprout Chips 51
172. Cauliflower Tots 51
173. Herbed Garlic Radishes 52
174. Jicama Fries 52
175. Zesty Salmon Jerky 52
176. Zucchini Bites 52
177. Pop Corn Broccoli 53
178. Rosemary Green Beans 53
179. Carrot Croquettes 53
180. Peppered Puff Pastry 53
181. Sautéed Green Beans 54
182. Horseradish Mayo & Gorgonzola Mushrooms ... 54
183. Scallion & Ricotta Potatoes 54
184. Crumbed Beans 55
185. Colby Potato Patties 55
186. Turkey Garlic Potatoes 55
187. Keto Croutons 56
188. Garlic Stuffed Mushrooms 56
189. Zucchini Sweet Potatoes 56
190. Cheese Lings 57
191. Potato Side Dish 57
192. Roasted Potatoes & Cheese 57
193. Vegetable & Cheese Omelet 57
194. Cabbage rolls stuffed with dried apricots 58
195. Squash pancakes 58
196. Avocado dip 58
197. Rice and Chicken Stuffed Tomatoes 58
198. Stuffed turnips 59
199. Apples stuffed with quark 59
200. Baked pumpkin oatmeal 59
201. Meringue cookies 59
202. Rose hip jelly 60
203. Easy Broccoli and Penne 60
204. Berry soufflé 60
205. White sponge cake 61
206. Roasted asparagus 61
207. Rigatoni with broccoli 61
208. Rutabaga Puree 61
209. Pan Seared Acorn Squash and Pecans 62
210. Shaved Brussels Sprouts with Walnuts 62
211. Honey Mustard Chicken Fillets 62
212. Grilled Pesto Shrimps 63
213. Rosemary Potato Shells 63
214. Basil Tomato Crostini 63

215. Cranberry Spritzer	63
216. Butternut Squash Fries	64

SEAFOOD 65

217. Paleo Salmon	65
218. Fish Dish	65
219. Thai Shrimp Delight	65
220. Salmon Skewers	66
221. Shrimp Dish	66
222. Salmon Tartar Delight	66
223. Salmon And Chili Sauce	67
224. Salmon With Avocado Sauce	67
225. Roasted Trout	68
226. Fish Tacos	68
227. Lobster And Sauce	69
228. Tuna Dish	69
229. Salmon And Lemon Relish	69
230. Salmon And Spicy Slaw	70
231. Grilled Salmon With Peaches	70
232. Wrapped Scallops	71
233. Tuna Cups	71
234. Tuna Skewers in Marinara Sauce	71
235. Piri-Piri Cod	71
236. Steamed Salmon with Lemon	72
237. Tilapia Stew	72
238. Grilled Hake	72
239. Glazed Salmon Fillet	73
240. Curry Fish	73
241. Tagine	73
242. Thyme Seabass	74
243. Fish Chowder	74
244. Coconut Pollock	75
245. Spicy Paella	75
246. Fennel Seabass with Peppercorns	75
247. Tuna Pie	76
248. Fish Cakes with Greens	76
249. Fish Bars	77
250. Pan-fried Cod	77
251. Crab Fat Bombs	77
252. Stuffed Salmon Fillets	78
253. Shrimp Burgers	78
254. Salmon Delight	79
255. Scallops Tartar	79
256. Shrimp Skewers	79
257. Infused Clams	80
258. Halibut And Tasty Salsa	80
259. Shrimp With Mango And Avocado Mix	80
260. Grilled Oysters	81
261. Stuffed Calamari	81
262. Shrimp Cocktail	82
263. Grilled Calamari	82
264. Grilled Salmon And Avocado Sauce	82
265. Crusted Salmon	83
266. Tuna with Chimichurri Sauce	83
267. Salmon and Chili Sauce	83
268. Infused Clams	84
269. Salmon and Apple Mix	84
270. Smoked Shrimp Mix	84
271. Scallops, Grapes and Spinach Bowls	85
272. Crab Cakes and Red Pepper Sauce	85
273. Grilled Oysters	86
274. Squid and Guacamole	86
275. Shrimp and Cauliflower Rice	86
276. Stuffed Salmon Fillets	87
277. Salmon and Coconut Sweet Potato Mash	87
278. Salmon and Spicy Slaw	88
279. Spicy Shrimp	88
280. Salmon and Lemon Relish	89
281. Mussels Mix	89
282. Mahi-Mahi and Cilantro Butter	89
283. Herbed Shrimp Mix	90
284. Grilled Salmon and Lime Sauce	90
285. Shrimp Pan	90
286. Shrimp and Cucumber Noodles	91
287. Walnut Crusted Salmon	91
288. Stuffed Calamari	91
289. Salmon and Chives	92
290. Shrimp Salsa	92
291. Salmon Bites	92
292. Avocado Salsa	93
293. Mussels and Shrimp Bowls	93
294. Calamari Bowls	93
295. Seafood Platter	93
296. Celery Dip	94
297. Creamy Shrimp Bowls	94
298. Herbed Fennel Salsa	94
299. Orange and Mango Salsa	94
300. Smoked Salmon Rolls	95
301. Hot Mussels Bowls	95
302. Tuna and Shrimp Bites	95
303. Tomato and Berries Salsa	96
304. Tomato and Carrot Dip	96
305. Cayenne Avocado and Shrimp Mix	96
306. Radish Bites	96
307. Avocado and Radish Dip	97
308. Orange and Olives Salsa	97
309. Peppers and Radishes Salsa	97
310. Beans Spread	97
311. Mint Avocado and Tomato Dip	98
312. Shrimp, Watermelon and Berries Mix	98
313. Berries Dip	98
314. Cilantro Squares	98
315. Spicy Baked Shrimp	99
316. Shrimp and Cilantro Meal	99
317. The Original Dijon Fish	99
318. Lemony Garlic Shrimp	100
319. Baked Zucchini Wrapped Fish	100
320. Heart-Warming Medi Tilapia	100
321. Baked Salmon and Orange Juice	101
322. Lemon and Almond butter Cod	101
323. Shrimp Scampi	101

324. Lemon and Garlic Scallops.................................. 102
325. Walnut Encrusted Salmon................................. 102
326. Roasted Lemon Swordfish................................ 102
327. Especial Glazed Salmon................................... 103
328. Generous Stuffed Salmon Avocado 103
329. Spanish Mussels 104
330. Tilapia Broccoli Platter...................................... 104
331. Salmon with Peas and Parsley Dressing............ 104
332. Mackerel and Orange Medley 105
333. Spicy Chili Salmon 105
334. Simple One Pot Mussels 105
335. Lemon Pepper and Salmon 106
336. Simple Sautéed Garlic and Parsley Scallops....... 106
337. Salmon and Cucumber Platter 106
338. Tuna Paté 107
339. Cinnamon Salmon... 107
340. Scallop and Strawberry Mix 107
341. Salmon and Orange Dish................................... 108
342. Mesmerizing Coconut Haddock......................... 108
343. Asparagus and Lemon Salmon Dish.................. 108
344. Ecstatic "Foiled" Fish 109
345. Brazilian Shrimp Stew....................................... 109
346. Inspiring Cajun Snow Crab 109
347. Grilled Lime Shrimp 110
348. Calamari Citrus 110
349. Spiced Up Salmon 110
350. Coconut Cream Shrimp 111
351. Shrimp and Avocado Platter 111
352. Calamari 111
353. Hearty Deep Fried Prawn and Rice Croquettes 112
354. Easy Garlic Almond butter Shrimp 112
355. Blackened Tilapia 112
356. Light Lobster Bisque 113
357. Herbal Shrimp Risotto 113
358. Thai Pumpkin Seafood Stew 114
359. Pistachio Sole Fish 114

POULTRY 115
360. Chicken with Tomato Rice 115
361. Turkey with Tomato Asparagus 115
362. Chicken Wings and Potatoes 115
363. Walnuts Chicken Mix 116
364. Chicken with Kidney Beans 116
365. Chicken Thighs and Green Beans Mix............... 116
366. Chicken with Sprouts and Beets........................ 116
367. Chicken with Grapes 117
368. Chicken with Bok Choy 117
369. Tarragon Turkey and Tomatoes.......................... 117
370. Chicken and Thyme Mushrooms 118
371. Chicken with Plums 118
372. Turkey with Apples and Peaches....................... 118
373. Chicken with Green Onions Quinoa.................. 118
374. Chicken with Blackberry Sauce 119
375. Turkey Curry 119
376. Chicken and Avocado 119
377. Ginger Chicken Thighs with Potatoes................ 120
378. Chili Turkey and Peppers 120
379. Chicken with Turmeric Mushrooms 120
380. Baked Turkey... 121
381. Maple Chicken Wings 121
382. Hot Chicken Wings with Artichokes 121
383. Chicken and Cilantro Sauce 121
384. Greek Style Chicken.. 122
385. Classic Whole Chicken with Herbs 122
386. Chicken Jalapeno Quesadillas............................ 122
387. Aromatic Tuscan Chicken 123
388. Baked Paprika Chicken Breast........................... 123
389. Stuffed Chicken Fillets...................................... 124
390. Grilled Chicken 124
391. Cajun Chicken 124
392. Hasselback Chicken Breast 125
393. Chicken Tenders 125
394. Chicken Balls with Coconut Sauce 125
395. Butter Chicken... 126
396. Hot Chicken Chowder.. 126
397. Coconut Chicken Tenders.................................. 127
398. Chicken Loaf 127
399. Chicken Bulgogi 127
400. Mustard Chicken 128
401. Fajitas 128
402. Glazed Duck Breast... 128
403. Duck Confit 129
404. Duck Drumsticks with Blackberry Sauce..........129
405. Oregano Roasted Duck...................................... 129
406. Crispy Duck Skin 130
407. Keto Duck de Marietta 130
408. Duck Pate 130
409. Soft Chicken Pate.. 131
410. Cardamom Chicken Breast 131
411. Balsamic Chicken Thighs 131

MEAT 133
412. Sausage Casserole... 133
413. Mexican Steaks.. 133
414. Beef Tenderloin With Special Sauce.................. 133
415. Roasted Duck Dish 134
416. Steaks And Scallops 134
417. Beef Stir Fry 135
418. Pork With Pear Salsa 135
419. Pork Tenderloin with Carrot Puree 135
420. Pork with Strawberry Sauce 136
421. Beef And Veggies.. 136
422. Chicken Meatballs... 137
423. Chicken And Veggies Stir Fry 137
424. Beef And Brussels Sprouts................................ 138
425. Steaks And Apricots.. 138
426. Beef And Wonderful Gravy............................... 138
427. Sheppard's Pie 139
428. Barbeque Ribs... 139
429. Souvlaki 140
430. Turkey Casserole... 140
431. Moroccan Lamb.. 141

- 432. Carne Asada 141
- 433. Steak And Blueberry Sauce 141
- 434. Filet Mignon And Special Sauce 142
- 435. Veal Rolls 142
- 436. Roasted Lamb 143
- 437. Beef Curry 143
- 438. Beef Teriyaki 143
- 439. Beef Skillet 144
- 440. Thai Curry 144
- 441. Beef Casserole 145
- 442. Grilled Lamb Chops 145
- 443. Lamb Casserole 145
- 444. Lamb Chops with Mint Sauce 146
- 445. Beef Tenderloin and Sauce 146
- 446. Beef Stir Fry 146
- 447. Pork with Blueberry Sauce 147
- 448. Pulled Pork 147
- 449. Barbeque Ribs 148
- 450. Flavored Pork Chops 148
- 451. Pork with Pear Salsa 148
- 452. Pork Tenderloin with Carrot Puree 149
- 453. Pork with Strawberry Sauce 149
- 454. Turkey Casserole 150
- 455. Greek Souvlaki 150
- 456. Mexican Steaks 151
- 457. `Grilled Steaks 151
- 458. Beef Lasagna 151
- 459. Steak and Apricots 152
- 460. Filet Mignon and Sauce 152
- 461. Beef Kabobs 153
- 462. Steak and Veggies 153
- 463. Beef Teriyaki 153
- 464. Beef and Gravy 154
- 465. Steak and Scallops 154
- 466. Sheppard's Pie 155
- 467. Ginger Lamb Chops 155
- 468. Hungarian Sausages 155
- 469. Sesame Pork Tenderloin 156
- 470. Kalua Pork 156
- 471. Pork Belly with Crunchy Crust 156
- 472. Sauteed Pork with Garlic Cloves 157
- 473. Eastern Aromatic Stew 157
- 474. Pork Rollatini 157
- 475. Chipotle Lamb Ribs 158
- 476. Sweet Spare Ribs 158
- 477. Grilled Beef Steaks 158
- 478. Indian Style Pork Saute 159
- 479. Lamb Fillet with Cream Sauce 159
- 480. Rosemary Lamb Roast 159
- 481. Lamb Ragu 160
- 482. Spiced Lamb Shoulder 160
- 483. Butter Lamb Shank 161
- 484. Lamb Vindaloo 161
- 485. Meat Bread 161
- 486. Saddle of Lamb 162
- 487. Herbed Beef Pie 162
- 488. Turmeric Rack of Lamb 163
- 489. Sausage Casserole 163
- 490. Cajun Pork Sliders 163
- 491. Stuffed Beef Loin in Sticky Sauce 164
- 492. BBQ Pork Tenders 164

VEGETABLES 166
- 493. Spinach Dip 166
- 494. Cauliflower Rice 166
- 495. Grilled Sprouts and Balsamic Glaze 166
- 496. Amazing Green Creamy Cabbage 166
- 497. Simple Rice Mushroom Risotto 167
- 498. Hearty Green Bean Roast 167
- 499. Almond and Blistered Beans 168
- 500. Tomato Platter 168
- 501. Lemony Sprouts 168
- 502. Cool Garbanzo and Spinach Beans 168
- 503. Delicious Garlic Tomatoes 169
- 504. Mashed Celeriac 169
- 505. Spicy Wasabi Mayonnaise 169
- 506. Mediterranean Kale Dish 170
- 507. Spicy Kale Chips 170
- 508. Seemingly Easy Portobello Mushrooms 170
- 509. The Garbanzo Bean Extravaganza 171
- 510. Classic Guacamole 171
- 511. Apple Slices 171
- 512. Elegant Cashew Sauce 172
- 513. Lovely Japanese Cabbage Dish 172
- 514. Almond Buttery Green Cabbage 172
- 515. Mesmerizing Brussels and Pistachios ... 172
- 516. Brussels's Fever 173
- 517. Hearty Garlic and Kale Platter 173
- 518. Acorn Squash with Mango Chutney 173
- 519. Satisfying Honey and Coconut Porridge 174
- 520. Pure Maple Glazed Carrots 174
- 521. Ginger and Orange "Beets" 174
- 522. Pineapple Rice 175
- 523. Creative Lemon and Broccoli Dish 175
- 524. Baby Potatoes 175
- 525. Cauliflower Cakes 176
- 526. Tender Coconut and Cauliflower Rice with Chili 176
- 527. Apple Slices 176
- 528. The Exquisite Spaghetti Squash 177
- 529. The Hearty Garlic and Mushroom Crunch 177
- 530. Easy Pepper Jack Cauliflower 177
- 531. The Brussels Platter 178
- 532. The Crazy Southern Salad 178
- 533. Kale and Carrot with Tahini Dressing ... 178
- 534. Crispy Kale 178
- 535. Juicy Summertime Veggies 179
- 536. Crazy Caramelized Onion 179
- 537. Kidney Beans and Cilantro 179
- 538. Broccoli Crunchies 180
- 539. Ultimate Buffalo Cashews 180
- 540. A Green Bean Mixture 180

541. Decisive Cauliflower and Mushroom Risotto ... 181
542. Authentic Zucchini Boats ... 181
543. Roasted Onions and Green Beans ... 181

SOUPS AND STEWS ... 183
544. Turkey Soup ... 183
545. Tomato and Basil Soup ... 183
546. Chicken and Mushroom Soup ... 183
547. Cauliflower Soup ... 184
548. Beef Soup ... 184
549. Root Vegetable Soup ... 184
550. Coconut Chicken Soup ... 185
551. Lemon Soup ... 185
552. Spinach and Watermelon Soup ... 185
553. Cream of Carrot Soup ... 186
554. Beef Stew ... 186
555. Slow Cooked Beef Stew ... 186
556. Veggie and Turkey Stew ... 187
557. Beef and Plantain Stew ... 187
558. Chicken Stew ... 187
559. Lamb and Coconut Stew ... 188
560. Veggie and Kale Stew ... 188
561. French Chicken Stew ... 189
562. Oxtail Stew ... 189
563. Eggplant Stew ... 189
564. Squash Soup ... 190
565. Broccoli Soup ... 190
566. Tomato Gazpacho ... 191
567. Veggie Soup ... 191
568. Jalapeno Chicken Soup ... 191

MEATLESS ... 193
569. Avocado Zucchini Noodles ... 193
570. Sweet & Tangy Green Beans ... 193
571. Tomato Cauliflower Rice ... 193
572. Spinach Pie ... 194
573. Zucchini Eggplant with Cheese ... 194
574. Turnips Mashed ... 194
575. Tasty Coconut Cauliflower Rice ... 195
576. Parmesan Zucchini Chips ... 195
577. Zucchini Carrot Patties ... 195
578. Cauliflower Mac n Cheese ... 196
579. Stir Fried Zucchini ... 196
580. Stir Fry Cauliflower & Cabbage ... 196
581. Avocado Salsa ... 197
582. Cabbage Stir Fry ... 197
588. Cauliflower Fried Rice ... 197
584. Basil Eggplant Casserole ... 198
585. Broccoli Fritters ... 198
586. Simple Stir Fry Brussels sprouts ... 199
587. Sautéed Mushrooms & Zucchini ... 199
588. Healthy Spinach Stir Fry ... 199
589. Roasted Carrots ... 200
590. Creamy Garlic Basil Mushrooms ... 200
591. Zucchini Noodles with Spinach ... 200
592. Parmesan Pepper Eggs ... 201
593. Vegetable Egg Scramble ... 201

SALADS ... 202
594. Shrimp and Asparagus Salad ... 202
595. Carrot and walnut salad ... 202
596. Pickled onion salad ... 202
597. Chicken Raisin Salad ... 202
598. Pickled Grape Salad with Pear, Taleggio and Walnuts ... 203
599. Mango salad ... 203
600. Fresh Fruit Salad ... 203
601. Dried apricot sauce ... 204
602. Tomato, Cucumber, and Basil Salad ... 204
603. Strawberries and Avocado Salad ... 204
604. Kelp salad ... 204
605. Chicken celery salad ... 205
606. Garlic Potato Salad ... 205
607. Spring salad ... 205
608. Appetizing Cucumber Salad ... 205
609. Tuna Caprese Salad ... 206
610. Cabbage and Carrot Salad ... 206
611. Warm Asparagus Salad with Oranges ... 206
612. Chicken in Orange Sauce ... 207
613. Pumpkin salad ... 207
614. Sweet Jicama Salad ... 207
615. Heart Healthy Chicken Salad ... 207
616. Cashews and Blueberries Salad ... 208
617. Radish Salad ... 208
618. Tarragon Tomatoes ... 208

SNACKS ... 209
619. Seeds Bowls ... 209
Snow Peas and Tomato Salsa ... 209
Apple Chips ... 209
622. Dill Cucumber Dip ... 209
623. Beans Salsa ... 209
624. Bell Peppers and Zucchinis Patties ... 210
625. Broccoli Bites ... 210
626. Balsamic Mushrooms Mix ... 210
627. Almond Artichoke Dip ... 211
628. Balsamic Pineapple Bites ... 211
629. Parsley Pearl Onions Mix ... 211
630. Clam Platter ... 211
631. Mustard Tuna Bites ... 212
632. Kale Chips ... 212
633. Avocado Salsa ... 212
634. Keto Marinated Eggs ... 212
635. Keto Bread Sticks ... 213
636. Special Keto Hummus ... 213
637. Keto Sausage And Cheese Dip ... 213
638. Chicken Egg Rolls ... 214
639. Easy Jalapeno Crisps ... 214
640. Keto Crab Dip ... 214
641. Keto Chili Lime Chips ... 215
642. Zucchini Rolls ... 215
643. Italian Style Meatballs ... 215
644. Keto Mushrooms Appetizer ... 216
645. Keto Broccoli Sticks ... 216
646. Caviar Salad ... 216

- 647. Tasty Bacon Delight 216
- 648. Delicious Corndogs 217
- 649. Keto Almond Butter Bars 217
- 650. Easy Keto Zucchini Snack 218
- 651. Green Crackers 218
- 652. Beef Jerky Snack 218
- 653. Spinach Garlic Dip 218
- 654. Marinated Keto Kebabs 219
- 655. Pesto And Cheese Terrine 219

DESSERTS 220
- 656. Low Carb Chocolate Coconut Fat Bombs 220
- 657. Crunchy Cherry Chocolate Confections 220
- 658. Low Carb Keto Caramels 220
- 659. Coconut Chocolate Bars 221
- 660. Keto Pumpkin Fudge 221
- 661. Low-Carb, Keto Strawberry Fat Bombs 222
- 662. Paleo Vegan Peppermint Patties 222
- 663. Keto Marshmallows 222
- 664. White Chocolate Butter Pecan Fat Bombs 223
- 665. Keto Low Carb Gummy Bears 223
- 666. Keto Chocolate Chip Cookies 224
- 667. Bakery-Style' Salted Chocolate Chip Cookies ... 224
- 668. Chocolate Chip Keto Cookie 225
- 669. Peanut Butter Cookies 225
- 670. Low Carb Keto Cream Cheese Cookies 226
- 671. Sugar-Free Paleo Pecan Snowball Cookies 226
- 672. Chocolate Chip Cookies with Coconut Flour 226
- 673. Cinnamon Keto French Toast Cookies 227
- 674. Gluten-free Flourless Chocolate Cookies 227
- 675. Low Carb Shortbread Cookies Recipe 228
- 676. Coconut Mousse 228
- 677. Blueberry Cream 228
- 678. Lemon Apple Mix 228
- 679. Minty Rhubarb 229
- 680. Nigella Mango Sweet Mix 229
- 681. Blueberry Compote 229
- 682. Lentils and Dates Brownies 229
- 683. Blueberry Curd 230
- 684. Almond Peach Mix 230
- 685. Coconut Cream 230
- 686. Cinnamon Apples 230
- 687. Green Tea Cream 231
- 688. Coconut Figs 231
- 689. Cocoa Banana Dessert Smoothie 231
- 690. Chocolate Pomegranate Fudge 231
- 691. Cheese Stuffed Apples 231
- 692. Green Apple Bowls 232
- 693. Peach Dip 232
- 694. Cashew Nut Cuppas 232
- 695. Pecan Granola 232
- 696. Walnut Green Beans 233
- 697. Banana Sashimi 233
- 698. Maple Malt 233
- 699. Parmesan Roasted Chickpeas 233
- 700. Apricot Nibbles 234
- 701. All Dressed Crispy Potato Skins 234
- 702. Delightful Coconut Shrimp 234
- 703. Creamy Peanuts with Apples 235

21-DAYS MEAL PLAN 236
CONCLUSION 237

Introduction

Recent studies have shown that a higher protein, low carbohydrate diet promotes improvements in blood lipid parameters, increased thermogenesis in individuals with obesity and superior results for fat reduction, insulin resistance and might help to solve the metabolic blocks which can prevent fat loss.

When starting a Ketogenic diet program, you may experience some distress such as headaches, fatigue, irritability, and hunger for your initial 2-7 days, nevertheless thereafter it is very simple to stick to this diet and it actually reduces appetite, increases energy levels and carbohydrate cravings.

The Ketogenic diet produces excellent results when followed consistently. Long term success is much more likely possible if a holistic approach is adopted that addresses exercise, daily diet, nutritional supplements and psychological factors in addition to some specific health challenges which are unique to the individual.

Even though ketosis is the foundation of the ketogenic diet type, in its strictest form it does not have to be maintained for very long. The state of ketosis may be held up until the weight is merely a couple of pounds higher than what is desired. Afterward, foods with higher quantities of carbs are slowly introduced (rice, beans,...).

In this particular period, it will be very helpful to keep a food consumption diary where regular amounts of taken carbs will be observed. The way you can discover the maximum amount of everyday carbs that nonetheless allows you never to gain weight. When you learn this particular parameter, you'll not have heavy related issues, because, until that moment, you'll definitely discover how to have an account of amounts and calories of carbohydrates, fats, and proteins which you eat every day.

The approach you will get to know the body much better, in the terminology of the optimum "allowable" daily intake. Due to that, we can say the ketogenic diet plan is, a process for learning habits which will see to it that you never ever go back to the existing tricky obese amounts. You will find numerous kinds of ketogenic diet programs which are available in different sources, though they almost all have in typical one fundamental concept - intake of high quantities of fats and proteins, and little amounts of carbs.

Breakfast

01. Breakfast Granola

Preparation Time: 55 minutes
Servings: 6

Ingredients:

- 2 tsp. cinnamon powder
- 1½ cups almond flour
- 2 tsp. nutmeg; ground
- 1/2 cup coconut flakes
- 2 tsp. vanilla extract
- 1/2 cup walnuts; chopped
- 1/3 cup coconut oil
- 1/4 cup hemp hearts

Instructions:

1. In a bowl; combine almond flour with coconut flakes, walnuts, cinnamon, nutmeg, vanilla, hemp and walnuts, stir well and spread on a baking sheet.
2. Bake in the oven at 275 °F and bake for 50 minutes, stirring every 10 minutes. Transfer to plates when the granola is cold and serve for breakfast.

Nutrition: Calories: 250; Fat: 23g; Fiber: 4g; Carbs: 5g; Protein: 6g

02 Green Smoothie

Preparation Time: 5 minutes
Servings: 3

Ingredients:

- 1 small cucumber; peeled and chopped
- 1 green apple; chopped
- Juice of 1/2 lemon
- Juice of 1/2 lime
- 1 tbsp. ginger; finely grated
- 1 tbsp. gelatin powder
- 1 cup kale; chopped
- 1 cup coconut water

Instructions:

1. In your kitchen blender, mix the apple with cucumber, ginger and kale and pulse a few times.
2. Add lime and lemon juice, coconut water and gelatin powder and blend a few more times. Transfer to glasses and serve right away.

Nutrition: Calories: 180; Fat: 1g; Carbs: 42g; Fiber: 7g; Sugar: 0g, protein: 7g

03. Muffins Breakfast

Preparation Time: 40 minutes
Servings: 4

Ingredients:

- 1 cup kale; chopped
- Some coconut oil for greasing the muffin cups
- 1/4 cup chives; finely chopped
- 1/2 cup almond milk
- 6 eggs
- Black pepper to the taste

Instructions:

1. In a bowl; mix eggs with chives and kale and whisk very well.
2. Add black pepper to the taste and almond milk and stir well.
3. Divide this into 8 muffin cups after you've greased it with some coconut oil.
4. Introduce this in preheated oven at 350 °F and bake for 30 minutes. Take muffins out of the oven, leave them to cool down, transfer them to plates and serve warm.

Nutrition: Calories: 100; Fat: 5g; Protein: 14; Sugar: 0

04. Special Burrito

Preparation Time: 25 minutes
Servings: 2

- **Ingredients:**
- 1/4 cup canned green chilies; chopped
- 1 small yellow onion; chopped
- 4 eggs; egg yolks and whites divided
- 1/4 cup cilantro; chopped
- 1 red bell pepper; finely cut in strips

- 2 tomatoes; chopped
- 1/2 cup beef; ground and browned for 10 minutes
- 1 avocado; peeled, pitted and chopped
- Some hot sauce for serving
- A drizzle of olive oil

Instructions:
1. Heat up a pan with a drizzle of olive oil over medium high heat, add half of the egg whites after you've whisked them in a bowl; spread evenly and cook for 1 minute.
2. Flip them cook for 1 minute more, transfer to a plate and repeat the action with the rest of the egg whites.
3. Heat up the same pan over medium high heat, add onions, stir and cook for 1 minute.
4. Add chilies, bell pepper, tomato, meat and cilantro, stir and cook for 5 minutes. Add egg yolks, stir well and cook until they are done.
5. Arrange egg whites tortillas on 2 plates, divide eggs and meat mix between them, add some chopped avocado and hot sauce, roll and serve them for breakfast.

Nutrition: Calories: 255; Fat: 23g; Fiber: 3g; Carbs: 7g; Protein: 12g

05. Coconut and Almonds Granola

Preparation Time: 45 minutes
Servings: 4

Ingredients:
- 3 cups coconut flakes
- 1½ cups almonds; chopped
- 1/2 cup sesame seeds
- 1/2 cup sunflower seeds
- 1/2 tsp. cinnamon; ground
- 2 tbsp. chia seeds
- 1/2 cup maple syrup
- A pinch of cardamom
- 1 tsp. vanilla extract
- 2 tbsp. olive oil

Instructions:
1. In a bowl; mix almonds with sunflower seeds, sesame seeds, coconut, chia seeds, cardamom and cinnamon and stir.
2. Meanwhile; heat up a small pot over medium heat, add oil, vanilla and maple syrup, stir well and cook for about 1 minute.
3. Pour this over almonds mix, stir everything, spread on a baking sheet, bake in the oven at 300 °F for 25 minutes, stirring the mixture after 15 minutes. Leave your special granola to cool down before dividing it between plates and serving it.

Nutrition: Calories: 270; Fat: 13g; Fiber: 5g; Carbs: 7g; Protein: 8g

06. Red Breakfast Smoothie

Preparation Time: 5 minutes
Servings: 2

Ingredients:

1 small red bell pepper; seeded and roughly chopped
- 5 strawberries; cut in halves
- 1 tomato; cut into 4 wedges
- 1 cup red cabbage; chopped
- 1/2 cup raspberries
- 8 oz. water
- 2 ice cubes for serving

Instructions:
1. In your food processor, mix cabbage with bell pepper, tomato, strawberries and raspberries and pulse well until you obtain cream.
2. Add water and pulse well a few more times. Transfer to glasses and serve with ice cubes.

Nutrition: Calories: 189; Fat: 2g; Carbs: 40g; Fiber: 7; Sugar: 1g; Protein: 5g

07. Tomato and Eggs Breakfast

Preparation Time: 40 minutes
Servings: 2

Ingredients:
- 2 tomatoes

- 2 eggs
- A pinch of black pepper
- 1 tsp. parsley; finely chopped
- Instructions:
- Cut tomatoes tops, scoop flesh and arrange them on a lined baking sheet.
- Crack an egg in each tomato.
- Season with salt and pepper. Introduce them in the oven at 350 °F and bake for 30 minutes.
- Take tomatoes out of the oven, divide between plates, season with pepper, sprinkle parsley at the end and serve.

Nutrition: Calories: 186g; Protein: 14; Fat: 10; Sugar: 6

08. Plantain Pancakes

Preparation Time: 20 minutes
Servings: 1

Ingredients:

- 1/2 plantain; peeled and chopped
- 1 tbsp. shaved coconut; toasted for serving
- 1 tbsp. coconut milk for serving
- 3 eggs
- 1/4 cup coconut flour
- 1/4 cup coconut water
- 1 tsp. coconut oil
- 1/4 tsp. cream of tartar
- 1/4 tsp. baking soda
- 1/4 tsp. chai spice

Instructions:

1. In your food processor, mix eggs with coconut water and flour, plantain, cream of tartar, baking soda and chai spice and blend well.
2. Heat up a pan with the coconut oil over medium heat, add 1/4 cup pancake batter, spread evenly, cook until it becomes golden, flip pancake and cook for 1 more minute and transfer to a plate.
3. Repeat this with the rest of the batter. Serve pancakes with shaved coconut and coconut milk.

Nutrition: Calories: 372; Fat: 17g; Carbs: 55g; Fiber: 12; Sugar: 21g; Protein: 23g

09. Strawberry and Kiwi Breakfast Smoothie

Preparation Time: 10 minutes
Servings: 2

Ingredients:

- 1½ cups kiwi; chopped
- 1½ cups frozen strawberries; chopped
- 8 mint leaves
- 2 cups crushed ice
- 2 oz. water

Instructions:

1. **In your blender, mix kiwi with strawberries and mint and pulse well.**
2. Add water and crushed ice and pulse again.
3. Transfer to glasses and serve right away.

Nutrition: Calories: 133; Fat: 1g; Carbs: 34g; Fiber: 4; Sugar: 9g; Protein: 1.3

10. Turkey Breakfast Sandwich

Preparation Time: 5 minutes
Servings: 1

Ingredients:

- 2 oz. turkey meat; roasted and thinly sliced
- 2 tbsp. pecans; toasted and chopped
- 2 slices paleo coconut bread
- 2 tbsp. cranberry chutney
- 1/4 cup arugula

Instructions:

1. In a bowl; mix pecans with chutney and stir well.
2. Spread this on bread slice, add turkey slices and arugula and top with the other bread slice. Serve right away.

Nutrition: Calories: 540; Fat: 11g; Carbs: 52g; Fiber: 4; Sugar: 13g; Protein: 32

11. Sweet Potato Breakfast

Preparation Time: 25 minutes

Servings: 4

Ingredients:

- 2 Italian sausages; casings removed
- 4 tbsp. coconut oil
- 1 small green bell pepper; chopped
- 1/2 cup onion; chopped
- 2 garlic cloves; minced
- 2 cups sweet potato; chopped
- 1 avocado; peeled, pitted, cut into halves and thinly sliced
- 3 eggs
- 2 cups spinach

Instructions:

1. Heat up a pan with the oil over medium high heat, add onion, stir and cook for 3 minutes.
2. Add garlic and bell pepper, stir and cook for 1 minute.
3. Add sausage meat, stir and brown for 4 minutes more.
4. Add sweet potato, stir and cook for 4 minutes.
5. Add spinach, stir and cook for 2 minutes.
6. Make 3 holes in this mix, crack an egg in each, introduce pan in preheated broiler and cook for 3 minutes. Divide this tasty mix on plates, add avocado pieces on the side and serve.

Nutrition: Calories: 200; Fat: 4g; Fiber: 2g; Carbs: 6g; Protein: 9g

12. Pork Skillet

Preparation Time: 30 minutes
Servings: 4

Ingredients:

- 8 oz. mushrooms; chopped
- 1 lb. pork; ground
- 1 tbsp. olive oil
- Black pepper to the taste
- 2 zucchinis; cut in halves and then in half moons
- 1/2 tsp. garlic powder
- 1/2 tsp. basil; dried
- A pinch of sea salt
- 2 tbsp. Dijon mustard

Instructions:

1. Heat up a pan with the oil over medium high heat, add mushrooms, stir and cook for 4 minutes.
2. Add zucchinis, a pinch of salt and black pepper, stir and cook for 4 minutes more.
3. Add pork, garlic powder and basil, stir and cook until meat is done. Add mustard, stir well, cook for a couple more minutes, divide between plates and serve.

Nutrition: Calories: 200; Fat: 4g; Fiber: 2g; Carbs: 5g; Protein: 12g

13. Squash Blossom Frittata

Preparation Time: 50 minutes
Servings: 4

Ingredients:

- 10 eggs; whisked
- Black pepper to the taste
- 1/4 cup coconut cream
- 1 yellow onion; finely chopped
- 1 leek; thinly sliced
- 2 scallions; thinly sliced
- 2 zucchinis; chopped
- 8 squash blossoms
- 2 tbsp. avocado oil

Instructions:

1. In a bowl; mix eggs with coconut cream and black pepper to the taste and stir well.
2. Heat up a pan with the oil over medium high heat, add leek and onions, stir and cook for 5 minutes.
3. Add zucchini, stir and cook for 10 more minutes.
4. Add eggs, spread, reduce heat to low, cook for 5 minutes.
5. Sprinkle scallions and arrange squash blossoms on frittata, press blossoms into eggs, introduce everything in the oven at 350 °F and bake for 20 minutes. Take frittata out of the oven, leave it to cool down, cut, arrange on plates and serve it.

Nutrition: Calories: 123; Fat: 8g; Protein: 7g; Carbs: 2; Sugar: 0

14. Maple Nut Porridge

Preparation Time: 10 minutes
Servings: 2

Ingredients:

- 2 tbsp. coconut butter
- 1/2 cup pecans; soaked
- 3/4 cup hot water
- 1 banana; peeled and chopped
- 1/2 tsp. cinnamon
- 2 tsp. maple syrup

Instructions:

1. In your food processor, mix pecans with water, coconut butter, banana, cinnamon and maple syrup and blend well.
2. Transfer this to a pan, heat up over medium heat until it thickens, pour into bowls and serve.

Nutrition: Calories: 170; Fat: 9g; Carbs: 20g; Fiber: 6g; Protein: 6g

15. Breakfast Waffles

Preparation Time: 20 minutes
Servings: 4

Ingredients:

- 2 eggs
- 1/2 cup almond milk
- 2 tbsp. coconut oil; melted
- 1/2 tsp. cinnamon; ground
- 1 tbsp. baking powder
- 1 tbsp. coconut flour
- 2 tbsp. honey
- 1½ cups almond flour
- 1/4 cup tapioca flour
- 1½ tsp. vanilla extract
- Pure maple syrup for serving

Instructions:

1. In your mixer bowl; combine coconut flour with almond flour, tapioca flour, baking powder and cinnamon and stir.
2. Add egg yolks, almond milk, coconut oil, honey and vanilla extract and blend very well.
3. In another bowl; whisk egg whites with your mixer.
4. Add them to waffles mix and stir everything very well.
5. Pour this into your waffle iron and make 8 waffles. Divide them on plates, top with maple syrup and serve.

Nutrition: Calories: 160; Fat: 11g; Fiber: 2g; Carbs: 7g; Protein: 6g

16. Nuts Porridge

Preparation Time: 15 minutes
Servings: 2

Ingredients:

- 1/2 cup pecans; soaked overnight and drained
- 1/2 banana; mashed
- 3/4 cup hot water
- 2 tbsp. coconut butter
- 1/2 tsp. cinnamon
- 2 tsp. maple syrup

Instructions:

1. In a blender, mix pecans, with water, banana, coconut butter, cinnamon and maple syrup, pulse really well and transfer to a small pot.
2. Heat everything up over medium heat, cook until it's creamy, transfer to serving bowls and serve.

Nutrition: Calories: 150; Fat: 2g; Fiber: 2g; Carbs: 4g; Protein: 6g

17. Eggplant French Toast

Preparation Time: 10 minutes
Servings: 2

Ingredients:

- 1 eggplant; peeled and sliced
- 1 tsp. vanilla extract
- 2 eggs
- Stevia to the taste
- 1 tsp. coconut oil
- A pinch of cinnamon

Instructions:

1. In a bowl; mix eggs with vanilla, stevia

and cinnamon and whisk well.
2. Heat up a pan with the coconut oil over medium-high heat.
3. Dip eggplant slices in eggs mix, add to heated pan and cook until they become golden on each side. Arrange them on plates and serve.

Nutrition: Calories: 125; Fat: 5g; Protein: 7.8g; Carbs: 13g; Fiber: 7.8

18. Blueberry Smoothie

Preparation Time: 5 minutes
Servings: 2

Ingredients:
- 2 cups blueberries
- 1 tsp. lemon zest
- 1/2 cup coconut milk
- A pinch of cinnamon
- Water as needed

Instructions:
1. In your kitchen blender, mix coconut milk with blueberries, lemon zest and a pinch of cinnamon and pulse a few times.
2. Add water as needed to thin your smoothie and pulse a few more times. Transfer to a tall glass and serve.

Nutrition: Calories: 177; Fat: 3g; Carbs: 45g; Fiber: 7; Sugar: 12g; Protein: 3g

19. Spinach Frittata

Preparation Time: 50 minutes
Servings: 4

Ingredients:
- 1/2 lb. sausage; ground
- 2 tbsp. ghee
- 1 cup mushrooms; thinly sliced
- 1 cup spinach leaves; chopped
- 10 eggs; whisked
- 1 small yellow onion; finely chopped
- Black pepper to the taste

Instructions:
1. Heat up a pan with the ghee over medium-high heat, add onion and some black pepper, stir and cook until it browns.
2. Add sausage, stir and also cook until it browns. Add spinach and mushrooms and cook for 4 minutes, stirring from time to time.
3. Take the pan off the heat, add eggs, spread evenly, introduce frittata in the oven at 350 °F and bake for 20 minutes.
4. Take frittata out of the oven, leave it aside for a few minutes to cool down, cut, arrange on plates and serve.

Nutrition: Calories: 233; Fat: 13g; Carbs: 4g; Fiber: 1.2; Sugar: 1g; Protein: 21g

20. Beef Burrito

Preparation time: 10 minutes
Cooking time: 15 minutes
Servings: 2

Ingredients:
- 0,5 oz green chilies, chopped
- 1 small yellow onion, chopped
- 4 eggs, egg yolks and whites separated
- ¼ cup cilantro, chopped
- 1 red bell pepper, finely cut into strips
- 2 tomatoes, chopped
- ½ cup beef meat, ground and browned for 10 minutes
- 1 avocado, peeled, pitted and chopped
- A drizzle of olive oil

Directions:
1. Heat up a pan with some olive oil over medium-high heat, add half of the egg whites after you've whisked them in a bowl, spread evenly, cook for 1 minute on each side and transfer to a plate.
2. Repeat the process with the rest of the egg whites and leave the egg "burritos" to one side.
3. Heat up the same pan over medium-high heat, add the onions, stir and sauté for 2 minutes.
4. Add chilies, bell pepper, tomato, meat, and cilantro, stir and cook for 5 minutes.
5. Add egg yolks, stir well and cook everything for 4-5 minutes more.

6. Divide the egg white burritos between 2 plates, divide the meat mixture, also divide the avocado, roll and serve for breakfast.
7. Enjoy!

Nutrition: calories 489, fat 37,4, fiber 9,8, carbs 22,2, protein 21,3

21. Eggs and Artichokes

Preparation time: 20 minutes
Cooking time: 30 minutes
Servings: 2

Ingredients:

- 1 egg white, whisked
- 4 eggs
- ¾ cup balsamic vinegar
- 4 ounces shallots, cooked and chopped
- 4 artichoke hearts, chopped
- A pinch of sea salt and black pepper
- For the sauce:
- 1 tablespoon lemon juice
- ¾ cup ghee, softened
- 4 egg yolks
- ¼ teaspoon sweet paprika

Directions:

1. Put artichoke hearts in a bowl, add the vinegar, toss well to combine and leave aside for 20 minutes
2. In a bowl, mix the egg yolks with paprika and lemon juice and whisk.
3. Put some water into a saucepan and bring to a simmer over medium heat.
4. Put the bowl with the egg yolks over the simmering water and stir constantly.
5. Add melted ghee gradually, stir until the sauce thickens and take off heat.
6. Drain artichokes, arrange them on a lined baking sheet, brush them with the egg white, sprinkle salt, pepper and the chopped shallots on top, and bake at 375 degrees F for 20 minutes.
7. Heat up a saucepan with some water, bring to a simmer over medium heat, crack the 4 whole eggs into the pan, poach them for 1 minute and divide them between plates.
8. Add the baked artichokes on the side, drizzle the egg yolk sauce all over and serve.

Nutrition: calories 1130, fat 94,9, fiber 17,6, carbs 46,7, protein 30,6

22. Italian Scrambled Eggs

Preparation time: 10 minutes
Cooking time: 10 minutes
Servings: 1

Ingredients:

- 2 eggs, whisked
- ¼ teaspoon rosemary, dried
- ½ cup cherry tomatoes halved
- 1 and ½ cups kale, chopped
- ½ teaspoon coconut oil, melted
- 3 tablespoons water
- 1 teaspoon balsamic vinegar
- ¼ avocado, peeled, pitted and chopped

Directions:

1. Heat up a pan with the oil over medium heat, add the water, kale, rosemary, and tomatoes, stir, cover and cook for 5 minutes.
2. Add the eggs, stir and scramble everything for 4 minutes more.
3. Add the vinegar, toss, transfer this to a plate, top with chopped avocado and serve.
4. Enjoy!

Nutrition: calories 403, fat 21,3, fiber 15,5, carbs 26,2, protein 24

23. Egg and Ham Muffins

Preparation time: 10 minutes
Cooking time: 15 minutes
Servings: 4

Ingredients:

- 4 eggs
- 10 ham slices
- 4 tablespoons scallions, chopped
- A pinch of black pepper
- ½ teaspoon sweet paprika
- 1 tablespoon melted ghee

Directions:
1. Grease a muffin pan with the melted ghee and divide the ham slices in each muffin mold to shape your cups.
2. In a bowl, mix the eggs with scallions, pepper, and paprika, whisk well, divide this into the ham cups, and bake at 400 degrees F for 15 minutes.
3. Divide between plates and serve for breakfast.

Nutrition: calories 214, fat 14,2, fiber 1,2, carbs 3,6, protein 17,3

24. Kale Frittata

Preparation time: 10 minutes
Cooking time: 30 minutes
Servings: 4

Ingredients:
- 3 small shallots, cooked and crumbled
- 1/3 cup yellow onion, chopped
- 1 tablespoon coconut oil, melted
- ½ cup red bell pepper, chopped
- 2 cups kale, torn
- ½ cup almond milk
- 8 eggs
- A pinch of black pepper

Directions:
1. In a bowl, mix the eggs with black pepper and the milk then whisk.
2. Heat up a pan with the oil over medium heat, add the bell pepper and onion, stir and sauté for 3 minutes.
3. Add kale, stir and cook for 5 minutes more.
4. Add the shallots and eggs, spread evenly into the pan, cook for 4 minutes and then bake at 350 degrees F for 15 minutes.
5. Divide between plates and serve.
6. Enjoy!

Nutrition: calories 264, fat 19,4, fiber 1,6, carbs 11,2, protein 13,5

25. Shallots Muffins

Preparation time: 10 minutes
Cooking time: 30 minutes
Servings: 4

Ingredients:
- 4 ounces shallots, sliced, chopped
- 3 garlic cloves, minced
- 1 small yellow onion, chopped
- 1 zucchini, sliced
- A handful spinach, torn
- 6 artichoke hearts, boiled, chopped
- 8 eggs, whisked
- ¼ teaspoon paprika
- A pinch of black pepper
- ¼ cup coconut cream

Directions:
1. Heat up a pan over medium-high heat, add the chopped shallots, cook until crispy, transfer to paper towels to drain excessive oil and leave aside for now.
2. Heat up the same pan over medium heat, add garlic and onion, stir and cook for 4 minutes.
3. In a bowl, mix eggs with coconut cream, onions, garlic, paprika, and black pepper and whisk well.
4. Add spinach, zucchini and artichokes and stir everything.
5. Divide the shallots in a muffin pan into four flat piles, add the egg mixture, place everything in the oven and bake at 400 degrees F for 20 minutes.
6. Cool down and serve for breakfast.
7. Enjoy!

Nutrition: calories 314, fat 12,9, fiber 14,6, carbs 36,1, protein 21,1

26. Turkey Frittata

Preparation time: 10 minutes
Cooking time: 30 minutes
Servings: 4

Ingredients:
- 10 eggs, whisked
- 2 tablespoons ghee, melted
- 1 cup spinach, chopped
- ½ pound turkey meat, minced
- 1 cup mushrooms, chopped

- 1 small yellow onion, chopped
- A pinch of sea salt and black pepper

Directions:
1. Heat up a pan with the ghee over medium-high heat, add the turkey mince, stir and brown for 2 minutes.
2. Add onion, mushroom, spinach, a pinch of salt and black pepper, stir and cook for 5 more minutes.
3. Add whisked eggs, spread evenly into the pan, toss, place in the oven and bake the frittata at 350 degrees F for 20 minutes.
4. Slice, divide between plates and serve.
5. Enjoy!

Nutrition: calories 322, fat 20,2, fiber 0,7, carbs 3,3, protein 31,4

27. Veggie and Egg Mix

Preparation time: 10 minutes
Cooking time: 25 minutes
Servings: 4

Ingredients:
- 4 ounces shallots, peeled, sliced, chopped
- 12 cherry tomatoes, halved
- ½ teaspoon turmeric powder
- ½ onion, chopped
- 5 eggs
- 2 Serrano peppers, chopped
- 1 green bell pepper, chopped
- A pinch of sea salt and black pepper

Directions:
1. In a bowl, mix the eggs with salt, black pepper, Serrano peppers, green pepper, and turmeric and whisk.
2. Heat up a pan over medium heat, add the shallots, stir and cook for 3 minutes.
3. Add the onion, stir and sauté for 2 minutes more.
4. Add eggs and tomatoes, stir, cook for 6 minutes and then bake in the oven at 350 degrees F for 15 minutes.
5. Divide between plates and serve.
6. Enjoy!

Nutrition: calories 182, fat 6,4, fiber 5,3, carbs 23,4, protein 11,4

28. Shallot and Egg Pancakes

Preparation time: 10 minutes
Cooking time: 30 minutes
Servings: 4

Ingredients:
- 12 small shallots, cooked and crumbled
- 8 eggs, whisked
- Black pepper to taste
- 1 tablespoon coconut oil
- 10 grain-free paleo pancakes
- For the pancakes:
- 1 cup almond flour
- 1 cup coconut flour
- ½ teaspoon baking soda
- 1 teaspoon cinnamon powder
- 1 cup almond milk
- 2 eggs, whisked
- 1 teaspoon vanilla extract
- 3 tablespoons maple syrup
- 2 tablespoons coconut oil, melted

Directions:
1. In a bowl, mix the almond flour with coconut flour, baking soda, cinnamon, milk, 2 eggs, maple syrup and vanilla extract and stir well until you obtain a smooth batter.
2. Heat up a pan with 2 tablespoons coconut oil over medium heat, add 1/10 of the batter, spread into the pan, cook for 2 minutes on each side and transfer to a plate.
3. Repeat with the rest of the batter and divide the pancakes between plates.
4. Heat up a pan with 1 tablespoon oil over medium high heat, add whisked eggs, shallots, and black pepper, cook for 5 minutes and take off the heat.
5. Divide this on top of the pancakes, roll them and serve for breakfast.
6. Enjoy!

Nutrition: calories 883, fat 54, fiber 18,5, carbs 75,4, protein 29,7

29. Pork and Turkey Mix

Preparation time: 10 minutes

Cooking time: 35 minutes
Servings: 8

Ingredients:

- 1 pound pork meat, ground
- 1 pound turkey meat, ground
- A pinch of sea salt and black pepper
- 8 eggs, whisked
- 3 tablespoons ghee, melted
- 1 avocado, pitted, peeled and chopped
- 1 tomato, chopped
- ½ cup red onion, chopped
- 2 tablespoons tomato sauce

Directions:

1. In a bowl, mix the pork with turkey, salt and black pepper and combine.
2. Spread this on a lined baking sheet, shape a circle, spread the tomato sauce all over and bake at 350 degrees F for 25 minutes.
3. Heat up a pan with the ghee over medium heat, add the eggs, stir and scramble them for 5 minutes
4. Spread this over the pork mix, add the onion, tomato, and avocado, divide between plates and serve.
5. Enjoy!

Nutrition: calories 456, fat 35, fiber 2, carbs 5, protein 29,9

30. Turkey Burger

Preparation time: 10 minutes
Cooking time: 20 minutes
Servings: 4

Ingredients:

- 5 small shallots, peeled, chopped and cooked
- 5 eggs
- 1 pound turkey meat, ground
- 3 sun-dried tomatoes, chopped
- 2 teaspoons basil, dried
- 2 tablespoons coconut oil, melted
- 1 teaspoon garlic, minced

Directions:

1. In a bowl, mix the turkey with tomatoes, basil and the garlic, mix together and shape 4 burgers.
2. Heat up a pan with half the oil over medium heat, add the burgers, cook for 4 minutes on each side, divide between plates and sprinkle the shallots over the burgers.
3. Heat up a pan with the rest of the coconut oil over medium heat, crack one egg at a time, fry them well, divide them on the burgers and serve for breakfast.
4. Enjoy!

Nutrition: calories 360, fat 18,1, fiber 1,1, carbs 7,2, protein 41,4

31. Turkey Balls

Preparation time: 10 minutes
Cooking time: 20 minutes
Servings: 8

- **Ingredients:**
- 2 eggs
- 1 teaspoon baking soda
- 1 pound turkey meat, ground
- ¼ cup coconut flour
- Black pepper to taste
- 1 teaspoon smoked paprika

Directions:

1. In a food processor, mix the turkey meat with eggs, baking soda, flour, pepper and paprika, pulse well and shape medium balls out of this mix.
2. Arrange them on a lined baking sheet, bake them in the oven at 350 degrees F for 35 minutes, divide between plates and serve.
3. Enjoy!

Nutrition: calories 166, fat 7,5, fiber 5,5, carbs 5,2, protein 19,8

32. Egg Cups

Preparation time: 10 minutes
Cooking time: 30 minutes
Servings: 2

Ingredients:

- 3 small shallots

- 4 eggs
- ½ yellow onion, chopped
- 1 sweet potato, peeled and chopped
- 1 tablespoon olive oil
- A pinch of sea salt and black pepper

Directions:
1. Heat up a pan over medium-high heat, add the shallots, cook for 5 minutes, drain excess oil on paper towels and fill 4 muffin molds with it.
2. Crack an egg into each shallot cup, season with salt and pepper, place in the oven at 375 degrees F and bake for 15 minutes.
3. Heat up a pan with the oil over medium-high heat, add the onion and sweet potato, stir and cook for 4 minutes.
4. Divide egg cups between plates and serve with the sweet potato mix on the side.
5. Enjoy!

Nutrition: calories 266, fat 15,9, fiber 2,5, carbs 19,3, protein 13,2

33. Blackberry Muffins

Preparation time: 10 minutes
Cooking time: 25 minutes
Servings: 10

Ingredients:
- ½ teaspoon baking soda
- 2 and ½ cups almond flour
- 1 tablespoon vanilla extract
- ¼ cup coconut oil, melted
- ¼ cup coconut milk
- 2 eggs, whisked
- ¼ cup maple syrup
- 3 tablespoons cinnamon powder
- 1 cup blackberries

Directions:
1. In a bowl, mix all the ingredients and combine them well.
2. Divide this into lined muffin cups, bake at 350 degrees F for 25 minutes, divide between plates and serve them for breakfast.
3. Enjoy!

Nutrition: calories 154, fat 7,8, fiber 0,9, carbs 7,2, protein 2,5

34. Pumpkin and Berry Muffins

Preparation time: 10 minutes
Cooking time: 25 minutes
Servings: 10

Ingredients:
- 1 and ¼ cup almond meal
- 3 tablespoons flax meal
- ¾ cup coconut flour
- 1 teaspoon baking soda
- 2 teaspoons pumpkin pie spice
- ½ teaspoon nutmeg, ground
- ½ teaspoon ginger powder
- 5 eggs, whisked
- ¼ cup coconut oil, melted
- ¼ cup coconut sugar
- 1 cup pumpkin puree
- 1 cup blueberries

Directions:
1. In a bowl, mix all the ingredients and combine them well.
2. Divide this into a lined muffin tray, place in the oven at 350 degrees F and bake for 25 minutes.
3. Leave your muffins to cool down, divide them between plates and serve.
4. Enjoy!

Nutrition: calories 179, fat 10,2, fiber 6,1, carbs 18,8, protein 5,3

35. Zucchini Muffins

Preparation time: 10 minutes
Cooking time: 30 minutes
Servings: 8

Ingredients:
- 4 eggs
- ¼ cup coconut sugar
- ¼ cup melted ghee
- ¼ cup coconut milk
- 1 cup coconut flour
- 1 teaspoon baking soda
- ¼ cup cocoa powder

- 1 zucchini, grated
- 3 ounces cocoa powder
- 1 ounce cocoa butter
- 1 teaspoon vanilla extract

Directions:
1. In a bowl, combine all the ingredients and stir well.
2. Divide into a lined muffin tray and bake in the oven at 350 degrees F for 30 minutes.
3. Serve your muffins for breakfast.
4. Enjoy!

Nutrition: calories 243, fat 11,6, fiber 11,6, carbs 26,7, protein 7,5

36. Avocado Muffins

Preparation time: 10 minutes
Cooking time: 25 minutes
Servings: 12

Ingredients:
- 6 small shallots, peeled, chopped
- 1 yellow onion, chopped
- 4 avocados, pitted, peeled and mashed
- 4 eggs
- ½ cup coconut flour
- 1 cup coconut milk
- ½ teaspoon baking soda
- A pinch of sea salt and black pepper

Directions:
1. Heat up a pan over medium-high heat, add the shallots and onion, stir and cook for 5 minutes.
2. In a bowl, mix the avocados with the eggs, salt, black pepper, milk, baking soda and coconut flour and stir.
3. Add the shallots and onions, stir well again and divide into muffin pans.
4. Place in the oven at 350 degrees F and bake for 20 minutes.
5. Divide the muffins between plates and serve.
6. Enjoy!

Nutrition: calories 252, fat 20,3, fiber 9,1, carbs 15,6, protein 5,2

37. Spinach Omelet

Preparation time: 10 minutes
Cooking time: 15 minutes
Servings: 4

Ingredients:
- 2 eggs, whisked
- 1 tablespoon ghee, melted
- A pinch of black pepper
- 1 handful baby spinach, torn
- 1 onion, chopped
- 4 thyme springs, chopped
- 3 garlic cloves, minced
- 1 red bell pepper, chopped
- 1 green bell pepper, chopped
- 3 tablespoon olive oil
- 1 cup cherry tomatoes, halved
- 1 red chili pepper, chopped

Directions:
1. Heat a pan with the ghee over medium-high heat, add the eggs and some black pepper, stir, cook for 5 minutes, the add the spinach. Stir, cook for 2-3 minutes more and divide between plates.
2. Heat up another pan with the oil over medium-high heat, add the onion, stir and cook for 3 minutes. Add garlic, thyme, tomatoes, red, yellow pepper, and chili pepper, stir, cook for 5 minutes more and divide over the omelet.
3. Serve hot for breakfast.
4. Enjoy!

Nutrition: calories 193, fat 16,2, fiber 3,1, carbs 10,4, protein 4,5

38. Pesto Omelet

Preparation Time: 10 mins
Servings: 2

Ingredients:
- Chopped cherry tomatoes
- 4 eggs
- 3 tbsps. Pistachio pesto
- 2 tsps. Essential organic olive oil
- ¼ tsp. black pepper

Directions:

1. In a bowl, combine the eggs with cherry tomatoes, black pepper and pistachio pesto and whisk well.
2. Heat up a pan while using oil over medium-high heat, add eggs mix, spread in the pan, cook for 3 minutes, flip, cook for 3 minutes more, divide between 2 plates and serve enjoying.
3. Enjoy!
4. **Nutrition:**

Calories: 199, Fat:2 g, Carbs:14 g, Protein:7 g, Sugars:16 g, Sodium:600 mg

39. Strawberry Sandwich

Preparation Time: 10 mins
Servings: 4

Ingredients:

- 1 tbsp. stevia
- 2 c. sliced strawberries
- 1 tsp. grated lemon zest
- 8 oz. soft low-fat cream cheese, soft
- 4 halved and toasted wheat grains English muffins

Directions:

1. In the meat processor, combine the cream cheese with the stevia and lemon zest and pulse well.
2. Spread 1 tablespoon with this mix on 1 muffin half and top with many of the sliced strawberries.
3. Repeat with all the rest from the muffin halves and serve enjoying.
4. Enjoy!

Nutrition:

Calories: 211, Fat:3 g, Carbs:8 g, Protein:4 g, Sugars:8 g, Sodium:70 mg

40. Irish Brown Bread

Preparation Time: 10 mins
Servings: 4

Ingredients:

- 4 tsps. Baking soda
- 3 c. all-purpose flour
- 4 c. low fat buttermilk
- 2 beaten eggs
- ½ tsp. salt
- 4 c. whole wheat flour
- 1 c. wheat germ

Directions:

1. Mix together all the dry Ingredients in a large bowl.
2. Add buttermilk and egg and mix until it forms a dough.
3. Transfer the dough onto a floured work area and knead gently.
4. Place on a nonstick baking sheet and form a large round. Cut an "X" shape in the center of the round, about 1/2 inch deep.
5. Bake in a preheated oven at 400 degree F for about 25-30 minutes or until the bread splits apart at the X cut.
6. When done, remove and place on a wire rack and cool completely.
7. Slice and serve.

Nutrition:

Calories: 92.1, Fat:1.2 g, Carbs:17.6 g, Protein:3.7 g, Sugars:2 g, Sodium:244 mg

41. Fresh Fruit Crunch

Preparation Time: 5 mins
Servings: 2

Ingredients:

- 2 tbsps. Toasted coconut
- 1 c. low fat vanilla yogurt
- ¼ c. low fat granola
- 2 c. mixed fresh fruits
- 1 tbsp. honey

Directions:

1. Divide the fruits into 2 tall glasses.
2. Divide the yogurt and spoon over the fruits.
3. Drizzle honey on top.
4. Top with granola and coconut. Refrigerate until chilled.
5. Serve cold.

Nutrition:

Calories: 358, Fat:5.4 g, Carbs:61.8 g, Protein:8.3 g, Sugars:6 g, Sodium:40 mg

42. Apple and Quinoa Breakfast Bake

Preparation Time: 10 mins
Servings: 6

Ingredients:

- 1 tsp. cinnamon powder
- 2 cored, peeled and chopped apples
- ¼ tsp. extra virgin organic olive oil
- ½ c. almond milk
- 2 tsps. Coconut sugar
- 1 c. cooked quinoa

Directions:

1. Grease a ramekin with all the current oil, add quinoa, apples, sugar, cinnamon and almond milk, stir, introduce inside oven, bake at 350 0F for 10 minutes, divide into bowls and serve.
2. Enjoy!

Nutrition:

Calories: 199, Fat:2 g, Carbs:14 g, Protein:8 g, Sugars:25 g, Sodium:170 mg

43. Banana and Pear Breakfast Salad

Preparation Time: 10 mins
Servings: 2

Ingredients:

- 1 cored and cubed Asian pear
- ½ tsp. cinnamon powder
- 1 peeled and sliced banana
- 2 oz. toasted pepitas
- ½ lime juice

Directions:

1. In a bowl, combine the banana using the pear, lime juice, cinnamon and pepitas, toss, divide between small plates and serve enjoying.
2. Enjoy!

Nutrition:

Calories: 188, Fat:2 g, Carbs:5 g, Protein:7 g, Sugars:10 g, Sodium:300 mg

44. Apple Cinnamon Crisp

Preparation Time: 10 mins
Servings: 4

Ingredients:

- 1 tsp. cinnamon
- 1 c. brown sugar
- 3 lbs. Granny Smith apples
- 2 tbsps. All-purpose flour
- 1 stick butter
- 1 c. oatmeal
- 1 tbsp. granulated sugar

Directions:

1. Peel and core the apples, slice thinly.
2. Mix granulated sugar with flour and add the apples. Toss to coat.
3. Put apples into the bottom of a 5-6 quart crock pot.
4. Combine brown sugar with oatmeal and butter. Mix until mixture is crumbly.
5. Sprinkle oatmeal mixture on top of the apples.
6. Cook apples fully on high heat.

Nutrition:

Calories: 549, Fat:27 g, Carbs:71 g, Protein:6 g, Sugars:43 g, Sodium:430 mg

45. Peanut butter & blueberry Parfait

Preparation Time: 5 mins
Servings: 2

Ingredients:

- ½ c. chopped almonds
- 1 tbsp. unsweetened peanut butter
- ½ tsp. cinnamon
- 1 tsp. honey
- 1 c. low fat vanilla yogurt
- 1 c. blueberries

Directions:

1. Combine the yogurt and peanut butter. Mix until blended and set aside.
2. Combine the blueberries, almonds, honey, and cinnamon. Toss to mix.
3. In two separate serving glasses, alternate layers of the yogurt and blueberry mixture

until all ingredients have been used.
4. Serve immediately or chill until ready to serve.

Nutrition:
Calories: 194.1, Fat:5.0 g, Carbs:31.1 g, Protein:6.8 g, Sugars:8.4 g, Sodium:48 mg

46. Quinoa Quiche

Preparation Time: 10 mins
Servings: 4

Ingredients:
- 1 c. fat-free ricotta cheese
- 2/3 c. grated low-fat parmesan
- 3 oz. chopped spinach
- 1 ½ tsps. Garlic powder
- 1 c. cooked quinoa
- 3 eggs

Directions:
1. In a bowl, combine the quinoa while using spinach, ricotta, eggs, garlic powder and parmesan, whisk well, pour into a lined pie pan, introduce inside oven and bake at 355 0F for 45 minutes.
2. Cool the quiche down, slice and serve enjoying.
3. Enjoy!

Nutrition:
Calories: 201, Fat:2 g, Carbs:12 g, Protein:7 g, Sugars:0 g, Sodium:130 mg

47. Sweet Rosemary Oats

Preparation Time: 5 mins
Servings: 2

Ingredients:
- 2 tbsps. Chopped fresh rosemary
- 1 tbsp. honey
- ½ c. chopped walnuts
- Fresh strawberries
- 2 c. low fat milk
- 2 c. old fashioned oats
- 1 tsp. ground pink peppercorns

Directions:
1. Combine the oats, walnuts, rosemary, and pink pepper in a bowl. Toss to mix and place in a mason jar or other lidded container.
2. Combine the milk and honey and pour over the oat mixture.
3. Cover and refrigerate for 12 hours, or overnight.
4. Warm for 1-2 minutes in the microwave before serving.
5. Top with fresh strawberries, if desired

Nutrition:
Calories: 305.3, Fat:13.1 g, Carbs:39.5 g, Protein:11.4 g, Sugars:1 g, Sodium:520 mg

48. Quinoa Breakfast Bars

Preparation Time: 2 hours
Servings: 6

Ingredients:
- 1/3 c. flaked coconut
- ½ tsp. cinnamon powder
- 2 tbsps. Coconut sugar
- 2 tbsps. Unsweetened chocolate chips
- ½ c. fat-free peanut butter
- 1 tsp. vanilla flavoring
- 1 c. quinoa flakes

Directions:
1. In a large bowl, combine the peanut butter with sugar, vanilla, cinnamon, quinoa, coconut and chocolate chips, stir well, spread about the bottom of the lined baking sheet, press well, cut in 6 bars, keep inside fridge for just two hours, divide between plates and serve.
2. Enjoy!

Nutrition:
Calories: 182, Fat:4 g, Carbs:13 g, Protein:11 g, Sugars:14.8 g, Sodium:69 mg

49. Granola Breakfast Pops

Preparation Time: 5 mins
Servings: 4-6

Ingredients:
- ½ c. chopped fresh pineapple
- ½ c. chopped mango

- 2 c. low fat vanilla yogurt
- ¼ c. sugar free granola
- ½ c. chopped strawberries

Directions:
1. Combine the yogurt, strawberries, pineapple, and mango in a bowl. Mix well.
2. Transfer the yogurt mixture to ice pop molds and then sprinkle a little bit of granola into each.
3. Place in the freezer and freeze for several hours or overnight.

Nutrition:
Calories: 133.8, Fat:1.4 g, Carbs:25.5 g, Protein:5.1 g, Sugars:13 g, Sodium:10 mg

50. Cinnamon Breakfast Quinoa

Preparation Time: 10 mins | Servings: 2

Ingredients:
- ¾ c. water
- ½ c. rinsed and drained quinoa
- Milk
- 2 tbsps. Chopped walnuts
- Honey
- 1/8 tsp. salt
- 1 stick cinnamon

Directions:
1. Place a heavy bottomed saucepan over a medium heat. Add quinoa, water, salt and cinnamon. Mix well and bring to a boil.
2. Lower the heat, cover and simmer until all the water is absorbed.
3. Remove from the heat. Do not uncover for 5 minutes.
4. Fluff the cooked quinoa with a fork and discard the cinnamon stick.
5. Divide the quinoa into individual serving bowls. Pour milk over the quinoa.
6. Drizzle honey over the quinoa, sprinkle walnuts on top and serve.

Nutrition:
Calories: 229.3, Fat:3.2 g, Carbs:35.6 g, Protein:6.1 g, Sugars:8 g, Sodium:69 mg

51. Cinnamon Walnut Breakfast Parfait

Preparation Time: 10 mins
Servings: 2

Ingredients:
- ¼ tsp. cinnamon
- 1 tsp. chia seeds
- ½ c. chopped walnuts
- 1 c. low fat vanilla yogurt
- 1 c. chopped granny smith apples
- 1 tsp. honey

Directions:
1. In a bowl, combine the yogurt and chia seeds. Set aside.
2. In another bowl, combine the apples, walnuts, honey, and cinnamon. Mix well.
3. In two separate serving glasses, alternate layers of apple walnut mixture and yogurt until all ingredients have been used.
4. Serve immediately or chill before serving.

Nutrition:
Calories: 364.2, Fat:23.4 g, Carbs:34.6 g, Protein:10.7 g, Sugars:6 g, Sodium:85 mg

52. Breakfast Taco

Preparation Time: 25 mins
Servings: 5

Ingredients:
- ¼ c. sliced bell peppers
- 3 warm tortillas
- 1 tsp. butter
- 3 portions lean meat
- Pepper and salt
- 4 large eggs
- 1 c. organic shredded cheese

Directions:
1. Preheat oven to 300°F. Wrap the tortillas in foil. Place in the oven. Heat for 5 minutes.
2. In a large skillet, cook the meat choice.
3. In a bowl, crack the eggs and mix. Add salt and pepper.
4. In another skillet, melt the butter. Cook the scrambled eggs.
5. Assemble the taco with scrambled egg, meat, bell pepper, cheese.

6. Serve immediately.

Nutrition:

Calories: 77, Fat:0.1 g, Carbs:40 g, Protein:0.6 g, Sugars:1 g, Sodium:300 mg

53. Egg Spinach Breakfast Muffins

Preparation Time: 40 mins
Servings: 6

Ingredients:

- 2 oz. chopped prosciutto
- 4 oz. chopped spinach
- Cooking spray
- ½ c. chopped roasted red pepper
- 1 c. crumbled low-fat cheese
- 6 eggs
- ½ c. skim milk

Directions:

1. In a mixing bowl, thoroughly mix the eggs, milk, cheese, spinach, red pepper, and prosciutto.
2. Grease the muffin tins with some cooking spray.
3. Pour the muffin mix in the tins.
4. Bake in the preheated oven at 350 0F for 25-30 minutes.
5. Serve warm.

Nutrition:

Calories: 98.9, Fat:6.7 g, Carbs:0.9 g, Protein:8.0 g, Sugars:1.5 g, Sodium:79 mg

54. Whole Grain Toast with Fruited Ricotta Spread

Preparation Time: 10 mins
Servings: 4

Ingredients:

- 2 tsps. Honey
- 1 c. low fat ricotta cheese
- ½ c. finely diced peaches
- 1 tsp. orange zest
- ¼ c. sliced almonds
- 4 toasted whole grain bread slices
- 1 tbsp. fresh chopped mint

Directions:

1. In a bowl, combine the ricotta cheese, orange zest, honey, mint, and peaches. Blend well.
2. Spread evenly on each piece of whole wheat toast and top with sliced almonds and additional fresh fruit, if desired.

Nutrition:

Calories: 196.1, Fat:8.9 g, Carbs:20.0 g, Protein:12.4 g, Sugars:7 g, Sodium:190 mg

55. Cherries Oatmeal

Preparation Time: 10 mins
Servings: 6

Ingredients:

- 2 c. pitted and sliced cherries
- 6 c. water
- 1 tsp. cinnamon powder
- 1 c. almond milk
- 2 c. old-fashioned oats
- 1 tsp. vanilla flavor

Directions:

1. In a little pot, combine the oats while using the water, milk, cinnamon, vanilla and cherries, toss, bring to a simmer over medium-high heat, cook for quarter-hour, divide into bowls and serve in the morning.
2. Enjoy!

Nutrition:

Calories 180, Fat 4g, Fiber 4g, Carbs 9g, Protein 7g, Sodium 98mg, Sugars 14g

56. Strawberry Chia Breakfast Pudding

Preparation Time: 5 mins
Servings: 4

Ingredients:

- 1 tbsp. honey
- 3 c. chopped strawberries
- 1 tsp. pure vanilla extract
- 2 c. unsweetened coconut milk
- ½ c. chia seeds

Directions:

1. Combine the coconut milk and strawberries in a blender and puree until smooth.
2. Add the chia seeds, vanilla extract, and honey. Stir well.
3. Cover and refrigerate at least 6 hours or overnight.

Nutrition:

Calories:314.8 , Fat:25.0 g, Carbs:22.1 g, Protein:4.5 g, Sugars:7.4 g, Sodium:46 mg

57. Banana Nutty Oats

Preparation Time: 30 mins.
Servings: 4

Ingredients:

- 2 c. water
- 2 tbsps. Chia seeds
- ¼ c. chopped walnuts
- 1 tsp. vanilla extract
- 2 peeled and mashed bananas
- 1 c. almond milk
- 1 c. steel-cut oats

Directions:

1. In a cooking pot, mix the water with the oats, milk, walnuts, chia seeds, bananas, and vanilla.
2. Combine well and boil the mix over medium flame.
3. Simmer for 15 minutes, stirring frequently.
4. Transfer to your serving bowls and serve warm.

Nutrition:

Calories: 425, Fat:17.5 g, Carbs:62.5 g, Protein:12.5 g, Sugars:22.5 g, Sodium:212.2 mg

58. Breakfast Apple and Raisin Oatmeal

Preparation Time: 10 mins
Servings: 2

Ingredients:

- 1 c. old fashioned oats
- 2 tbsps. Honey
- ¼ c. raisins
- ½ tsp. ground cinnamon
- 2 drops vanilla essence
- 2 c. milk low-fat milk
- 1 tbsp. light butter
- 1 c. chopped apples

Directions:

1. Use a Crock Pot Liner or spray the inside of a 5-quart slow cooker with non-stick cooking spray
2. Combine all ingredients to the slow cooker and stir well to combine.
3. Cover and cook on LOW overnight, ideally no more than 6 hours or it will dry out.
4. Stir well in the morning before serving.

Nutrition:

Calories: 240, Fat:3.9 g, Carbs:49 g, Protein:4.6 g, Sugars:38 g, Sodium:62 mg

59. Fast Punch

Preparation Time: 5 mins
Servings: 6

Ingredients:

- 4 tbsps. Lemon juice
- 2 c. peeled citrus fruits
- 1 c. ice
- 8 oz. cranberry juice
- 1 ½ c. chopped pineapple

Directions:

1. Place all ingredients in a food blender.
2. Puree until smooth.
3. Serve immediately.

Nutrition:

Calories: 116.6, Fat:0 g, Carbs:29.6 g, Protein:0 g, Sugars:28 g, Sodium:94.2 mg

60. Chocolate Covered Banana Quinoa

Preparation Time: 5 mins
Servings: 4

Ingredients:

- 1 tbsp. honey
- ¼ c. dark chocolate shavings
- 2 tsps. Dark cocoa powder
- 1 c. sliced banana

- 2 c. low fat milk
- 1 c. uncooked quinoa

Directions:
1. In a saucepan, combine the milk with the dark cocoa powder and honey. Heat over medium to medium high heat until mixture bubbles, stirring frequently.
2. Add the quinoa and reduce heat to low. Cover and simmer for 15-20 minutes, or until most of the liquid is absorbed and grain is tender.
3. Serve warm garnished with sliced banana and chocolate shavings, if desired.

Nutrition:
Calories: 256.5, Fat:4.4 g, Carbs:49.4 g, Protein:7.4 g, Sugars:5 g, Sodium:155 mg

61. Egg Parsley Omelet

Preparation Time: 15 mins
Servings: 5-6

Ingredients:
- ¼ tsp. black pepper
- 2 tsps. Olive oil
- 2 tbsps. Chopped parsley
- 1 tbsp. shredded low-fat cheddar cheese
- 6 whisked eggs
- 2 tbsps. almond milk

Directions:
1. In a bowl of medium-large size, thoroughly stir the eggs, milk, pepper, parsley, and cheese.
2. Heat some olive oil in a pan over medium flame; add the eggs mix, spreading evenly along the pan.
3. Cook for 2-3 minutes, flip, cook for 3 minutes more.
4. Serve warm.

Nutrition:
Calories: 238, Fat:20.6 g, Carbs:2.7 g, Protein:11.9 g, Sugars:0.5 g, Sodium:804.2 mg

Mains

62. Lime Chicken Soup

Preparation time: 10 minutes
Cooking time: 1 hour
Servings: 8

Ingredients:

- 1 yellow onion, chopped
- 1 pound chicken breast, skinless, boneless and cubed
- 1 tablespoon olive oil
- 2 carrots, sliced
- 3 garlic cloves, minced
- A pinch of salt and black pepper
- 6 cups veggie stock
- 2 teaspoons turmeric powder
- Juice of 1 lime
- Zest of 1 lime, grated
- 1 tablespoon cilantro, chopped

Directions:

1. Heat up a pot with the oil over medium heat, add the onion, carrots and the garlic and sauté for 5 minutes.
2. Add the meat and brown it for 5 minutes more.
3. Add the stock and the other ingredients except the cilantro, toss, bring to a simmer and cook over medium heat for 50 minutes.
4. Divide the soup into bowls, sprinkle the cilantro on top and serve.

Nutrition: calories 271, fat 8, fiber 11, carbs 16, protein 8

63. Spinach Soup

Preparation time: 10 minutes
Cooking time: 20 minutes
Servings: 4

Ingredients:

- 1 pound spinach leaves
- 1 yellow onion, chopped
- 1 tablespoon olive oil
- 4 cups chicken stock
- 4 cherry tomatoes, halved
- 1 red bell pepper, chopped
- 1 tablespoon parsley, chopped

Directions:

1. Heat up a pot with the oil over medium-high heat, add the onion and the bell pepper and sauté for 5 minutes.
2. Add the spinach and the other ingredients, toss, bring to a simmer and cook over medium heat for 15 minutes.
3. Ladle the soup into bowls and serve for lunch.

Nutrition: calories 148, fat 2, fiber 6, carbs 8, protein 5

64. Hot Turkey Meatballs

Preparation time: 10 minutes
Cooking time: 10 minutes
Servings: 4

Ingredients:

- 1 pound turkey meat, ground
- 1 yellow onion, chopped
- 1 egg, whisked
- 1 tablespoon cilantro, chopped
- 2 tablespoons olive oil
- 1 red chili pepper, minced
- 2 teaspoons lime juice
- Zest of 1 lime, grated
- A pinch of salt and black pepper
- 1 teaspoon turmeric powder

Directions:

1. In a bowl, combine the turkey meat with the onion and the other ingredients except the oil, stir and shape medium meatballs out of this mix.
2. Heat up a pan with the oil over medium-high heat, add the meatballs, cook them for 5 minutes on each side, divide between plates and serve for lunch.

Nutrition: calories 200, fat 12, fiber 5, carbs 12, protein 7

65. Cauliflower Soup

Preparation time: 10 minutes
Cooking time: 35 minutes
Servings: 4

Ingredients:

- 1 yellow onion, chopped
- 1 carrot, chopped
- ½ cup celery, chopped
- 1 tablespoon olive oil
- 1 pound cauliflower florets
- A pinch of salt and black pepper
- 1 red bell pepper, chopped
- 5 cups vegetable stock
- 15 ounces canned tomatoes, chopped
- 1 tablespoon cilantro, chopped

Directions:

1. Heat up a pot with the oil over medium-high heat, add the onion, celery, carrot and the bell pepper and sauté for 10 minutes.
2. Add the cauliflower and the other ingredients, toss, bring to a simmer and cook over medium heat for 25 minutes more.
3. Ladle the soup into bowls and serve.

Nutrition: calories 210, fat 1, fiber 5, carbs 14, protein 6

66. Tarragon Cod with Olives

Preparation time: 10 minutes
Cooking time: 25 minutes
Servings: 4

Ingredients:

- 4 cod fillets, skinless
- 2 garlic cloves, minced
- 2 shallots, chopped
- Salt and black pepper to the taste
- 2 tablespoons olive oil
- 2 tablespoons tarragon, chopped
- ½ cup black olives, pitted and halved
- Juice of 1 lemon
- ¼ cup chicken stock
- 1 tablespoon chives, chopped

Directions:

1. Heat up a pan with the oil over medium-high heat, add the shallots and the garlic and sauté for 5 minutes.
2. Add the fish and sear it for 2 minutes on each side.
3. Add the remaining ingredients, put the pan in the oven and cook at 360 degrees F for 15 minutes.
4. Divide the mix between plates and serve for lunch.

Nutrition: calories 173, fat 3, fiber 4, carbs 9, protein 12

67. Kale Soup

Preparation time: 10 minutes
Cooking time: 15 minutes
Servings: 4

Ingredients:

- 1 pound kale, chopped
- Salt and black pepper to the taste
- 5 cups vegetable stock
- 2 carrots, sliced
- 1 yellow onion, chopped
- 1 tablespoon olive oil
- 1 tablespoon parsley, chopped
- 1 tablespoon lemon juice

Directions:

1. Heat up a pot with the oil over medium heat, add the carrots and the onion, stir and sauté for 5 minutes.
2. Add the kale and the other ingredients, toss, bring to a simmer and cook over medium heat for 10 minutes more.
3. Ladle the soup into bowls and serve.

Nutrition: calories 210, fat 7, fiber 2, carbs 10, protein 8

68. Salmon with Balsamic Fennel

Preparation time: 10 minutes
Cooking time: 20 minutes
Servings: 4

Ingredients:

- 4 salmon fillets, boneless

- 1 tablespoon olive oil
- 2 fennel bulbs, shredded
- 1 tablespoon balsamic vinegar
- 1 tablespoon lime juice
- ½ teaspoon cumin, ground
- ½ teaspoon oregano, dried
- 1 tablespoon chives, chopped
- Salt and black pepper to the taste

Directions:
1. Heat up a pan with the oil over medium heat, add the fennel, stir and sauté for 5 minutes.
2. Add the fish and sear it for 2 minutes on each side.
3. Add the remaining ingredients, cook everything for 10 minutes more, divide between plates and serve.

Nutrition: calories 200, fat 2, fiber 4, carbs 10, protein 8

69. Carrot Soup

Preparation time: 10 minutes
Cooking time: 25 minutes
Servings: 4

Ingredients:
- 1 pound carrots, peeled and sliced
- 2 tablespoons olive oil
- 1 yellow onion, chopped
- 1 teaspoon rosemary, dried
- 1 teaspoon cumin, ground
- 2 garlic cloves, minced
- A pinch of salt and black pepper
- 5 cups vegetable stock
- ½ teaspoon turmeric powder
- 1 cup coconut milk
- 1 tablespoon chives, chopped

Directions:
1. Heat up a pot with the oil over medium heat, add the onion and the garlic and sauté for 5 minutes.
2. Add the carrots, the stock and the other ingredients except the chives, stir, bring to a simmer and cook over medium heat for 20 minutes more.
3. Divide the soup into bowls, sprinkle the chives on top and serve for lunch.

Nutrition: calories 210, fat 8, fiber 6, carbs 10, protein 7

70. Leeks Cream Soup

Preparation time: 10 minutes
Cooking time: 20 minutes
Servings: 4

Ingredients:
- 4 leeks, sliced
- 1 yellow onion, chopped
- 1 tablespoon avocado oil
- A pinch of salt and black pepper
- 2 garlic cloves, minced
- 4 cups vegetable soup
- ½ cup coconut milk
- ½ teaspoon nutmeg, ground
- ¼ teaspoon red pepper, crushed
- ½ teaspoon rosemary, dried
- 1 tablespoon parsley, chopped

Directions:
1. Heat up a pot with the oil over medium-high heat, add the onion and the garlic and sauté for 2 minutes.
2. Add the leeks, stir and sauté for 3 minutes more.
3. Add the stock and the rest of the ingredients except the parsley, bring to a simmer and cook over medium heat for 15 minutes more.
4. Blend the soup with an immersion blender, divide the soup into bowls, sprinkle the parsley on top and serve.

Nutrition: calories 268, fat 11.8, fiber 4.5, carbs 37.4, protein 6.1

71. Turkey and Artichokes

Preparation time: 10 minutes
Cooking time: 40 minutes
Servings: 4

Ingredients:
- 1 yellow onion, sliced
- 1 pound turkey breast, skinless, boneless

- and roughly cubed
- 2 tablespoons olive oil
- Salt and black pepper to the taste
- 1 cup canned artichoke hearts, drained and halved
- ½ teaspoon nutmeg, ground
- ½ teaspoon sweet paprika
- 1 teaspoon cumin, ground
- 1 tablespoon cilantro, chopped

Directions:
1. In a roasting pan, combine the turkey with the onion, artichokes and the other ingredients, toss and at 350 degrees F for 40 minutes.
2. Divide everything between plates and serve.

Nutrition: calories 345, fat 12, fiber 3, carbs 12, protein 14

72. Smoked Salmon Salad

Preparation time: 10 minutes
Cooking time: 0 minutes
Servings: 4

Ingredients:
- 2 cups smoked salmon, skinless, boneless and cut into strips
- 1 yellow onion, chopped
- 1 avocado, peeled, pitted and cubed
- 1 cup cherry tomatoes, halved
- 1 tablespoon olive oil
- 2 cups baby spinach
- A pinch of salt and cayenne pepper
- 1 tablespoon balsamic vinegar

Directions:
1. In a salad bowl, mix the salmon with the onion, the avocado and the other ingredients, toss, divide between plates and serve for lunch.

Nutrition: calories 260, fat 2, fiber 8, carbs 17, protein 11

73. Shrimp with Zucchini

Preparation time: 10 minutes
Cooking time: 17 minutes
Servings: 4

Ingredients:
- 1 pound shrimp, peeled and deveined
- 1 tablespoon lemon juice
- 2 zucchinis, sliced
- 1 yellow onion, roughly chopped
- 1 tablespoon olive oil
- 1 teaspoon turmeric powder
- A pinch of salt and black pepper
- 1 tablespoons capers, drained
- 2 tablespoons pine nuts

Directions:
1. Heat up a pan with the oil over medium-high heat, add the onion and the zucchini, stir and sauté for 5 minutes.
2. Add the shrimp and the other ingredients, toss, cook everything for 12 minutes more, divide into bowls and serve for lunch.

Nutrition: calories 162, fat 3, fiber 4, carbs 12, protein 7

74. Turmeric Broccoli and Leeks Stew

Preparation time: 10 minutes
Cooking time: 25 minutes
Servings: 4

Ingredients:
- 1 tablespoon olive oil
- 1 pound broccoli florets
- ½ teaspoon coriander, ground
- 1 yellow onion, chopped
- 2 leeks, sliced
- 4 garlic cloves, minced
- ½ teaspoon turmeric powder
- A pinch of cayenne pepper
- 1 cup tomato passata
- A pinch of salt and black pepper
- 1 tablespoon lemon juice
- 1 tablespoon cilantro, chopped

Directions:
1. Heat up a pot with the oil over medium heat, add the onion, garlic, leeks and the turmeric and sauté for 5 minutes.

2. Add the broccoli and the other ingredients, toss, bring to a simmer and cook over medium heat for 25 minutes more.
3. Divide into bowls and serve for lunch.

Nutrition: calories 113, fat 4.1, fiber 4.5, carbs 17.7, protein 4.4

75. Salmon and Green Beans

Preparation time: 10 minutes
Cooking time: 26 minutes
Servings: 4

Ingredients:
- 2 tablespoons olive oil
- 1 yellow onion, chopped
- 4 salmon fillets, boneless
- 1 cup green beans, trimmed and halved
- 2 garlic cloves, minced
- ½ cup chicken stock
- 1 teaspoon chili powder
- 1 teaspoon sweet paprika
- A pinch of salt and black pepper
- 1 tablespoon cilantro, chopped

Directions:
1. Heat up a pan with the oil over medium heat, add onion, stir and sauté for 2 minutes.
2. Add the fish and sear it for 2 minutes on each side.
3. Add the rest of the ingredients, toss gently and bake everything at 360 degrees F for 20 minutes.
4. Divide everything between plates and serve for lunch.

Nutrition: calories 322, fat 18.3, fiber 2, carbs 5.8, protein 35.7

76. Chicken Stew

Preparation time: 10 minutes
Cooking time: 45 minutes
Servings: 4

Ingredients:
- 1 tablespoon olive oil
- 1 pound chicken thighs, skinless, boneless and cubed
- 2 garlic cloves, minced
- 1 small yellow onion, chopped
- 1 green bell pepper, chopped
- 1 red bell pepper, chopped
- ½ teaspoon cumin, ground
- ½ teaspoon sweet paprika
- 2 cups chicken stock
- A pinch of salt and black pepper
- 1 tablespoon lemon juice
- 1 cup coconut milk
- 1 tablespoon cilantro, chopped

Directions:
1. Heat up a pot with the oil over medium heat, add the onion, garlic and the meat and brown for 10 minutes stirring often.
2. Add the rest of the ingredients except the coconut milk and the cilantro, stir, bring to a simmer and cook over medium for 30 minutes more.
3. Add the coconut milk and the cilantro, stir, simmer the stew for 5 minutes more, divide into bowls and serve for lunch.

Nutrition: calories 419, fat 26.8, fiber 2.7, carbs 10.7, protein 35.5

77. Spiced Turkey Stew

Preparation time: 10 minutes
Cooking time: 45 minutes
Servings: 6

Ingredients:
- 1 pound turkey breast, skinless, boneless and cubed
- 1 yellow onion, chopped
- 2 tablespoons olive oil
- ½ teaspoon mustard seeds
- 1 teaspoon ginger, grated
- 2 garlic cloves, minced
- 1 green chili pepper, chopped
- 1 teaspoon sweet paprika
- 1 teaspoon coriander, ground
- ½ teaspoon cardamom, ground
- ½ teaspoon turmeric powder
- A pinch of salt and black pepper

- 1 teaspoon lemon juice
- 1 cup chicken stock
- 1 tablespoon parsley, chopped

Directions:
1. Heat up a pot with the oil over medium-high heat, add the onion, the meat, mustard seeds, ginger, garlic, paprika, coriander, cardamom and the turmeric, stir and brown for 10 minutes.
2. Add all the other ingredients, toss, simmer over medium heat for 35 minutes more, divide into bowls and serve.

Nutrition: calories 202, fat 9.4, fiber 1.7, carbs 9.3, protein 20.3

78. Beans and Salmon Pan

Preparation time: 10 minutes
Cooking time: 25 minutes
Servings: 4

Ingredients:
- 1 cup canned black beans, drained and rinsed
- 4 garlic cloves, minced
- 1 yellow onion, chopped
- 2 tablespoons olive oil
- 4 salmon fillets, boneless
- ½ teaspoon coriander, ground
- 1 teaspoon turmeric powder
- 2 tomatoes, cubed
- ½ cup chicken stock
- A pinch of salt and black pepper
- ½ teaspoon cumin seeds
- 1 tablespoon chives, chopped

Directions:
1. Heat up a pan with the oil over medium heat, add the onion and the garlic and sauté for 5 minutes.
2. Add the fish and sear it for 2 minutes on each side.
3. Add the beans and the other ingredients, toss gently and cook for 10 minutes more.
4. Divide the mix between plates and serve right away for lunch.

Nutrition: calories 219, fat 8, fiber 8, carbs 12, protein 8

79. Turmeric Cauliflower and Cod Stew

Preparation time: 5 minutes
Cooking time: 30 minutes
Servings: 4

Ingredients:
- ½ pound cauliflower florets
- 1 pound cod fillets, boneless, skinless and cubed
- 1 tablespoons olive oil
- 1 yellow onion, chopped
- ½ teaspoon cumin seeds
- 1 green chili, chopped
- ¼ teaspoon turmeric powder
- 2 tomatoes chopped
- A pinch of salt and black pepper
- ½ cup chicken stock
- 1 tablespoon cilantro, chopped

Directions:
1. Heat up a pot with the oil over medium heat, add the onion, chili, cumin and turmeric, stir and cook for 5 minutes.
2. Add the cauliflower, the fish and the other ingredients, toss, bring to a simmer and cook over medium heat for 25 minutes more.
3. Divide the stew into bowls and serve.

Nutrition: calories 281, fat 6, fiber 4, carbs 8, protein 12

80. Chicken Chili

Preparation time: 10 minutes
Cooking time: 1 hour
Servings: 6

Ingredients:
- 1 yellow onion, chopped
- 2 tablespoons olive oil
- 2 garlic cloves, minced
- 1 pound chicken breast, skinless, boneless and cubed
- 1 green bell pepper, chopped
- 2 cups chicken stock
- 1 tablespoon cocoa powder

- 2 tablespoons chili powder
- 1 teaspoon smoked paprika
- 1 cup canned tomatoes, chopped
- 1 tablespoon cilantro, chopped
- A pinch of salt and black pepper

Directions:
1. Heat up a pot with the oil over medium heat, add the onion and the garlic and sauté for 5 minutes.
2. Add the meat and brown it for 5 minutes more.
3. Add the rest of the ingredients, toss, cook over medium heat for 40 minutes.
4. Divide the chili into bowls and serve for lunch.

Nutrition: calories 300, fat 2, fiber 10, carbs 15, protein 11

81. Green Beans Soup

Preparation time: 10 minutes
Cooking time: 35 minutes
Servings: 6

Ingredients:
- 1 yellow onion, chopped
- 1 pound green beans, trimmed and halved
- 1 carrot, peeled and grated
- 2 tomatoes, cubed
- 1 tablespoon olive oil
- 2 teaspoons cumin, ground
- 6 cups veggie stock
- ¼ teaspoon chipotle chili powder
- 1 tablespoon cilantro, chopped

Directions:
1. Heat up a pot with the oil over medium heat, add the onion and the carrot and sauté for 5 minutes.
2. Add the green beans and the rest of the ingredients, toss, bring to a simmer and cook over medium heat for 30 minutes.
3. Ladle the soup into bowls and serve.

Nutrition: calories 224, fat 2, fiber 12, carbs 10, protein 17

82. Mashed Garlic Turnips

Preparation Time: 10 minutes
Servings: 2

Ingredients
- 3 cups diced turnip
- 2 cloves garlic, minced
- ¼ cup heavy cream
- 3 tbsp melted butter
- Salt and pepper to season

Directions:
1. Boil the turnips until tender.
2. Drain and mash the turnips.
3. Add the cream, butter, salt, pepper and garlic. Combine well.
4. Serve!

83. Lasagna Spaghetti Squash

Preparation Time: 90 minutes
Servings: 6

Ingredients
- 25 slices mozzarella cheese
- 1 large jar (40 oz Rao's Marinara sauce
- 30 oz whole-milk ricotta cheese
- 2 large spaghetti squash, cooked (44 oz
- 4 lbs ground beef

Direction
1. Preheat your oven to 375°F/190°C.
2. Slice the spaghetti squash and place it face down inside an oven proof dish. Fill with water until covered.
3. Bake for 45 minutes until skin is soft.
4. Sear the meat until browned.
5. In a large skillet, heat the browned meat and marinara sauce. Set aside when warm.
6. Scrape the flesh off the cooked squash to resemble strands of spaghetti.
7. Layer the lasagna in a large greased pan in alternating layers of spaghetti squash, meat sauce, mozzarella, ricotta. Repeat until all increased have been used.
8. Bake for 30 minutes and serve!

84. Blue Cheese Chicken Wedges

Preparation Time: 45 minutes
Servings: 4

Ingredients

- Blue cheese dressing
- 2 tbsp crumbled blue cheese
- 4 strips of bacon
- 2 chicken breasts (boneless
- 3/4 cup of your favorite buffalo sauce

Direction

1. Boil a large pot of salted water.
2. Add in two chicken breasts to pot and cook for 28 minutes.
3. Turn off the heat and let the chicken rest for 10 minutes. Using a fork, pull the chicken apart into strips.
4. Cook and cool the bacon strips and put to the side.
5. On a medium heat, combine the chicken and buffalo sauce. Stir until hot.
6. Add the blue cheese and buffalo pulled chicken. Top with the cooked bacon crumble.
7. Serve and enjoy.

85. 'Oh so good' Salad

Preparation Time: 10 minutes
Servings: 2

Ingredients

- 6 brussels sprouts
- ½ tsp apple cider vinegar
- 1 tsp olive/grapeseed oil
- 1 grind of salt
- 1 tbsp freshly grated parmesan

Direction

1. Slice the clean brussels sprouts in half.
2. Cut thin slices in the opposite direction.
3. Once sliced, cut the roots off and discard.
4. Toss together with the apple cider, oil and salt.
5. Sprinkle with the parmesan cheese, combine and enjoy!

86. 'I Love Bacon'

Preparation Time: 90 minutes
Servings: 4

Ingredients

- 30 slices thick-cut bacon
- 12 oz steak
- 10 oz pork sausage
- 4 oz cheddar cheese, shredded

Direction

1. Lay out 5 x 6 slices of bacon in a woven pattern and bake at 400°F/200°C for 20 minutes until crisp.
2. Combine the steak, bacon and sausage to form a meaty mixture.
3. Lay out the meat in a rectangle of similar size to the bacon strips. Season with salt/peppe.
4. Place the bacon weave on top of the meat mixture.
5. Place the cheese in the center of the bacon.
6. Roll the meat into a tight roll and refrigerate.
7. Make a 7 x 7 bacon weave and roll the bacon weave over the meat, diagonally.
8. Bake at 400°F/200°C for 60 minutes or 165°F/75°C internally.
9. Let rest for 5 minutes before serving.

87. Lemon Dill Trout

Preparation Time: 10 minutes
Servings: 1

Ingredients

- 2 lb pan-dressed trout (or other small fish, fresh or frozen
- 1 ½ tsp salt
- ½ cup butter or margarine
- 2 tbsp dill weed
- 3 tbsp lemon juice

Direction

1. Cut the fish lengthwise and season the with pepper.
2. Prepare a skillet by melting the butter and dill weed.
3. Fry the fish on a high heat, flesh side down, for 2-3 minutes per side.
4. Remove the fish. Add the lemon juice to the butter and dill to create a sauce.
5. Serve the fish with the sauce.

88. 'No Potato' Shepherd's Pie

Preparation Time: 70 minutes
Servings: 6

Ingredients

- 1 lb lean ground beef
- 8 oz low-carb mushroom sauce mix
- ¼ cup ketchup
- 1 lb package frozen mixed vegetables
- 1 lb Aitkin's low-carb bake mix or equivalent

Direction

1. Preheat your oven to 375°F/190°C.
2. Prepare the bake mix according to package instructions. Layer into the skillet base.
3. Cut the dough into triangles and roll them from base to tip. Set to the side.
4. Brown the ground beef with the salt. Stir in the mushroom sauce, ketchup and mixed vegetables.
5. Bring the mixture to the boil and reduce the heat to medium, cover and simmer until tender.
6. Put the dough triangles on top of the mixture, tips pointing towards the center.
7. Bake for 60 minutes until piping hot and serve!

89. Easy Slider

Preparation Time: 70 minutes
Servings: 6

Ingredients

- 1 lb Ground Beef
- 1 Egg
- Garlic/salt/pepper/onion powder to taste
- Several dashes of Worcestershire sauce
- 8 oz cheddar cheese (½ oz per patty

Direction

1. Mix the beef, eggs and spices together.
2. Divide the meat into 1.5 oz patties.
3. Add a half-ounce of cheese to each patty and combine two patties to make one burger, like a sandwich. Heat the oil on high and fry the burgers until cooked as desired. Serve.

90. Dijon Halibut Steak

Preparation Time: 20 minutes
Servings: 1

Ingredients

- 1 6-oz fresh or thawed halibut steak
- 1 tbsp butter
- 1 tbsp lemon juice
- ½ tbsp Dijon mustard
- 1 tsp fresh basil

Direction

1. Heat the butter, basil, lemon juice and mustard in a small saucepan to make a glaze.
2. Brush both sides of the halibut steak with the mixture.
3. Grill the fish for 10 minutes over a medium heat until tender and flakey.

91. Cast-Iron Cheesy Chicken

Preparation Time: 10 minutes
Servings: 4

Ingredients

- 4 chicken breasts
- 4 bacon strips
- 4 oz ranch dressing
- 2 green onions
- 4 oz cheddar cheese

Direction

1. Pour the oil into a skillet and heat on high. Add the chicken breasts and fry both sides until piping hot.
2. Fry the bacon and crumble it into bits.
3. Dice the green onions.
4. Put the chicken in a baking dish and top with soy sauce.
5. Toss in the ranch, bacon, green onions and top with cheese.
6. Cook until the cheese is browned, for around 4 minutes.
7. Serve.

92. Cauliflower Rice Chicken Curry

Preparation Time: 40 minutes
Servings: 4

Ingredients

- 2 lb chicken (4 breasts
- 1 packet curry paste
- 3 tbsp ghee (can substitute with butter
- ½ cup heavy cream
- 1 head cauliflower (around 1 kg/2.2 lb

Direction

1. Melt the ghee in a pot. Mix in the curry paste.
2. Add the water and simmer for 5 minutes.
3. Add the chicken, cover, and simmer on a medium heat for 20 minutes or until the chicken is cooked.
4. Shred the cauliflower florets in a food processor to resemble rice.
5. Once the chicken is cooked, uncover, and incorporate the cream.
6. Cook for 7 minutes and serve over the cauliflower.

93. Bacon Chops

Preparation Time: 20 minutes
Servings: 2

Ingredients

- 2 pork chops (I prefer bone-in, but boneless chops work great as well
- 1 bag shredded brussels sprouts
- 4 slices of bacon
- Worcestershire sauce
- Lemon juice (optional

Direction

1. Place the pork chops on a baking sheet with the Worcestershire sauce inside a preheated grill for 5 minutes.
2. Turnover and cook for another 5 minutes. Put to the side when done.
3. Cook the chopped bacon in a large pan until browned. Add the shredded brussels sprouts and cook together.
4. Stir the brussels sprouts with the bacon and grease and cook for 5 minutes until the bacon is crisp.

94. Chicken in a Blanket

Preparation Time: 60 minutes
Servings: 3

Ingredients

- 3 boneless chicken breasts
- 1 package bacon
- 1 8-oz package cream cheese
- 3 jalapeno peppers
- Salt, pepper, garlic powder or other seasonings

Direction

1. Cut the chicken breast in half lengthwise to create two pieces.
2. Cut the jalapenos in half lengthwise and remove the seeds.
3. Dress each breast with a half-inch slice of cream cheese and half a slice of jalapeno. Sprinkle with garlic powder, salt and pepper.
4. Roll the chicken and wrap 2 to 3 pieces of bacon around it—secure with toothpicks.
5. Bake in a preheated 375°F/190°C oven for 50 minutes.
6. Serve!

95. Stuffed Chicken Rolls

Preparation Time: 45 minutes
Servings: 4

Ingredients

- 4 boneless, skinless chicken breasts
- 7 oz cream cheese
- ¼ cup green onions, chopped
- 4 slices bacon, partially cooked

Direction

1. Partially cook your strips of bacon, about 5 minutes for each side and set aside.
2. Pound the chicken breasts to a quarter-inch thick.
3. Mix the cream cheese and green onions together. Spread 2 tablespoons of the mixture onto each breast. Roll and wrap them with the strip of bacon, then secure with a toothpick.
4. Place the chicken on a baking sheet and bake in a preheated oven at 375°F/190°C

for 30 minutes.
5. Broil for 5 minutes to crisp the bacon.
6. Serve.

96. Duck Fat Ribeye

Preparation Time: 20 minutes
Servings: 1

Ingredients

- One 16-oz ribeye steak (1 - 1 ¼ inch thick
- 1 tbsp duck fat (or other high smoke point oil like peanut oil
- ½ tbsp butter
- ½ tsp thyme, chopped
- Salt and pepper to taste

Direction

1. Preheat a skillet in your oven at 400°F/200°C.
2. Season the steaks with the oil, salt and pepper. Remove the skillet from the oven once pre-heated.
3. Put the skillet on your stove top burner on a medium heat and drizzle in the oil.
4. Sear the steak for 1-4 minutes, depending on if you like it rare, medium or well done.
5. Turn over the steak and place in your oven for 6 minutes.
6. Take out the steak from your oven and place it back on the stove top on low heat.
7. Toss in the butter and thyme and cook for 3 minutes, basting as you go along.
8. Rest for 5 minutes and serve.

97. Easy Zoodles & Turkey Balls

Preparation Time: 35 minutes
Servings: 2

Ingredients

- 1 zucchini, cut into spirals
- 1 can vodka pasta sauce
- 1 package frozen Armour Turkey meatballs
- Direction
- Cook the meatballs and sauce on a high heat for 25 minutes, stirring occasionally.
- Wash the zucchini and put through a vegetable spiral maker.
- Boil the water and blanch the raw zoodles for 60 seconds. Remove and drain.
- Combine the zoodles and prepared saucy meatballs.
- Serve!

98. Sausage Balls

Preparation Time: 25 minutes
Servings: 6

Ingredients

- 12 oz Jimmy Dean's Sausage
- 6 oz. shredded cheddar cheese
- 10 cubes cheddar (optional

Direction

1. Mix the shredded cheese and sausage.
2. Divide the mixture into 12 equal parts to be stuffed.
3. Add a cube of cheese to the center of the sausage and roll into balls.
4. Fry at 375°F/190°C for 15 minutes until crisp.
5. Serve!

99. Bacon Scallops

Preparation Time: 10 minutes
Servings: 6

Ingredients

- 12 scallops
- 12 thin bacon slices
- 12 toothpicks
- Salt and pepper to taste
- ½ tbsp oil

Direction

1. Heat a skillet on a high heat while drizzling in the oil.
2. Wrap each scallop with a piece of thinly cut bacon—secure with a toothpick.
3. Season to taste.
4. Cook for 3 minutes per side.
5. Serve!

100. Buffalo Chicken Salad

Preparation Time: 40 minutes
Servings: 1

Ingredients

- 3 cups salad of your choice
- 1 chicken breast
- 1/2 cup shredded cheese of your choice
- Buffalo wing sauce of your choice
- Ranch or blue cheese dressing

Direction

1. Preheat your oven to 400°F/200°C.
2. Douse the chicken breast in the buffalo wing sauce and bake for 25 minutes. In the last 5 minutes, throw the cheese on the wings until it melts.
3. When cooked, remove from the oven and slice into pieces.
4. Place on a bed of lettuce.
5. Pour the salad dressing of your choice on top.
6. Serve!

101. Meatballs

Preparation Time: 30 minutes
Servings: 6

Ingredients

- 1 lb ground beef (or ½ lb beef, ½ lb pork
- ½ cup grated parmesan cheese
- 1 tbsp minced garlic (or paste
- ½ cup mozzarella cheese
- 1 tsp freshly ground pepper

Direction

1. Preheat your oven to 400°F/200°C.
2. In a bowl, mix all the ingredients together.
3. Roll the meat mixture into 5 generous meatballs.
4. Bake inside your oven at 170°F/80°C for about 18 minutes.
5. Serve with sauce!

102. Fat Bombs

Preparation Time: 100 minutes
Servings: 2

Ingredients

- 1 cup coconut butter
- 1 cup coconut milk (full fat, canned
- 1 tsp vanilla extract (gluten free
- ½ tsp nutmeg
- ½ cup coconut shreds

Direction

1. Pour some water into pot and put a glass bowl on top.
2. Add all the ingredients except the shredded coconut into the glass bowl and cook on a medium heat.
3. Stir and melt until they start melting.
4. Then, take them off of the heat.
5. Put the glass bowl into your refrigerator until the mix can be rolled into doughy balls. Usually this happens after around 30 minutes.
6. Roll the dough into 1-inch balls through the coconut shreds.
7. Place the balls on a plate and refrigerate for one hour.
8. Serve!

103. Cabbage & Beef Casserole

Preparation Time: 40 minutes
Servings: 6

Ingredients

- ½ lb ground beef
- ½ cup chopped onion
- ½ bag coleslaw mix
- 1-1/2 cups tomato sauce
- 1 tbsp lemon juice

Direction

1. In a skillet, cook the ground beef until browned and to the side.
2. Mix in the onion and cabbage to the skillet and sauté until soft.
3. Add the ground beef back in along with the tomato sauce and lemon juice.
4. Bring the mixture to a boil, then cover and simmer for 30 minutes.
5. Enjoy!

104. Roast Beef Lettuce Wraps

Preparation Time: 10 minutes
Servings: 4

Ingredients

- 8 large iceberg lettuce leaves
- 8 oz (8 slices rare roast beef
- ½ cup homemade mayonnaise
- 8 slices provolone cheese
- 1 cup baby spinach

Direction

1. Wash the lettuce leaves and sake them dry. Try not to rip them.
2. Place 1 slice of roast beef inside each wrap.
3. Smother 1 tablespoon of mayonnaise on top of each piece of roast beef.
4. Top the mayonnaise with 1 slice of provolone cheese and 1 cup of baby spinach.
5. Roll the lettuce up around the toppings.
6. Serve & enjoy!

105. Turkey Avocado Rolls

Preparation Time: 10 minutes
Servings: 6

Ingredients

- 12 slices (12 oz turkey breast
- 12 slices Swiss cheese
- 2 cups baby spinach
- 1 large avocado, cut into 12 slices
- 1 cup homemade mayonnaise (see recipe in Chapter 9

Direction

1. Lay out the slices of turkey breast flat and place a slice of Swiss cheese on top of each one.
2. Top each slice with 1 cup baby spinach and 3 slices of avocado.
3. Drizzle the mayonnaise on top.
4. Sprinkle each "sandwich" with lemon pepper.
5. Roll up the sandwiches and secure with toothpicks.
6. Serve immediately or refrigerate until ready to serve.

106. Nearly Pizza

Preparation Time: 30 minutes
Servings: 4

Ingredients

- 4 large portobello mushrooms
- 4 tsp olive oil
- 1 cup marinara sauce
- 1 cup shredded mozzarella cheese
- 10 slices sugar-free pepperoni

Direction

1. Preheat your oven to 375°F/190°C.
2. De-steam the 4 mushrooms and brush each cap with the olive oil, one spoon for each cap.
3. Place on a baking sheet and bake stem side down for 8 minutes.
4. Take out of the oven and fill each cap with 1 cup marinara sauce, 1 cup mozzarella cheese and 3 slices of pepperoni.
5. Cook for another 10 minutes until browned.
6. Serve hot.

107. Taco Stuffed Peppers

Preparation Time: 30 minutes
Servings: 4

Ingredients

- 1 lb. ground beef
- 1 tbsp. taco seasoning mix
- 1 can diced tomatoes and green chilis
- 4 green bell peppers
- 1 cup shredded Monterey jack cheese, divided

Direction

1. Set a skillet over a high heat and cook the ground beef for seven to ten minutes. Make sure it is cooked through and brown all over. Drain the fat.
2. Stir in the taco seasoning mix, as well as the diced tomatoes and green chilis. Allow the mixture to cook for a further three to five minutes.
3. In the meantime, slice the tops off the green peppers and remove the seeds and membranes.
4. When the meat mixture is fully cooked,

spoon equal amounts of it into the peppers and top with the Monterey jack cheese. Then place the peppers into your fryer.
5. Cook at 350°F for fifteen minutes.
6. The peppers are ready when they are soft, and the cheese is bubbling and brown. Serve warm and enjoy!

108. Beef Tenderloin & Peppercorn Crust

Preparation Time: 45 minutes
Servings: 6

Ingredients

- 2 lb. beef tenderloin
- 2 tsp. roasted garlic, minced
- 2 tbsp. salted butter, melted
- 3 tbsp. ground 4-peppercorn blender

Direction

1. Remove any surplus fat from the beef tenderloin.
2. Combine the roasted garlic and melted butter to apply to your tenderloin with a brush.
3. On a plate, spread out the peppercorns and roll the tenderloin in them, making sure they are covering and clinging to the meat.
4. Cook the tenderloin in your fryer for twenty-five minutes at 400°F, turning halfway through cooking.
5. Let the tenderloin rest for ten minutes before slicing and serving.

109. Bratwursts

Preparation Time: 18 minutes
Servings: 4

Ingredients

- 4 x 3-oz. beef bratwursts

Direction

1. Place the beef bratwursts in the basket of your fryer and cook for fifteen minutes at 375°F, turning once halfway through.
2. Enjoy with the low-carb toppings and sides of your choice.

110. Bacon-Wrapped Hot Dog

Preparation Time: 25 minutes
Servings: 4

Ingredients

- 4 slices sugar-free bacon
- 4 beef hot dogs

Direction

1. Take a slice of bacon and wrap it around the hot dog, securing it with a toothpick. Repeat with the other pieces of bacon and hot dogs, placing each wrapped dog in the basket of your fryer.
2. Cook at 370°F for ten minutes, turning halfway through to fry the other side.
3. Once hot and crispy, the hot dogs are ready to serve. Enjoy!

111. Herb Shredded Beef

Preparation Time: 25 minutes
Servings: 6

Ingredients

- 1 tsp. dried dill
- 1 tsp. dried thyme
- 1 tsp. garlic powder
- 2 lbs. beefsteak
- 3 tbsp. butter

Directions:

1. Pre-heat your fryer at 360°F.
2. Combine the dill, thyme, and garlic powder together, and massage into the steak.
3. Cook the steak in the fryer for twenty minutes, then remove, shred, and return to the fryer. Add the butter and cook for a further two minutes at 365°F. Make sure the beef is coated in the butter before serving.

112. Herbed Butter Rib Eye Steak

Preparation Time: 60 minutes
Servings: 4

Ingredients

- 4 ribeye steaks

- Olive oil
- ¾ tsp. dry rub
- ½ cup butter
- 1 tsp. dried basil
- 3 tbsp. lemon garlic seasoning

Directions:
1. Massage the olive oil into the steaks and your favorite dry rub. Leave aside to sit
5.
   for thirty minutes.
2. In a bowl, combine the button, dried basil, and lemon garlic seasoning, then refrigerate.
3. Pre-heat the fryer at 450°F and set a rack inside. Place the steaks on top of the rack and allow to cook for fifteen minutes.
4. Remove the steaks from the fryer when cooked and serve with the herbed butter.

Sides

113. Grilled Artichokes

Servings: 4
Preparation time: 10 minutes
Cooking time: 30 minutes

Ingredients:

- Juice of 1 lemon
- A pinch of salt and black pepper
- 2 artichokes, trimmed and halved lengthwise
- 4 garlic cloves, minced
- ¾ cup extra virgin olive oil

Directions:

1. Put water in a bowl, add half of the lemon juice and artichoke halves, leave aside for 10 minutes and drain them.
2. Put some water in a large saucepan, bring to a simmer over medium heat, add the artichokes, cook for 15 minutes, drain them again, transfer to a bowl, add the rest of the ingredients and toss well.
3. Place the artichokes on preheated grill and cook them over medium heat for 5 minutes on each side.
4. Divide between plates and serve as a side dish.
5. Put artichokes in a bowl, add the rest of the lemon juice, the oil, a pinch of salt, black pepper to the taste and garlic and toss to coat.
6. Enjoy!

Nutritional value: calories 370, fat 28, fiber 4,5, carbs 10,6, protein 2,9

114. Mashed Yams

Preparation time: 10 minutes
Cooking time: 1 hour
Servings: 6

Ingredients:

- ¼ cup coconut oil, melted
- 3 pounds yams, peeled and cubed
- A pinch of sea salt and black pepper

Directions:

1. Arrange the yams on a lined baking sheet and bake at 375 degrees F for 1 hour.
2. In a bowl, mix the yams with salt, pepper and the oil, mash using a potato masher and whisk well.
3. Serve as a side dish.
4. Enjoy!

Nutrition: calories 341, fat 9,4, fiber 8,9, carbs 62,3, protein 3,4

115. Balsamic Roasted Beets

Preparation time: 10 minutes
Cooking time: 1 hour
Servings: 4

Ingredients:

- 2 tablespoons balsamic vinegar
- 8 beets, cut into quarters
- 1 tablespoon melted coconut oil
- A pinch of black pepper

Directions:

1. In a bowl, mix all the ingredients, toss, spread to a lined baking sheet and bake at 350 degrees F for 1 hour.
2. Divide the beets between plates and serve them.
3. Enjoy!

Nutrition: calories 120, fat 3,9, fiber 4, carbs 20, protein 3,4

116. Kale Mix

Preparation time: 10 minutes
Cooking time: 8 minutes
Servings: 4

Ingredients:

- 1 bunch kale, roughly chopped
- ½ cup veggie stock
- A drizzle of olive oil
- 1 tablespoon lemon juice
- 1 garlic clove, minced

- Black pepper to taste

Directions:
1. Heat up a pan with the oil over medium heat, add the kale, the stock, lemon juice, black pepper and garlic, toss, cook for 8 minutes, divide between plate and serve as a side dish.
2. Enjoy!

Nutrition: calories 44, fat 3,8, fiber 0,4, carbs 2,8, protein 0,7

117. Pumpkin Fries

Preparation time: 10 minutes
Cooking time: 35 minutes
Servings: 4

Ingredients:
- 1 big pumpkin, peeled and cut in medium fries
- 1 tablespoon maple syrup
- 1 tablespoon coconut oil, melted

Directions :
1. Drizzle the oil on a lined baking sheet, add pumpkin fries and toss.
2. Add maple syrup, toss to coat well again, place in the oven at 400 degrees F and bake for 35 minutes.
3. Divide the fries between plates and serve them as a side dish.
4. Enjoy!

Nutrition: calories 95, fat 3,6, fiber 1, carbs 16,6, protein 2

118. Pumpkin and Bok Choy

Preparation time: 10 minutes
Cooking time: 15 minutes
Servings: 4

Ingredients:
- 2 tablespoons olive oil
- 3 tablespoons coconut aminos
- 1-inch ginger, grated
- A pinch of red pepper flakes
- 4 bok choy heads, cut into quarters
- 2 garlic cloves, minced
- 1 small pumpkin, peeled, seeded and thinly sliced
- 1 tablespoon sesame seeds, toasted

Directions:
1. Heat up a pan with the oil over medium heat, add coconut aminos, garlic, pepper flakes and ginger, stir, cook for 1 minute and take off heat.
2. Heat up another pan, add some water, bring to a simmer over medium heat, add pumpkin pieces, cook for 10 minutes, drain and transfer them to a platter.
3. Add bok choy to the pan with the water, heat it up again over medium heat, cover, cook for 5 minutes, drain as well and add to the platter with the pumpkin.
4. Add the coconut mix from the pan, add sesame seeds as well, toss and serve as a side dish.
5. Enjoy!

Nutrition: calories 223, fat 10, fiber 9,5, carbs 28,6, protein 14,4

119. Pumpkin Mash

Preparation time: 10 minutes
Cooking time: 45 minutes
Servings: 4

Ingredients:
- 1 teaspoon cinnamon powder
- 1 cup unsweetened coconut, shredded
- 1 pumpkin, peeled, seeded and cubed
- ½ cup coconut oil, melted
- A pinch of sea salt and white pepper

Directions:
1. Put water in a large saucepan, add pumpkin cubes, heat up over medium high heat, cover and cook for 30 minutes.
2. Drain the pumpkin, add a pinch of salt and pepper, oil and coconut to the pan, stir and cook everything for 3 minutes more.
3. Mash using a potato masher, add the cinnamon, stir well, cook for 2 minutes more, divide between plates and serve.
4. Enjoy!

Nutrition: calories 343, fat 34,1, fiber 2,5, carbs 12,5, protein 2,1

120. Pumpkin Salad

Preparation time: 10 minutes
Cooking time: 30 minutes
Servings: 6

Ingredients:

- 2 tablespoons olive oil + 2 teaspoons olive oil
- 21 ounces pumpkin, peeled, seeded and cubed
- 2 teaspoons sesame seeds
- 1 tablespoon lemon juice
- 2 teaspoons mustard
- 4 ounces baby spinach
- 2 tablespoons pine nuts, toasted
- A pinch of sea salt and black pepper

Directions:

1. In a bowl, mix pumpkin with salt, black pepper and 2 teaspoons oil, toss to coat well, spread on a lined baking sheet, place in the oven at 400 degrees F and bake for 25 minutes.
2. Leave pumpkin pieces to cool down a bit, add sesame seeds, toss to coat, place in the oven again and bake for 5 minutes more.
3. In a bowl, mix lemon juice with the rest of the oil and mustard and whisk.
4. Leave pumpkin to completely cool down and transfer it to a salad bowl.
5. Add baby spinach, pine nuts and the salad dressing, toss to coat well, divide between plates and serve as a side salad.
6. Enjoy!

Nutrition: calories 149, fat 12,5, fiber 3,7, carbs 9,8, protein 2,5

121. Turnips and Sauce

Preparation time: 10 minutes
Cooking time: 15 minutes
Servings: 4

Ingredients:

- 1 tablespoon lemon juice
- Zest of 2 oranges
- 16 ounces turnips, thinly sliced
- 3 tablespoons coconut oil
- 1 tablespoon rosemary, chopped
- A pinch of sea salt
- Black pepper to taste

Directions:

1. Heat up a pan with the oil over medium-high heat, add turnips, stir and cook for 4 minutes.
2. Add lemon juice, a pinch of salt, black pepper, and rosemary, stir and cook for 10 minutes more.
3. Take off the heat, add orange zest, stir, divide between plates and serve.
4. Enjoy!

Nutrition: calories 125, fat 10,4, fiber 2,3, carbs 8,2, protein 1

122. Lemon Fennel

Preparation time: 10 minutes
Cooking time: 0 minutes
Servings: 4

Ingredients:

- 3 tablespoons lemon juice
- 1 pound fennel, chopped
- A pinch of sea salt and black pepper
- 2 tablespoons olive oil

Directions:

1. In a salad bowl, mix fennel with a pinch of salt and black pepper and toss,
2. In another bowl, mix the oil with a pinch of salt, pepper and lemon juice and whisk well.
3. Add this to the salad bowl, toss to coat well, divide between plates and serve as a side dish.
4. Enjoy!

Nutrition: calories 98, fat 7,3, fiber 3,6, carbs 8,5, protein 1,5

123. Plantain Fries

Preparation time: 10 minutes
Cooking time: 10 minutes

Servings: 4

Ingredients:

- ½ cup ghee, melted
- 2 green plantains, peeled and sliced
- A pinch of sea salt and black pepper

Directions:

1. Heat up a pan with the ghee over medium-high heat, season plantain slices with salt and black pepper, add half of them to the pan, cook for 5 minutes and transfer to paper towels.
2. Fry the second batch of plantain slices, drain grease as well, divide them between plates and serve them as a side.
3. Enjoy!

Nutrition: calories 334, fat 25,8, fiber 2,1, carbs 28,5, protein 1,2

124. Roasted Broccoli

Preparation time: 10 minutes
Cooking time: 30 minutes
Servings: 4

Ingredients:

- 8 garlic cloves, minced
- ¼ cup avocado oil
- 8 cups broccoli florets
- Zest of 1 lemon, grated
- ¼ cup parsley, chopped
- A pinch of sea salt and black pepper

Directions:

1. In a bowl, mix broccoli with salt, pepper, oil, garlic and lemon zest, toss to coat, spread on a lined baking sheet, place in the oven at 450 degrees F and bake for 30 minutes.
2. Divide between plates, sprinkle parsley on top and serve as a side.
3. Enjoy!

Nutrition: calories 92, fat 2,4, fiber 5,6, carbs 15,1, protein 5,8

125. Kumquat Side Salad

Preparation time: 10 minutes
Cooking time: 0 minutes
Servings: 2

Ingredients:

- 2 cups arugula leaves
- 1 tablespoon olive oil
- 1 tablespoon balsamic vinegar
- 2 cups kale, torn
- 3 tablespoons red onion, chopped
- 4 kumquats, sliced
- 1 small avocado, pitted, peeled and cubed
- ½ cup walnuts, chopped

Directions:

1. In a bowl, combine all the ingredients, toss, divide between plates and serve as a side dish.
2. Enjoy!

Nutrition: calories 531, fat 45,5, fiber 13, carbs 27, protein 12,8

126. Baked Brussels Sprouts

Preparation time: 10 minutes
Cooking time: 30 minutes
Servings: 4

Ingredients:

- ¼ cup avocado oil
- 4 pounds Brussels sprouts, halved
- A pinch of sea salt and black pepper

Directions:

1. In a bowl, mix Brussels sprouts with oil, salt, and pepper, toss to coat well, spread on a lined baking sheet, place in the oven at 375 degrees F and bake for 30 minutes.
2. Divide between plates and serve as a side dish.
3. Enjoy!

Nutrition: calories 215, fat 3,3, fiber 17,6, carbs 42, protein 15,6

127. Squash and Sweet Potato Mix

Preparation time: 10 minutes
Cooking time: 1 hour and 30 minutes
Servings: 8

Ingredients:

- 1 pound yellow squash, peeled and chopped
- 1 yellow onion, chopped
- 3 tablespoons olive oil
- 2 garlic cloves, minced
- 4 pounds mixed sweet potatoes, cubed
- 1 cup veggie stock
- A pinch of black pepper

Directions:
1. In a baking dish, combine all the ingredients, toss and bake at 400 degrees F and bake for 1 hour.
2. Divide between plates and serve warm as a side dish.
3. Enjoy!

Nutrition: calories 555, fat 6,2, fiber 17,5, carbs 120,5, protein 7,2

128. Tapioca Root Fries

Preparation time: 10 minutes
Cooking time: 1 hour
Servings: 4

Ingredients:
- 2 and ½ pound tapioca root, cut in medium fries
- ½ cup ghee, melted
- Black pepper to taste

Directions:
1. Put some water in a large saucepan, bring to a boil over medium high heat, add tapioca fries, boil for 10 minutes and drain them well.
2. Spread the fries on a lined baking sheet, add black pepper and the ghee, toss everything to coat well, place in the oven at 375 degrees F and bake for 45 minutes.
3. Divide them between plates and serve as a side.
4. Enjoy!

Nutrition: calories 905, fat 25,5, fiber 1,7, carbs 168,5, protein 0,4

129. Cauliflower and Turnips

Preparation time: 10 minutes
Cooking time: 30 minutes
Servings: 4

Ingredients:
- 6 cups cauliflower florets
- 1 and ½ pounds turnips, thinly sliced
- 1 cup chicken stock
- 2 tablespoons avocado oil
- A pinch of sea salt and black pepper

Directions:
1. In a baking dish, toss well to combine all the ingredients, and bake at 375 degrees F for 30 minutes.
2. Divide between plates and serve.
3. Enjoy!

Nutrition: calories 140, fat 1,5, fiber 9,9, carbs 29,4, protein 6,2

130. Roasted Broccoli

Preparation time: 10 minutes
Cooking time: 20 minutes
Servings: 4

Ingredients:
- 1 and ½ pounds broccoli
- 2 tablespoons lemon juice
- A pinch of sea salt
- 3 tablespoons avocado oil

Directions:
1. In a bowl, mix broccoli with a pinch of salt, oil and lemon juice, toss to coat well, spread on a lined baking sheet, place in the oven at 450 degrees F and roast for 20 minutes.
2. Divide them between plates and serve.
3. Enjoy!

Nutrition: calories 76, fat 1,9, fiber 5,2, carbs 12,7, protein 5,2

131. Roasted Cauliflower

Preparation time: 10 minutes
Cooking time: 30 minutes
Servings: 4

Ingredients:
- 1 cauliflower head, florets separated

- ¼ cup coconut oil, melted
- ¼ cup parsley, chopped
- 2 teaspoons lemon zest, grated
- A pinch of sea salt and black pepper
- 10 garlic cloves, minced

Directions:
1. Spread cauliflower florets on a lined baking sheet, add oil and toss to coat.
2. Add a pinch of salt and black pepper, garlic, and lemon zest, toss again, place in the oven at 450 degrees F and bake for 30 minutes.
3. Sprinkle the parsley on top, toss, divide between plates and serve.
4. Enjoy!

Nutrition: calories 147, fat 13,8, fiber 1,9, carbs 6,2, protein 1,9

132. Garlic Plantain Mash

Preparation time: 10 minutes
Cooking time: 30 minutes
Servings: 4

Ingredients:
- 6 ounces shallots, chopped
- 3 green bananas, peeled, halved lengthwise
- 4 garlic cloves, minced
- 1 yellow onion, chopped
- 2 tablespoons coconut oil, melted
- A pinch of sea salt

Directions:
1. Put the water in a large saucepan, bring to a boil over medium-high heat, add plantain halves, cover, cook them for 20 minutes and drain the water.
2. Heat up a pan over medium high heat, add shallots, stir and cook for 5 minutes.
3. Add garlic and onion, stir, cook for 5 minutes more, drain excess grease and transfer everything to a blender.
4. Add plantains and 2 tablespoons oil and pulse well.
5. Add a pinch of sea salt, blend again, divide between plates and serve.
6. Enjoy!

Nutrition: calories 183, fat 7,2, fiber 3, carbs 30,9, protein 2,5

133. Sage Kohlrabi

Preparation time: 10 minutes
Cooking time: 17 minutes
Servings: 3

Ingredients:
- 4 tablespoons ghee
- 3 kohlrabi, peeled and cubed
- 1 tablespoon sage, chopped
- A pinch of sea salt and black pepper

Directions:
1. Heat up a pan with the ghee over medium-high heat, add kohlrabi, a pinch of salt and black pepper, stir and cook for 15 minutes.
2. Add sage, stir again, cook for 2 minutes more, divide between plates and serve as a side dish.
3. Enjoy!

Nutrition: calories 212, fat 17,3, fiber 8,4, carbs 14,4, protein 4

134. Spaghetti Squash Mix

Preparation time: 10 minutes
Cooking time: 55 minutes
Servings: 4

Ingredients:
- 1 spaghetti squash, cut in halves and seeded
- 12 sage leaves, chopped
- 3 tablespoons ghee, melted
- A pinch of sea salt
- Black pepper to taste

Directions:
1. Place spaghetti squash on a lined baking sheet, place in the oven at 375 degrees F, bake for 40 minutes, and scoop strings of flesh into a bowl.
2. Heat up a pan with the ghee over medium heat, add sage, cook for 5 minutes and transfer them to paper towels.
3. Heat up the pan again over medium heat,

add spaghetti squash, salt and black pepper to the taste, stir and cook for 3 minutes.
4. Add the sage, stir, divide between plates and serve as a side.
5. Enjoy!

Nutrition: calories 108, fat 10,3, fiber 2, carbs 4,8, protein 0,7

135. Coconut Butternut Squash

Preparation time: 10 minutes
Cooking time: 35 minutes
Servings: 6

Ingredients:

- 2 tablespoons coconut oil, melted
- 2 pounds butternut squash, peeled, seeded and cubed
- 2 teaspoons thyme, chopped
- A pinch of black pepper

Directions

1. In a bowl, mix squash cubes with oil, thyme, and pepper and toss to combine.
2. Spread them on a lined baking sheet, place in the oven at 425 degrees F and bake for 35 minutes.
3. Divide between plates and serve as a side dish.
4. Enjoy!

Nutrition: calories 108, fat 4,7, fiber 3,1, carbs 17,9, protein 1,5

136. Cinnamon Butternut Squash

Preparation time: 10 minutes
Cooking time: 30 minutes
Servings: 4

Ingredients:

- ½ teaspoon cinnamon powder
- 2 tablespoons olive oil
- 2 apples, peeled, cored and cubed
- 1 and ½ pounds butternut squash, peeled, seeded and cubed

Directions:

1. In a baking dish, toss well to combine all ingredients, place in the oven at 350 degrees F and roast for 30 minutes.
2. Divide between plates and serving.
3. Enjoy!

Nutrition: calories 221, fat 7,5, fiber 11, carbs 42,3, protein 2,6

137. Stir Fried Veggies

Preparation time: 10 minutes
Cooking time: 15 minutes
Servings: 4

Ingredients:

- 1 teaspoon ginger, grated
- 1 pound white mushrooms, sliced
- 1 bunch turnip greens, trimmed
- 2 garlic cloves, minced
- Black pepper to taste
- A pinch of sea salt
- ½ cup raw almonds, chopped
- ¼ cup lime juice
- 2 tablespoons coconut oil, melted
- 1 tablespoon coconut aminos

Directions:

1. Heat up a pan with the oil over medium high heat, add mushrooms and turnips greens, stir and cook for 2 minutes.
2. Add ginger and garlic, stir and cook for 2 minutes more.
3. Add lime juice, almonds, coconut aminos, salt and black pepper, stir and cook for 10 minutes more.
4. Divide between plates and serve.
5. Enjoy!

Nutrition: calories 164, fat 13,2, fiber 3,2, carbs 9,4, protein 6,5

138. Flavored Carrots

Preparation time: 10 minutes
Cooking time: 30 minutes
Servings: 4

Ingredients:

- 2 teaspoons rosemary, dried
- 2 pounds baby carrots, trimmed
- 3 tablespoons coconut oil
- ½ teaspoon garlic powder

- A pinch of sea salt
- Black pepper to taste

Directions:
1. In a baking dish, toss well to combine all the ingredients, and bake at 375 degrees F for 30 minutes.
2. Divide between plates and serve as a side dish.
3. Enjoy!

Nutrition: calories 170, fat 10,6, fiber 6,9, carbs 19,3, protein 1,5

139. Quinoa and Spinach Mix

Preparation time: 10 minutes
Cooking time: 0 minutes
Servings: 4

Ingredients:
- 1 cup quinoa, cooked
- 1 cup baby spinach
- A pinch of sea salt and black pepper
- 1 cucumber, chopped
- 1 teaspoon chili powder
- 2 tablespoons balsamic vinegar
- 2 tablespoons cilantro, chopped

Directions:
1. In a bowl, mix the quinoa with the spinach and the other ingredients, toss and serve as a side dish.

Nutrition: calories 100, fat 0.5, fiber 2, carbs 6, protein 6

140. Minty Asparagus

Preparation time: 10 minutes
Cooking time: 10 minutes
Servings: 4

Ingredients:
- 1 pound asparagus, trimmed
- 2 tablespoons olive oil
- 3 garlic cloves, minced
- Salt and black pepper to the taste
- 1 teaspoon lemon zest, grated
- ¼ cup lemon juice
- ¼ cup mint leaves, chopped

Directions:
1. Heat up a pan with the oil over medium heat, add the garlic and sauté for 2 minutes.
2. Add the asparagus and the other ingredients, toss, cook for 8 minutes more, divide between plates and serve as a side dish.

Nutrition: calories 100, fat 1, fiber 6, carbs 8, protein 6

141. Chard Mix

Preparation time: 10 minutes
Cooking time: 15 minutes
Servings: 4

Ingredients:
- 2 spring onions, chopped
- 4 cups red chard, shredded
- 2 tablespoons olive oil
- 2 teaspoons ginger, grated
- ½ teaspoon red pepper flakes, crushed
- 2 tablespoons balsamic vinegar
- 1 tablespoon chives, chopped

Directions:
1. Heat up a pan with the oil over medium heat, add the spring onions and the ginger and sauté for 5 minutes.
2. Add the chard and the other ingredients, toss, cook for 10 minutes more, divide between plates and serve as a side dish.

Nutrition: calories 160, fat 10, fiber 3, carbs 10, protein 5

142. Cabbage and Tomatoes

Preparation time: 10 minutes
Cooking time: 0 minutes
Servings: 4

Ingredients:
- 1 cup green cabbage, shredded
- 1 cup tomatoes, cubed
- 2 tablespoons walnuts, chopped
- 1 bunch green onions, chopped
- ¼ cup balsamic vinegar
- 2 tablespoons olive oil

- 1 tablespoon chives, chopped
- A pinch of salt and black pepper

Directions:
1. In a salad bowl, mix the cabbage with the tomatoes, the walnuts and the other ingredients, toss and serve as a side dish.

Nutrition: calories 140, fat 3, fiber 3, carbs 8, protein 6

143. Carrots Salad

Preparation time: 10 minutes
Cooking time: 0 minutes
Servings: 4

Ingredients:
- 3 scallions, chopped
- 1 pound carrots, peeled and sliced
- ½ cup cilantro, chopped
- 3 tablespoons sesame seeds
- 2 tablespoons balsamic vinegar
- 2 tablespoons olive oil
- A pinch of salt and black pepper

Directions:
1. In a salad bowl, mix the carrots with the scallions and the other ingredients, toss well and serve as a side dish.

Nutrition: calories 140, fat 4, fiber 3, carbs 5, protein 6

144. Sweet Potatoes and Raisins Mix

Preparation time: 10 minutes
Cooking time: 30 minutes
Servings: 4

Ingredients:
- 2 sweet potatoes, peeled and cut into wedges
- 2 tablespoons raisins
- 2 garlic cloves, minced
- 2 tablespoons walnuts, chopped
- Juice of ½ lemon
- 2 tablespoons olive oil
- A pinch of salt and black pepper

Directions:
1. In a roasting pan, combine the sweet potatoes with the raisins and the other ingredients, toss and bake at 370 degrees F for 30 minutes.
2. Divide everything between plates and serve.

Nutrition: calories 120, fat 1, fiber 2, carbs 3, protein 5

145. Turmeric Okra

Preparation time: 10 minutes
Cooking time: 30 minutes
Servings: 4

Ingredients:
- 2 cups okra, sliced
- 1 teaspoon turmeric powder
- A pinch of salt and black pepper
- 1 teaspoon thyme, dried
- 2 tablespoons olive oil
- 1 tablespoon coconut aminos
- 1 tablespoon cilantro, chopped

Directions:
1. In a baking dish, combine the okra with the turmeric, salt, pepper and the other ingredients, toss and cook at 360 degrees F for 30 minutes.
2. Divide the mix between plates and serve as a side dish.

Nutrition: calories 87, fat 7.2, fiber 1.8, carbs 5, protein 1

146. Creamy Green Beans

Preparation time: 10 minutes
Cooking time: 30 minutes
Servings: 4

Ingredients:
- 1 pound green beans, trimmed and halved
- 2 tablespoons olive oil
- 2 garlic cloves, minced
- 1 yellow onion, chopped
- ½ cup coconut cream
- 1 teaspoon coriander, ground
- 1 teaspoon cumin, ground
- A pinch of red pepper flakes

- A pinch of salt and black pepper

Directions:
1. Heat up a pan with the oil over medium heat, add the onion and the garlic and sauté for 5 minutes.
2. Add the green beans and the other ingredients, toss, cook over medium heat for 25 minutes more, divide between plates and serve.

Nutrition: calories 180, fat 14.5, fiber 5.2, carbs 13.1, protein 3.3

147. Radish and Cabbage Salad

Preparation time: 10 minutes
Cooking time: 0 minutes
Servings: 4

Ingredients:
- 2 cups green cabbage, shredded
- ½ cup radishes, sliced
- 1 tablespoon olive oil
- 4 scallions, chopped
- A pinch of salt and black pepper
- 1 tablespoon chives, chopped
- 1 teaspoon sesame seeds

Directions:
1. In a bowl, combine the radishes with the cabbage and the other ingredients, toss and serve.

Nutrition: calories 121, fat 3, fiber 4, carbs 8.30, protein 3

148. Baked Beets Mix

Preparation time: 10 minutes
Cooking time: 40 minutes
Servings: 4

Ingredients:
- 1 pound red beets, peeled and roughly cubed
- 1 red onion, cut into wedges
- 1 tablespoon smoked paprika
- 1 teaspoon red pepper flakes, crushed
- 3 garlic cloves, minced
- A pinch of salt and black pepper
- 3 tablespoons olive oil
- 2 tablespoon chives, chopped

Directions:
1. In a baking dish, mix the beets with the onion, the paprika and the other ingredients, toss and bake at 380 degrees F for 40 minutes.
2. Divide everything between plates and serve as a side dish.

Nutrition: calories 162, fat 4, fiber 7, carbs 11, protein 7

149. Roasted Sprouts and Carrots

Preparation time: 5 minutes
Cooking time: 30 minutes
Servings: 4

Ingredients:
- 1 pound Brussels sprouts, trimmed and halved
- 2 carrots, grated
- 2 tablespoons avocado oil
- 1 tablespoon rosemary, chopped
- 2 tablespoons walnuts, chopped
- A pinch of salt and black pepper

Directions:
1. In a baking dish, mix the sprouts with the carrots, the oil and the other ingredients, toss and bake at 380 degrees F for 30 minutes.
2. Divide everything between plates and serve as a side dish.

Nutrition: calories 191, fat 2, fiber 4, carbs 13, protein 7

150. Coconut Corn and Tomatoes

Preparation time: 10 minutes
Cooking time: 20 minutes
Servings: 4

Ingredients:
- 2 cups corn
- 2 cups cherry tomatoes, halved
- 1 cup coconut milk
- 1 tablespoon mint, chopped

- 1 teaspoon turmeric powder
- 1 teaspoon chili powder
- A pinch of salt and black pepper
- 2 tablespoons green onions, chopped

Directions:
1. In a pan, combine the corn with the cherry tomatoes, the milk and the other ingredients, toss, bring to a simmer and cook over medium heat for 20 minutes.
2. Divide the mix between plates and serve as a side dish.

Nutrition: calories 199, fat 2, fiber 3, carbs 8, protein 6

151. Squash Mix

Preparation time: 10 minutes
Cooking time: 25 minutes
Servings: 4

Ingredients:
- 1 butternut squash, peeled and roughly cubed
- 2 spring onions, chopped
- 1 tablespoon avocado oil
- A pinch of salt and black pepper
- 1 tablespoon balsamic vinegar
- 1 tablespoon cilantro, chopped
- ½ cup pecans, toasted and chopped

Directions:
1. In a roasting pan, combine the squash with the spring onions and the other ingredients, toss and bake at 400 degrees F for 25 minutes.
2. Divide the mix between plates and serve.

Nutrition: calories 211, fat 3, fiber 4, carbs 9, protein 6

152. Cinnamon Carrots Mix

Preparation time: 10 minutes
Cooking time: 30 minutes
Servings: 4

Ingredients:
- 1 pound baby carrots, peeled
- 1 tablespoon ginger, grated
- 3 tablespoons cinnamon powder
- 1 tablespoon coconut oil, melted
- 1 tablespoon chives, chopped

Directions:
1. Spread the carrots on a baking sheet lined with parchment paper, add the ginger and the other ingredients, toss and bake at 380 degrees F for 30 minutes.
2. Divide everything between plates and serve.

Nutrition: calories 198, fat 2, fiber 4, carbs 11, protein 6

153. Brown Rice Salad

Preparation time: 10 minutes
Cooking time: 0 minutes
Servings: 4

Ingredients:
- 2 tablespoons olive oil
- 2 cups brown rice, cooked
- ½ cup cherry tomatoes, halved
- 2 teaspoons cumin, ground
- ¼ cup cilantro, chopped
- A pinch of salt and black pepper
- 2 tablespoons olive oil

Directions:

In a bowl, combine the rice with the oil and the other ingredients, toss and serve.

Nutrition: calories 122, fat 4, fiber 3, carbs 8, protein 5

154. Curry Green Beans

Preparation time: 10 minutes
Cooking time: 25 minutes
Servings: 4

Ingredients:
- 2 tablespoons olive oil
- 1 yellow onion, chopped
- 1 pound green beans, trimmed
- 2 teaspoons garlic, minced
- A pinch of salt and black pepper
- 2 teaspoons curry powder
- ½ cup vegetable stock

- ½ teaspoon brown mustard seeds
- 1 tablespoon lime juice

Directions:
1. Heat up a large pan with the oil over medium-high heat, add the onion and the garlic and sauté for 5 minutes.
2. Add the green beans and the other ingredients, toss, cook over medium heat for 20 minutes, divide between plates and serve.

Nutrition: calories 181, fat 3, fiber 6, carbs 12, protein 6

155. Onion and Avocado Salad

Preparation time: 10 minutes
Cooking time: 0 minutes
Servings: 4

Ingredients:
- 2 red onions, sliced
- 2 avocados, peeled, pitted and roughly sliced
- 1 tablespoon olive oil
- 1 tablespoon balsamic vinegar
- 1 tablespoon dill, chopped
- 1 teaspoon chili powder
- A pinch of salt and black pepper

Directions:
1. In a bowl, combine the avocado with the onions and the other ingredients, toss, and serve.

Nutrition: calories 171, fat 2, fiber 7, carbs 13, protein 6

156. Chili Green Beans and Radish

Preparation time: 10 minutes
Cooking time: 20 minutes
Servings: 4

Ingredients:
- 1 pound green beans, trimmed and halved
- 1 cup radishes, sliced
- 2 tablespoons olive oil
- 1 yellow onion, chopped
- A pinch of salt and black pepper
- 4 scallions, chopped
- 1 teaspoon chili flakes
- 1 tablespoon cilantro, chopped

Directions:
1. Heat up a pan with the oil over medium heat, add the onion and the scallions and sauté for 5 minutes.
2. Add the green beans and the other ingredients, toss, cook over medium heat for 15 minutes, divide between plates and serve.

Nutrition: calories 60, fat 3, fiber 2, carbs 5, protein 1

157. Broccoli and Peas

Preparation time: 10 minutes
Cooking time: 20 minutes
Servings: 4

Ingredients:
- 1 pound broccoli florets
- 1 cup green peas
- 1 teaspoon cumin, ground
- A pinch of salt and black pepper
- 1 tablespoon mint leaves, chopped
- 2 tablespoons olive oil
- 1 tablespoon coriander, chopped

Directions:
1. In a roasting pan, combine the broccoli with the peas, the mint and the other ingredients, toss and bake at 390 degrees F for 20 minutes.
2. Divide everything between plates and serve.

Nutrition: calories 120, fat 6, fiber 1, carbs 5, protein 6

158. Bok Choy Mix

Preparation time: 10 minutes
Cooking time: 20 minutes
Servings: 4

Ingredients:
- 1 pound bok choy, torn
- 1 yellow onion, chopped

- 1 tablespoon olive oil
- A pinch of salt and black pepper
- 1 tablespoon red pepper flakes, crushed
- 3 garlic cloves, minced
- ¼ cup cilantro, chopped

Directions:
1. Heat up a pan with the oil over medium heat, add the onion and the garlic and sauté for 5 minutes.
2. Add the bok choy and the other ingredients, toss, cook over medium heat for 15 minutes more, divide between plates and serve as a side dish.

Nutrition: calories 143, fat 3, fiber 4, carbs 3, protein 6

159. Garlic Kale and Bok Choy

Preparation time: 5 minutes
Cooking time: 20 minutes
Servings: 4

Ingredients:
- 2 tablespoons olive oil
- 1 yellow onion, chopped
- 1 cup kale, torn
- 2 cups bok boy, torn
- 2 garlic cloves, minced
- 1 teaspoon turmeric powder
- 3 tablespoons lemon juice
- A pinch of salt and black pepper

Directions:
1. Heat up a pan with the oil over medium heat, add the onion and the garlic and sauté for 5 minutes.
2. Add the kale, bok choy and the other ingredients, toss, cook over medium heat for 15 minutes, divide between plates and serve.

Nutrition: calories 180, fat 2, fiber 7, carbs 6, protein 8

160. Endives and Watercress Salad

Preparation time: 10 minutes
Cooking time: 0 minutes
Servings: 4

Ingredients:
- 2 endives, trimmed and thinly sliced
- 2 tablespoons olive oil
- 4 scallions, chopped
- 2 ounces watercress, chopped
- 1 tablespoon balsamic vinegar
- A pinch of salt and black pepper
- 1 tablespoon tarragon, chopped
- 1 tablespoon chives, chopped
- 1 tablespoon pine nuts, toasted
- 1 tablespoon walnuts, chopped

Directions:
1. In a bowl, mix the endives with the scallions, the watercress and the other ingredients, toss well and serve as a side salad.

Nutrition: calories 140, fat 10.3, fiber 8.8, carbs 10.5, protein 4.8

161. Zucchini and Kale Mix

Preparation time: 5 minutes
Cooking time: 20 minutes
Servings: 4

Ingredients:
- 1 cup kale, torn
- 2 zucchinis, sliced
- 1 yellow onion, chopped
- 2 tablespoons olive oil
- 1 teaspoon chili powder
- 1 teaspoon turmeric powder
- 1 tablespoon mint, chopped
- 1 tablespoon lemon juice
- A pinch of salt and black pepper

Directions:
1. Heat up a pan with the oil over medium heat, add the onion and sauté for 5 minutes.
2. Add the zucchinis, the kale and the other ingredients, toss, cook over medium heat for 15 minutes more, divide between plates and serve.

Nutrition: calories 140, fat 1, fiber 2, carbs 11, protein 7

162. Chili Corn and Zucchinis

Preparation time: 10 minutes
Cooking time: 15 minutes
Servings: 4

Ingredients:

- 1 cup corn
- 2 zucchinis, roughly sliced
- 1 yellow onion, thinly sliced
- 2 tablespoon olive oil
- 2 teaspoons chili paste
- ¼ cup vegetable stock
- 1 tablespoon rosemary, chopped
- ½ teaspoon cumin, ground
- 4 green onions, chopped

Directions:

1. Heat up a pan with the oil over medium-high heat, add the onion and the chili paste, stir and sauté for 5 minutes
2. Add the corn, zucchinis and the other ingredients, toss well, cook over medium heat for 10 minutes more, divide between plates and serve as a side dish.

Nutrition: calories 142, fat 7, fiber 4, carbs 5, protein 3

163. Spinach and Radish Salad

Preparation time: 5 minutes
Cooking time: 0 minutes
Servings: 4

Ingredients:

- 1 pound baby spinach
- 1 cucumber, sliced
- 1 tomato, cubed
- 1 yellow onion, sliced
- 3 tablespoons olive oil
- ¼ cup pine nuts, toasted
- 2 tablespoons balsamic vinegar
- A pinch of salt and black pepper
- A pinch of red pepper, crushed

Directions:

1. In a bowl, combine the spinach with the cucumber, tomato and the other ingredients, toss and serve as a side salad.

Nutrition: calories 120, fat 1, fiber 2, carbs 3, protein 6

164. Low-Carb Pizza Crust

Preparation Time: 20 minutes
Servings: 4

Ingredients

- 1 tbsp. full-fat cream cheese
- ½ cup whole-milk mozzarella cheese, shredded
- 2 tbsp. keto almond flour
- 1 egg white

Directions:

1. In a microwave-safe bowl, combine the cream cheese, mozzarella, and almond flour and heat in the microwave for half a minute. Mix well to create a smooth consistency. Add in the egg white and stir to form a soft ball of dough.
2. With slightly wet hands, press the dough into a pizza crust about six inches in diameter.
3. Place a sheet of parchment paper in the bottom of your fryer and lay the crust on top. Cook for ten minutes at 350°F, turning the crust over halfway through the cooking time.
4. Top the pizza base with the toppings of your choice and enjoy!

165. Bacon-Wrapped Onion Rings

Preparation Time: 15 minutes
Servings: 8

Ingredients

- 1 large onion, peeled
- 8 slices sugar-free bacon
- 1 tbsp. sriracha

Directions:

1. Chop up the onion into slices a quarter-inch thick. Gently pull apart the rings. Take a slice of bacon and wrap it around an onion ring. Repeat with the rest of the ingredients. Place each onion ring in your fryer.
2. Cut the onion rings at 350°F for ten

minutes, turning them halfway through to ensure the bacon crisps up.
3. Serve hot with the sriracha.

166. Smoked BBQ Toasted Almonds

Preparation Time: 10 minutes
Servings: 1

Ingredients

- 2 tsp. coconut oil, melted
- ¼ tsp. smoked paprika
- 1 tsp. chili powder
- ¼ tsp. cumin
- 1 cup raw almonds

Directions:

1. Mix the melted coconut oil with the paprika, chili powder, and cumin. Place the almonds in a large bowl and pour the coconut oil over them, tossing them to cover them evenly.
2. Place the almonds in the basket of your fryer and spread them out across the base.
3. Cook for six minutes at 320°F, giving the basket an occasional shake to make sure everything is cooked evenly.
4. Leave to cool and serve.

167. Roasted Eggplant

Preparation Time: 20 minutes
Servings: 1

Ingredients

- 1 large eggplant
- 2 tbsp. olive oil
- ¼ tsp. salt
- ½ tsp. garlic powder

Directions:

1. Prepare the eggplant by slicing off the top and bottom and cutting it into slices around a quarter-inch thick.
2. Apply olive oil to the slices with a brush, coating both sides. Season each side with sprinklings of salt and garlic powder.
3. Place the slices in the fryer and cook for fifteen minutes at 390°F.
4. Serve right away.

168. Low-Carb Pita Chips

Preparation Time: 15 minutes
Servings: 1

Ingredients

- 1 cup mozzarella cheese, shredded
- 1 egg
- ¼ cup blanched finely ground keto almond flour
- ½ oz. pork rinds, finely ground

Directions:

1. Melt the mozzarella in the microwave. Add the egg, almond flour, and pork rinds and combine together to form a smooth paste. Microwave the cheese again if it begins to set.
2. Put the dough between two sheets of parchment paper and use a rolling pin to flatten it out into a rectangle. The thickness is up to you. With a sharp knife, cut into the dough to form triangles. It may be necessary to complete this step-in multiple batches.
3. Place the chips in the fryer and cook for five minutes at 350°F. Turn them over and cook on the other side for another five minutes, or until the chips are golden and firm.
4. Allow the chips to cool and harden further. They can be stored in an airtight container.

169. Keto Flatbread

Preparation Time: 20 minutes
Servings: 1

Ingredients

- 1 cup mozzarella cheese, shredded
- ¼ cup blanched finely ground keto almond flour
- 1 oz. full-fat cream cheese, softened

Directions:

1. Microwave the mozzarella for half a minute until melted. Combine with the almond flour to achieve a smooth consistency, before adding the cream cheese. Keep mixing to create a dough,

microwaving the mixture again if the cheese begins to harden.
2. Divide the dough into two equal pieces. Between two sheets of parchment paper, roll out the dough until it is about a quarter-inch thick. Cover the bottom of your fryer with another sheet of parchment.
3. Transfer the dough into the fryer and cook at 320°F for seven minutes. You may need to complete this step in two batches. Make sure to turn the flatbread halfway through cooking. Take care when removing it from the fryer and serve warm.

170. Buffalo Cauliflower

Preparation Time: 10 minutes
Servings: 1

Ingredients

- ½ packet dry ranch seasoning
- 2 tbsp. salted butter, melted
- Cauliflower florets
- ¼ cup buffalo sauce

Directions:

1. In a bowl, combine the dry ranch seasoning and butter. Toss with the cauliflower florets to coat and transfer them to the fryer.
2. Cook at 400°F for five minutes, shaking the basket occasionally to ensure the florets cook evenly.
3. Remove the cauliflower from the fryer, pour the buffalo sauce over it, and enjoy.

171. Brussels Sprout Chips

Preparation Time: 15 minutes
Servings: 1

Ingredients

- 1 lb. Brussels sprouts
- 1 tbsp. coconut oil, melted
- 1 tbsp. unsalted butter, melted

Directions:

1. Prepare the Brussels sprouts by halving them, discarding any loose leaves.
2. Combine with the melted coconut oil and transfer to your air fryer.
3. Cook at 400°F for ten minutes, giving the basket a good shake throughout the cooking time to brown them up if desired.
4. The sprouts are ready when they are partially caramelized. Remove them from the fryer and serve with a topping of melted butter before serving.

172. Cauliflower Tots

Preparation Time: 20 minutes
Servings: 8

Ingredients

- 1 large head cauliflower
- ½ cup parmesan cheese, grated
- 1 cup mozzarella cheese, shredded
- 1 tsp. seasoned salt
- 1 egg

Directions:

1. Place a steamer basket over a pot of boiling water, ensuring the water is not high enough to enter the basket.
2. Cut up the cauliflower into florets and transfer to the steamer basket. Cover the pot with a lid and leave to steam for seven minutes, making sure the cauliflower softens.
3. Place the florets on a cheesecloth and leave to cool. Remove as much moisture as possible. This is crucial as it ensures the cauliflower will harden.
4. In a bowl, break up the cauliflower with a fork.
5. Stir in the parmesan, mozzarella, seasoned salt, and egg, incorporating the cauliflower well with all of the other ingredients. Make sure the mixture is firm enough to be moldable.
6. Using your hand, mold about two tablespoons of the mixture into tots and repeat until you have used up all of the mixture. Put each tot into your air fryer basket. They may need to be cooked in multiple batches.
7. Cook at 320°F for twelve minutes, turning them halfway through. Ensure

they are brown in color before serving.

173. Herbed Garlic Radishes

Preparation Time: 15 minutes
Servings: 2

Ingredients

- 1 lb. radishes
- 2 tbsp. unsalted butter, melted
- ¼ tsp. dried oregano
- ½ tsp. dried parsley
- ½ tsp. garlic powder

Directions:

1. Prepare the radishes by cutting off their tops and bottoms and quartering them.
2. In a bowl, combine the butter, dried oregano, dried parsley, and garlic powder. Toss with the radishes to coat.
3. Transfer the radishes to your air fryer and cook at 350°F for ten minutes, shaking the basket at the halfway point to ensure the radishes cook evenly through. The radishes are ready when they begin to turn brown.

174. Jicama Fries

Preparation Time: 25 minutes
Servings: 1

Ingredients

- 1 small jicama, peeled
- ¼ tsp. onion powder
- ¾ tsp. chili powder
- ¼ tsp. garlic powder
- ¼ tsp. ground black pepper

Directions:

1. To make the fries, cut the jicama into matchsticks of your desired thickness.
2. In a bowl, toss them with the onion powder, chili powder, garlic powder, and black pepper to coat. Transfer the fries into the basket of your air fryer.
3. Cook at 350°F for twenty minutes, giving the basket an occasional shake throughout the cooking process. The fries are ready when they are hot and golden in color. Enjoy!

175. Zesty Salmon Jerky

Preparation Time: 6 hours
Servings: 2

Ingredients

- 1 lb. boneless skinless salmon
- ½ tsp. liquid smoke
- ½ tsp. ground ginger
- ¼ cup soy sauce
- ¼ tsp. red pepper flakes

Directions:

1. Cut the salmon into strips about four inches long and a quarter-inch thick.
2. Put the salmon in an airtight container or bag along with the liquid smoke, ginger, soy sauce, and red pepper flakes, combining everything to coat the salmon completely. Leave the salmon in the refrigerator for at least two hours.
3. Transfer the salmon slices in the fryer, taking care not to overlap any pieces. This step may need to be completed in multiple batches.
4. Cook at 140°F for four hours.
5. Take care when removing the salmon from the fryer and leave it to cool. This jerky makes a good snack and can be stored in an airtight container.

176. Zucchini Bites

Preparation Time: 15 minutes
Servings: 4

Ingredients

- 4 zucchinis
- 1 egg
- ½ cup parmesan cheese, grated
- 1 tbsp. Italian herbs
- 1 cup coconut, grated

Directions:

1. Thinly grate the zucchini and dry with a cheesecloth, ensuring to remove all of the moisture.
2. In a bowl, combine the zucchini with the egg, parmesan, Italian herbs, and grated coconut, mixing well to incorporate

everything. Using your hands, mold the mixture into balls.
3. Pre-heat the fryer at 400°F and place a rack inside. Lay the zucchini balls on the rack and cook for ten minutes. Serve hot.

177. Pop Corn Broccoli

Preparation Time: 10 minutes
Servings: 1

Ingredients

- egg yolks
- ¼ cup butter, melted
- 2 cups keto coconut flower
- Salt and pepper
- 2 cups broccoli florets

Directions:

1. In a bowl, whisk the egg yolks and melted butter together. Throw in the keto coconut flour, salt and pepper, then stir again to combine well.
2. Pre-heat the fryer at 400°F.
3. Dip each broccoli floret into the mixture and place in the fryer. Cook for six minutes, in multiple batches if necessary. Take care when removing them from the fryer and enjoy!

178. Rosemary Green Beans

Preparation Time: 10 minutes
Servings: 1

Ingredients

- 1 tbsp. butter, melted
- 2 tbsp. rosemary
- ½ tsp. salt
- 3 cloves garlic, minced
- ¾ cup green beans, chopped

Directions:

1. Pre-heat your fryer at 390°F.
2. Combine the melted butter with the rosemary, salt, and minced garlic. Toss in the green beans, making sure to coat them well.
3. Cook in the fryer for five minutes.

179. Carrot Croquettes

Preparation Time: 10 minutes
Servings: 4

Ingredients

- 2 medium-sized carrots, trimmed and grated
- 2 medium-sized celery stalks, trimmed and grated
- ½ cup of leek, finely chopped
- 1 tbsp. garlic paste
- ¼ tsp. freshly cracked black pepper
- 1 tsp. fine sea salt
- 1 tbsp. fresh dill, finely chopped
- 1 egg, lightly whisked
- ¼ cup keto almond flour
- ¼ tsp. baking powder
- ½ cup keto bread crumbs [seasoned or regular]
- Chive mayo to serve

Directions:

- Drain any excess liquid from the carrots and celery by placing them on a paper towel.
- Stir together the vegetables with all of the other ingredients, save for the bread crumbs and chive mayo.
- Use your hands to mold 1 tablespoon of the vegetable mixture into a ball and repeat until all of the mixture has been used up. Press down on each ball with your hand or a palette knife. Cover completely with bread crumbs. Spritz the croquettes with a non-stick cooking spray.
- Arrange the croquettes in a single layer in your Air Fryer and fry for 6 minutes at 360°F.
- Serve warm with the chive mayo on the side.

180. Peppered Puff Pastry

Preparation Time: 25 minutes
Servings: 4

Ingredients

- 1 ½ tbsp. sesame oil

- 1 cup white mushrooms, sliced
- 2 cloves garlic, minced
- 1 bell pepper, seeded and chopped
- ¼ tsp. sea salt
- ¼ tsp. dried rosemary
- ½ tsp. ground black pepper, or more to taste
- 11 oz. puff pastry sheets
- ½ cup crème fraiche
- 1 egg, well whisked
- ½ cup parmesan cheese, preferably freshly grated

Directions:
1. Pre-heat your Air Fryer to 400°F.
2. In a skillet, heat the sesame oil over a moderate heat and fry the mushrooms, garlic, and pepper until soft and fragrant.
3. Sprinkle on the salt, rosemary, and pepper.
4. In the meantime, unroll the puff pastry and slice it into 4-inch squares.
5. Spread the crème fraiche across each square.
6. Spoon equal amounts of the vegetables into the puff pastry squares. Enclose each square around the filling in a triangle shape, pressing the edges with your fingertips.
7. Brush each triangle with some whisked egg and cover with grated Parmesan.
8. Cook for 22-25 minutes.

181. Sautéed Green Beans

Preparation Time: 12 minutes
Servings: 4

Ingredients
- ¾ lb. green beans, cleaned
- 1 tbsp. balsamic vinegar
- ¼ tsp. kosher salt
- ½ tsp. mixed peppercorns, freshly cracked
- 1 tbsp. butter
- Sesame seeds to serve

Directions:
1. Pre-heat your Air Fryer at 390°F.
2. Combine the green beans with the rest of the ingredients, except for the sesame seeds. Transfer to the fryer and cook for 10 minutes.
3. In the meantime, heat the sesame seeds in a small skillet to toast all over, stirring constantly to prevent burning.
4. Serve the green beans accompanied by the toasted sesame seeds.

182. Horseradish Mayo & Gorgonzola Mushrooms

Preparation Time: 15 minutes
Servings: 5

Ingredients
- ½ cup of keto bread crumbs
- 2 cloves garlic, pressed
- 2 tbsp. fresh coriander, chopped
- ⅓ tsp. kosher salt
- ½ tsp. crushed red pepper flakes
- 1 ½ tbsp. olive oil
- 20 medium-sized mushrooms, stems removed
- ½ cup Gorgonzola cheese, grated
- ¼ cup low-fat mayonnaise
- 1 tsp. prepared horseradish, well-drained
- tbsp. fresh parsley, finely chopped

Directions:
1. Combine the bread crumbs together with the garlic, coriander, salt, red pepper, and the olive oil.
2. Take equal-sized amounts of the bread crumb mixture and use them to stuff the mushroom caps. Add the grated Gorgonzola on top of each.
3. Put the mushrooms in the Air Fryer grill pan and transfer to the fryer.
4. Grill them at 380°F for 8-12 minutes, ensuring the stuffing is warm throughout.
5. In the meantime, prepare the horseradish mayo. Mix together the mayonnaise, horseradish and parsley.
6. When the mushrooms are ready, serve with the mayo.

183. Scallion & Ricotta Potatoes

Preparation Time: 15 minutes
Servings: 4

Ingredients

- baking potatoes
- 2 tbsp. olive oil
- ½ cup Ricotta cheese, room temperature
- 2 tbsp. scallions, chopped
- 1 heaped tbsp. fresh parsley, roughly chopped
- 1 heaped tbsp. coriander, minced
- 2 oz. Cheddar cheese, preferably freshly grated
- 1 tsp. celery seeds
- ½ tsp. salt
- ½ tsp. garlic pepper

Directions:

1. Pierce the skin of the potatoes with a knife.
2. Cook in the Air Fryer basket for roughly 13 minutes at 350°F. If they are not cooked through by this time, leave for 2 – 3 minutes longer.
3. In the meantime, make the stuffing by combining all the other ingredients.
4. Cut halfway into the cooked potatoes to open them.
5. Spoon equal amounts of the stuffing into each potato and serve hot.

184. Crumbed Beans

Preparation Time: 10 minutes
Servings: 4

Ingredients

- ½ cup keto almond flour
- 1 tsp. smoky chipotle powder
- ½ tsp. ground black pepper
- 1 tsp. sea salt flakes
- 2 eggs, beaten
- ½ cup crushed saltines
- 10 oz. wax beans

Directions:

1. Combine the keto almond flour, chipotle powder, black pepper, and salt in a bowl. Put the eggs in a second bowl. Place the crushed saltines in a third bowl.
2. Wash the beans with cold water and discard any tough strings.
3. Coat the beans with the flour mixture, before dipping them into the beaten egg. Lastly cover them with the crushed saltines.
4. Spritz the beans with a cooking spray.
5. Air-fry at 360°F for 4 minutes. Give the cooking basket a good shake and continue to cook for 3 minutes. Serve hot.

185. Colby Potato Patties

Preparation Time: 15 minutes
Servings: 8

Ingredients

- 2 lb. white potatoes, peeled and grated
- ½ cup scallions, finely chopped
- ½ tsp. freshly ground black pepper, or more to taste
- 1 tbsp. fine sea salt
- ½ tsp. hot paprika
- 2 cups Colby cheese, shredded
- ¼ cup canola oil
- 1 cup crushed crackers

Directions:

1. Boil the potatoes until soft. Dry them off and peel them before mashing thoroughly, leaving no lumps.
2. Combine the mashed potatoes with scallions, pepper, salt, paprika, and cheese.
3. Mold the mixture into balls with your hands and press with your palm to flatten them into patties.
4. In a shallow dish, combine the canola oil and crushed crackers. Coat the patties in the crumb mixture.
5. Cook the patties at 360°F for about 10 minutes, in multiple batches if necessary.
6. Serve with tabasco mayo or the sauce of your choice.

186. Turkey Garlic Potatoes

Preparation Time: 45 minutes
Servings: 2

Ingredients

- 3 unsmoked turkey strips
- small potatoes
- 1 tsp. garlic, minced
- 2 tsp. olive oil
- Salt to taste
- Pepper to taste

Directions:

1. Peel the potatoes and cube them finely.
2. Coat in 1 teaspoon of oil and cook in the Air Fryer for 10 minutes at 350°F.
3. In a separate bowl, slice the turkey finely and combine with the garlic, oil, salt and pepper. Pour the potatoes into the bowl and mix well.
4. Lay the mixture on some silver aluminum foil, transfer to the fryer and cook for about 10 minutes.
5. Serve with raita.

187. Keto Croutons

Preparation Time: 25 minutes
Servings: 4

Ingredients

- 2 slices keto friendly bread
- 1 tbsp. olive oil

Directions:

1. Cut the slices of bread into medium-size chunks.
2. Coat the inside of the Air Fryer with the oil. Set it to 390°F and allow it to heat up.
3. Place the chunks inside and shallow fry for at least 8 minutes.
4. Serve with hot soup.

188. Garlic Stuffed Mushrooms

Preparation Time: 25 minutes
Servings: 4

Ingredients

- small mushrooms
- 1 oz. onion, peeled and diced
- 1 tbsp. keto friendly bread crumbs
- 1 tbsp. olive oil
- 1 tsp. garlic, pureed
- 1 tsp. parsley
- Salt and pepper to taste

Directions:

1. Combine the keto bread crumbs, oil, onion, parsley, salt, pepper and garlic in a bowl. Cut out the mushrooms' stalks and stuff each cap with the crumb mixture.
2. Cook in the Air Fryer for 10 minutes at 350°F.
3. Serve with a side of mayo dip.

189. Zucchini Sweet Potatoes

Preparation Time: 20 minutes
Servings: 4

Ingredients

- 2 large-sized sweet potatoes, peeled and quartered
- 1 medium-sized zucchini, sliced
- 1 Serrano pepper, deveined and thinly sliced
- 1 bell pepper, deveined and thinly sliced
- 1 – 2 carrots, cut into matchsticks
- ¼ cup olive oil
- 1 ½ tbsp. maple syrup
- ½ tsp. porcini powder
- ¼ tsp. mustard powder
- ½ tsp. fennel seeds
- 1 tbsp. garlic powder
- ½ tsp. fine sea salt
- ¼ tsp. ground black pepper
- Tomato ketchup to serve

Directions:

1. Put the sweet potatoes, zucchini, peppers, and the carrot into the basket of your Air Fryer. Coat with a drizzling of olive oil.
2. Pre-heat the fryer at 350°F.
3. Cook the vegetables for 15 minutes.
4. In the meantime, prepare the sauce by vigorously combining the other ingredients, save for the tomato ketchup, with a whisk.
5. Lightly grease a baking dish small enough to fit inside your fryer.
6. Move the cooked vegetables to the baking dish, pour over the sauce and make sure

to coat the vegetables well.
7. Raise the temperature to 390°F and cook the vegetables for an additional 5 minutes.
8. Serve warm with a side of ketchup.

190. Cheese Lings

Preparation Time: 25 minutes
Servings: 6

Ingredients

- 1 cup keto almond flour
- small cubes cheese, grated
- ¼ tsp. chili powder
- 1 tsp. butter
- Salt to taste
- 1 tsp. baking powder

Directions:

1. Combine all the ingredients to form a dough, along with a small amount water as necessary.
2. Divide the dough into equal portions and roll each one into a ball.
3. Pre-heat Air Fryer at 360°F.
4. Transfer the balls to the fryer and air fry for 5 minutes, stirring periodically.

191. Potato Side Dish

Preparation Time: 30 minutes
Servings: 2

Ingredients

- 2 medium potatoes
- 1 tsp. butter
- 3 tbsp. sour cream
- 1 tsp. chives
- 1 ½ tbsp. cheese, grated
- Salt and pepper to taste

Directions:

1. Pierce the potatoes with a fork and boil them in water until they are cooked.
2. Transfer to the Air Fryer and cook for 15 minutes at 350°F.
3. In the meantime, combine the sour cream, cheese and chives in a bowl. Cut the potatoes halfway to open them up and fill with the butter and toppings.
4. Serve with salad.

192. Roasted Potatoes & Cheese

Preparation Time: 55 minutes
Servings: 4

Ingredients

- 4 medium potatoes
- 1 asparagus bunch
- ⅓ cup cottage cheese
- ⅓ cup low-fat crème fraiche
- 1 tbsp. wholegrain mustard

Directions:

1. Pour some oil into your Air Fryer and pre-heat to 390°F.
2. Cook potatoes for 20 minutes.
3. Boil the asparagus in salted water for 3 minutes.
4. Remove the potatoes and mash them with rest of ingredients. Sprinkle on salt and pepper.
5. Serve with rice.

193. Vegetable & Cheese Omelet

Preparation Time: 15 minutes
Servings: 2

Ingredients

- 3 tbsp. plain milk
- 4 eggs, whisked
- 1 tsp. melted butter
- Kosher salt and freshly ground black pepper, to taste
- 1 red bell pepper, deveined and chopped
- 1 green bell pepper, deveined and chopped
- 1 white onion, finely chopped
- ½ cup baby spinach leaves, roughly chopped
- ½ cup Halloumi cheese, shaved

Directions:

1. Grease the Air Fryer baking pan with some canola oil.
2. Place all of the ingredients in the baking pan and stir well.
3. Transfer to the fryer and cook at 350°F

for 13 minutes.
4. Serve warm.

194. Cabbage rolls stuffed with dried apricots

Preparation Time: 30 mins
Servings: 4

Ingredients:

- 4 tbsps. Rinsed and chopped dried apricots,
- 2 peeled, cored and grated apples
- 1/3 tsp. cinnamon
- 1 boiled cabbage head
- 2 tbsps. Rinsed raisins
- 1 tbsp. sugar

Directions:

1. Combine the grated apples, raisins, dried apricots, sugar and cinnamon.
2. Prepare the cabbage leaves: place the head of cabbage into water and bring to a boil. As the cabbage softens take it out, remove the outer leaves and carefully peel the leaves off one by one.
3. Spread the leaves out on paper towels and fill with apricot stuffing. Roll them up.
4. Place the rolls into preheated to 400F oven for 40 minutes.

Nutrition:
Calories: 175, Fat:0.4 g, Carbs:16.6 g, Protein:10.8 g, Sugars:2.9 g, Sodium:980.4 mg

195. Squash pancakes

Preparation Time: 10 mins
Servings: 4

Ingredients:

- 2 beaten eggs
- Salt
- Sour cream
- 2 peeled, deseeded and grated medium summer squashes
- 1 tbsp. flour

Directions:

1. Drain the liquid from the grated squashes.
2. Add eggs, flour and season with salt. Mix well. Form this mixture into pancakes.
3. Line a baking sheet with parchment paper and scoop the pancakes onto it.
4. Bake in the oven at 400F for 20-30 minutes.
5. Serve with sour cream.

Nutrition:
Calories: 31, Fat:0.4 g, Carbs:12.7 g, Protein:5.8 g, Sugars:3.4 g, Sodium:41.7 mg

196. Avocado dip

Preparation Time: 5 mins
Servings: 2

Ingredients:

- ½ c. low-fat sour cream
- 2 tsps. minced onions
- 1/8 tsp. hot sauce
- 1 peeled, pitted and mashed avocado

Directions:

1. Mix all the ingredients together in a blender and blend until smooth.
2. Serve with tortilla chips.

Nutrition:
Calories: 217, Fat:17.3 g, Carbs:7 g, Protein:1.6 g, Sugars:0.6 g, Sodium:44.5 mg

197. Rice and Chicken Stuffed Tomatoes

Preparation Time: 10 mins
Servings: 4

Ingredients:

- 1 pack grilled and sliced chicken breast
- 2 tbsps. Chopped basil leaf
- 2 c. cooked brown rice
- 1 tbsp. olive oil
- 4 large tomatoes
- ½ c. grated parmesan cheese
- 2 minced garlic cloves

Directions:

1. Set the oven at 350F.
2. Take the top of the tomatoes off and then carefully scoop the seeds using a spoon.
3. In a large bowl, mix together the cooked

brown rice, chicken, basil, garlic, and parmesan (leave about 1 tsp. of parmesan. Use this mixture to stuff the tomatoes.
4. Sprinkle the stuffed tomatoes with the remaining parmesan. Place them in an oven-safe dish and brush with the olive oil.
5. Place in the oven to cook for 25 minutes.
6. Let it cool down before serving.

Nutrition:

Calories: 230, Fat:4.1 g, Carbs:27.3 g, Protein:21.5 g, Sugars:2.9 g, Sodium:407.7 mg

198. Stuffed turnips

Preparation Time: 5 mins
Servings: 4

Ingredients:

- 2 peeled and grated carrots
- 2 tbsps. Olive oil
- 2 tbsps. Honey
- 4 rinsed turnips.
- 2 peeled and grated apples

Directions:

1. Preheat the oven to 400°F.
2. Mix grated carrots with grated apples in honey.
3. Boil the turnips until half-done.
4. When the turnips are cool enough to handle, cut off the tops and scoop out some of the flesh.
5. Rub the turnips inside with olive oil and fill with vegetable stuffing.
6. Bake for 1 hr.

Nutrition:

Calories: 197, Fat:7.3 g, Carbs:8 g, Protein:4 g, Sugars:3.5 g, Sodium:61.3 mg

199. Apples stuffed with quark

Preparation Time: 5 mins
Servings: 4

Ingredients:

- oz. cottage cheese
- 1 tsp. confectioners' sugar
- 2 tbsps. Sugar
- 4 cored apples
- 1 whisked egg
- 1 tbsp. raisins

Directions:

1. Combine the quark with egg, sugar and raisins. Mix well.
2. Scrape out the some of the apples' flesh and fill with quark mixture.
3. Place on a baking sheet and bake at 400F for 20 minutes.

Nutrition:

Calories: 189, Fat:0.6 g, Carbs:9 g, Protein:12 g, Sugars:20 g, Sodium:108 mg

200. Baked pumpkin oatmeal

Preparation Time: 30 mins
Servings: 4

Ingredients:

- 3¼ c. water
- 2 tbsps. Sour cream
- 1 c. peeled, cored and grated pumpkin
- 2 tbsps. Sugar
- 2 c. oats
- 1 c. milk
- 2 egg whites

Directions:

1. In a medium saucepan prepare the oatmeal: bring 3¼ cups water to a boil and stir in the oats. Add sugar. Stir constantly until thick.
2. In a skillet add ½ cup milk, grated pumpkin and simmer until the pumpkin is half-cooked.
3. Combine oatmeal with pumpkin.
4. Whisk the egg whites until smooth. Add to pumpkin-oatmeal mixture.
5. Pour the mixture into a baking pan and bake at 400F for 30 minutes.
6. Serve with sour cream.

Nutrition:

Calories: 189, Fat:3.1 g, Carbs:57 g, Protein:6.3 g, Sugars:14.2 g, Sodium:224.2 mg

201. Meringue cookies

Preparation Time: 5 mins
Servings: 4

Ingredients:

- 2 tbsps. Sugar
- 3 beaten egg whites

Directions:

1. Using a blender beat the cooled egg whites on high.
2. Constantly blending add sugar little by little.
3. Line a baking sheet with parchment paper. Using an icing bag, squeeze our portions of the egg mixture unto the parchment paper.
4. Place into a preheated to 155°F oven for 15 min.

Nutrition:

Calories: 35, Fat:0 g, Carbs:6 g, Protein:0.4 g, Sugars:6 g, Sodium:10.7 mg

202. Rose hip jelly

Preparation Time: 7 hours
Servings: 2

Ingredients:

- 2 c. water
- 1 tsp. gelatin
- 2 tbsps. Sugar
- 2 tbsps. Rinsed and crushed rose-hip berries
- 2 lemon slices

Directions:

1. Bring the 2 cups water to a boil, add the crushed rose hips and boil for 5 minutes.
2. Leave the hips in the liquid to infuse for 6 hours. Then strain the infusion through a sieve, retaining the liquid.
3. Dissolve sugar in ½ cup of rose-hip water and bring to boil. Add the remaining rose-hip water and lemon slices.
4. Soak the gelatin in cool water for 25-30 minutes.
5. Add the gelatin to the rose-hip extract and bring to a boil. Take it from the heat immediately and pour into molds or jars
6. Place in the fridge to cool and thicken.

Nutrition:

Calories: 45, Fat:0 g, Carbs:11 g, Protein:0 g, Sugars:2.6 g, Sodium:4 mg

203. Easy Broccoli and Penne

Preparation Time: 10 mins
Servings: 3

Ingredients:

- 3 chopped garlic cloves
- 6 oz. uncooked whole-wheat penne
- Ground pepper
- 3 c. roughly chopped broccoli florets
- 1 tbsp. olive oil
- 2 tbsps. Grated Romano cheese

Directions:

1. Cook the penne in a pot according to the package instructions. Add the florets to cook with the pasta.
2. Before draining, take ¼ cup of the pasta water and set aside.
3. Place the pot back to the stove and heat the olive oil over high heat. Sauté the garlic for about a minute.
4. Reduce the heat and then add the pasta and broccoli to the pot. Stir well.
5. Add the Romano and ¼ cup of the pasta water. Mix well. Season with pepper.

Nutrition:

Calories: 419.8, Fat:12.9 g, Carbs:52 g, Protein:32.2 g, Sugars:2.4 g, Sodium:540.5 mg

204. Berry soufflé

Preparation Time: 15 mins
Servings: 2

Ingredients:

- 2 tbsps. sugar
- ½ c. water
- 3 oz. rinsed berries
- 3 egg whites

Directions:

1. Combine the berries sugar and water in a saucepan and boil until thick.
2. Using an electric beater beat the egg whites until foamy.

3. Constantly stirring, combine the berry mixture with egg whites.
4. Pour the soufflé mixture into a mold.
5. Bake at 390°F for 15 minutes.
6. Serve immediately, sprinkled with confectioners' sugar if desired.

Nutrition:
Calories: 79, Fat:0.4 g, Carbs:28.6 g, Protein:8.3 g, Sugars:8.3 g, Sodium:36.7 mg

205. White sponge cake

Preparation Time: 15 mins
Servings: 4

Ingredients:
- 1 tbsp. sugar
- 1 tbsp. flour
- 2 egg whites

Directions:
1. Using an electric mixer beat the egg whites until foamy.
2. Slowly add sugar, continuing to whisk.
3. Slowly add the flour, constantly stirring.
4. Pour the mixture into a silicone mold.
5. Bake at 400F for 20 min. Check for doneness with a toothpick.

Nutrition:
Calories: 23, Fat:0.1 g, Carbs:36.4 g, Protein:4.6 g, Sugars:46 g, Sodium:144 mg

206. Roasted asparagus

Preparation Time: 1 hour
Servings: 2

Ingredients:
- Black pepper
- 1 tsp. olive oil
- 2 c. quartered mushrooms
- Zest of 1 lemon
- 1 lb. sliced asparagus
- 2 tbsps. Balsamic vinegar

Directions:
1. In a bowl combine all ingredients until well coated.
2. Place into the fridge for 1 hour to marinate.
3. Broil the asparagus mixture under high heat until lightly browned.

Nutrition:
Calories: 143, Fat:7.6 g, Carbs:3.9 g, Protein:22 g, Sugars:1.2 g, Sodium:74 mg

207. Rigatoni with broccoli

Preparation Time: 5 mins
Servings: 2

Ingredients:
- 3 minced garlic cloves
- 2 tbsps. grated parmesan cheese
- Pepper.
- 1/3 lb. rigatoni pasta
- 2 c. broccoli florets
- 2 tsps. olive oil

Directions:
1. Fill a large saucepan with water and bring to a boil. Following the Directions:on the package add the pasta and cook until al dente.
2. In a separate pot add 1 inch water and bring to boil. Put the broccoli florets into a steamer basket and steam for 10 minutes.
3. In a large bowl combine the cooked pasta with broccoli. Toss with garlic, olive oil, Parmesan cheese, and black pepper.

Nutrition:
Calories: 46.2, Fat:14.9 g, Carbs:25 g, Protein:14 g, Sugars:2 g, Sodium:640 mg

208. Rutabaga Puree

Preparation Time: 10 mins
Servings: 4

Ingredients:
- 2 c. low sodium vegetable broth
- 1 tbsp. fresh tarragon
- 4 c. chopped rutabaga
- 2 tsps. fresh thyme
- 2 c. unsweetened coconut milk
- ½ c. low-fat sour cream

Directions:
1. In a large saucepan, bring the coconut milk and vegetable broth to a boil.
2. Add the rutabaga, reduce heat, and let simmer for 30 minutes.
3. Remove from heat and strain the rutabaga, reserving the liquid.
4. Using a blender or immersion blender, blend until smooth, adding the reserved liquid as desired to reach preferred consistency.
5. Season with tarragon and thyme.
6. Serve immediately.

Nutrition:
Calories: 207.2, Fat:16.7 g, Carbs:11.8 g, Protein:3.4 g, Sugars:10.8 g, Sodium:39 mg

209. Pan Seared Acorn Squash and Pecans

Preparation Time: 5 mins
Servings: 6

Ingredients:
- 1 tsp. chopped rosemary
- 1 c. sliced sweet yellow onion
- 2 tbsps. vegetable oil
- 4 c. cubed acorn squash
- 1 tbsp. honey
- 1 c. chopped pecans

Directions:
1. Add the vegetable oil to a sauté pan over medium high heat.
2. Add the onion and sauté until tender, 2-3 minutes.
3. Add the acorn squash, tossing gently for 5-7 minutes.
4. Add the honey, pecans, and rosemary. Stir to coat and cook an additional 3 minutes.
5. Serve warm.

Nutrition:
Calories: 222.3, Fat:17.6 g, Carbs:17.4 g, Protein:2.7 g, Sugars:0.9 g, Sodium:92.5 mg

210. Shaved Brussels Sprouts with Walnuts

Preparation Time: 10 mins
Servings: 4

Ingredients:
- ½ c. fresh shaved parmesan
- 1 tsp. thyme
- 2 tbsps. olive oil
- 1 tsp. black pepper
- ½ c. chopped walnuts
- ½ c. diced red onion
- 4 c. shaved Brussels sprouts

Directions:
1. Heat the olive oil in a skillet over medium heat. Add the onions and sauté until tender, approximately 2-3 minutes.
2. Add the Brussels sprouts and cook for 5 minutes. Season with thyme and black pepper.
3. Remove from heat and stir in the walnuts.
4. Garnish with fresh Parmesan for serving.

Nutrition:
Calories: 173.0, Fat:12.8 g, Carbs:10.0 g, Protein:5.7 g, Sugars:2.7 g, Sodium:220 mg

211. Honey Mustard Chicken Fillets

Preparation Time: 10 mins
Servings: 4

Ingredients:
- ¼ c. Dijon mustard
- 3 tsps. raw honey
- 4 packs chicken fillets
- ½ juice of lime
- ¼ c. toasted slivered almonds
- 1 minced garlic clove

Directions:
1. Pre-heat grill to medium-high heat.
2. In a small bowl, combine the Dijon mustard, honey and lime juice. Whisk well.
3. Using this mixture, brush the chicken fillets on each side.
4. When the grill is hot, cook the chicken fillets for 12-15 minutes turning and brushing with the sauce occasionally.
5. Garnish with the toasted slivered almonds

on top before serving.

Nutrition:
Calories: 192.7, Fat:2.5 g, Carbs:10.2 g, Protein:27.3 g, Sugars:8.6 g, Sodium:122.1 mg

212. Grilled Pesto Shrimps

Preparation Time: 10 mins
Servings: 2

Ingredients:
- Kosher salt
- 1 garlic clove
- ¼ kg. peeled and deveined large shrimp
- ½ c. chopped basil
- Ground pepper
- Skewers
- 2 tbsps. olive oil
- 2 tbsps. parmesan cheese

Directions:
1. Place the fresh basil, garlic, cheese, salt and pepper in a food processor and pulse. Gradually add the oil to the mixture until you create a pesto sauce.
2. Place the shrimps in a bowl and pour over the pesto sauce. Toss gently and let it marinate in t fridge for at least an hour.
3. When you're ready to cook, pre-heat your grill to medium-low heat.
4. Thread the shrimps into the skewers and cook on the grill for about 3-4 minutes on each side.
5. Serve warm with a bowl of yogurt and fresh fruits.

Nutrition:
Calories: 219.7, Fat:7.8 g, Carbs:22.2 g, Protein:15.1 g, Sugars:1.7 g, Sodium:238.7 mg

213. Rosemary Potato Shells

Preparation Time: 5 mins
Servings: 2

Ingredients:
- Butter-flavored cooking spray
- 2 medium russet potatoes
- 1/8 tsp. freshly ground black pepper
- 1 tbsp. minced fresh rosemary

Directions:
1. Switch on the oven and set it to 375 0F to preheat.
2. Pierce the mashed potatoes with a fork and place them in a baking sheet.
3. Bake for 1 hour until crispy.
4. Allow the potatoes to cool for handling then cut them in half.
5. Scoop out the pulp leaving the 1/8-inch-thick shell.
6. Brush the shells with melted butter and season with pepper and rosemary.
7. Bake for another 5 minutes.
8. Serve.

Nutrition:
Calories: 167, Fat:0 g, Carbs:27 g, Protein:7.6 g, Sugars:1.5 g, Sodium:200.7 mg

214. Basil Tomato Crostini

Preparation Time: 10 mins
Servings: 4

Ingredients:
- ¼ c. minced fresh basil
- ¼ lb. sliced and toasted Italian bread
- 4 chopped plum tomatoes
- 2 tsps. olive oil
- Freshly ground pepper
- 1 minced garlic clove

Directions:
1. Toss tomatoes with oil, garlic, pepper, and basil in a bowl.
2. Cover and allow them sit for 30 minutes.
3. Top the toasts with this mixture.
4. Serve.

Nutrition:
Calories: 104, Fat:3.5 g, Carbs:15 g, Protein:3 g, Sugars:0.3 g, Sodium:7.5 mg

215. Cranberry Spritzer

Preparation Time: 10 mins
Servings: 4

Ingredients:
- 1 c. raspberry sherbet
- 1-quart sugar-free cranberry juice

- ¼ c. sugar
- lemon wedges
- ½ c. fresh lemon juice
- 1-quart carbonated water

Directions:
1. Refrigerate carbonated water, lemon juice, and cranberry juice until cold.
2. Mix cranberry juice with sugar, sherbet, lemon juice, and carbonated water.
3. Garnish with a lemon wedge.
4. Serve.

Nutrition:
Calories: 50, Fat:0 g, Carbs:15.1 g, Protein:1.2 g, Sugars:45 g, Sodium:65 mg

216. Butternut Squash Fries

Preparation Time: 10 mins
Servings: 4

Ingredients:

- 1 tbsp. olive oil
- 1 tbsp. chopped fresh thyme
- 1 medium butternut squash
- ½ tsp. salt
- 1 tbsp. chopped fresh rosemary

Directions:
1. Switch on the oven and set it to 425 0F to preheat.
2. Layer a baking sheet with cooking spray.
3. Peel the squash and slice into 3-inch-long and ½ inch wide.
4. Place the pieces in a large bowl and toss with oil, thyme, salt, and rosemary.
5. Spread the squash in the baking sheet and bake for 10 minutes.
6. Toss the fries well and bake again for 5 minutes or more until golden brown.
7. Serve.

Nutrition:
Calories: 62, Fat:2 g, Carbs:11 g, Protein:11 g, Sugars:5 g, Sodium:164.1 mg

Seafood

217. Paleo Salmon

Preparation Time: 30 minutes
Servings: 4

Ingredients:

- 6 cabbage leaves; sliced in half
- 4 medium salmon steaks; skinless
- 2 red bell peppers; chopped
- Some coconut oil
- 1 yellow onion; chopped
- A pinch of sea salt
- Black pepper to the taste

Instructions:

1. Put water in a pot, bring to a boil over medium high heat, add cabbage leaves, blanch them for 2 minutes, transfer to a bowl filled with cold water and pat dry them.
2. Season salmon steaks with a pinch of sea salt and black pepper to the taste and wrap each in 3 cabbage leaf halves.
3. Heat up a pan with some coconut oil over medium high heat, add onion and bell pepper, stir and cook for 4 minutes.
4. Add wrapped salmon, introduce pan in the oven at 350 °F and bake for 12 minutes. Divide salmon and veggies between plates and serve.

Nutrition: Calories: 140; Fat: 3g; Fiber: 1g; Carbs: 2g; Protein: 15g

218. Fish Dish

Preparation Time: 20 minutes
Servings: 4

Ingredients:

- 1/4 cup ghee; melted
- 4 halibut fish fillets
- 4 garlic cloves; minced
- 2 tbsp. parsley; chopped
- Zest and juice from 1 lemon
- 1 lemon; sliced
- A pinch of sea salt
- Black pepper to the taste

Instructions:

1. In a bowl; mix garlic with ghee, lemon zest, juice, parsley, a pinch of sea salt and pepper and stir well.
2. Arrange fish in a baking dish, season with pepper to the taste, drizzle the mix you've made, top with lemon slices, introduce in the oven at 425 °F and bake for 15 minutes. Divide between plates and serve warm.

Nutrition: Calories: 150; Fat: 19g; Carbs: 5g; Fiber: 0.4g; Protein: 31

219. Thai Shrimp Delight

Preparation Time: 60 minutes
Servings: 4

Ingredients:

- 1 lb. shrimp; peeled and deveined
- 2 shallots; chopped
- 1 spaghetti squash; cut in halves and seedless
- Juice from 1 lime
- 2 tbsp. coconut aminos
- 1 tbsp. chili sauce
- 1 tsp. ginger; grated
- 3 garlic cloves; minced
- 3 cups mung beans sprouts
- 3 tbsp. coconut oil
- 2 tbsp. almond butter
- 2 eggs; whisked
- 1 cup carrots; chopped
- 1/4 cup nuts; roasted and chopped
- 1/4 cup cilantro; chopped
- 4 green onions; chopped
- A pinch of sea salt
- Black pepper to the taste

Instructions:

1. Brush squash halves with 1 tbsp. coconut oil, arrange pieces on a lined baking sheet, place in the oven at 400 °F and bake for

40 minutes.
2. Leave squash to cool down and make squash noodles using a fork.
3. Heat up a pan over medium heat, add coconut aminos, lime juice, almond butter and chili sauce and stir well until everything combines.
4. Heat up another pan with the rest of the oil over medium high heat, add shrimp, cook for 4 minutes and transfer to a plate.
5. Heat up the pan again over medium high heat, add ginger, shallots and garlic, stir and cook for 2 minutes.
6. Add carrots and sprouts, stir and cook for 1 minute. Add eggs and stir everything.
7. Add almond butter sauce you've made earlier, squash noodles, cilantro, green onions, nuts, shrimp, a pinch of salt and black pepper, stir well, divide between plates and serve right away.

Nutrition: Calories: 150; Fat: 3g; Fiber: 2g; Carbs: 3g; Protein: 14g

220. Salmon Skewers

Preparation Time: 25 minutes
Servings: 4

Ingredients:

- 1 lb. wild salmon; skinless, boneless and cubed
- 2 Meyer lemons; sliced
- 1/4 cup balsamic vinegar
- 1/4 cup orange juice
- 1/3 cup Paleo orange marmalade
- A pinch of pink salt
- Black pepper to the taste

Instructions:

1. Heat up a small pot with the vinegar over medium heat, add marmalade and orange juice, stir; bring to a simmer for 1 minute and take off heat.
2. Skewer salmon cubes and lemon slices, season with a pinch of salt and black pepper, brush them with half of the vinegar mix, place on preheated grill over medium heat, cook for 4 minutes on each side.
3. Brush skewers with the rest of the vinegar mix, grill for 1 minute more, divide between plates and serve.

Nutrition: Calories: 150; Fat: 1g; Fiber: 2g; Carbs: 4g; Protein: 10g

221. Shrimp Dish

Preparation Time: 20 minutes
Servings: 4

Ingredients:

- 1 small red bell pepper; chopped
- 1 small yellow onion; chopped
- 20 shrimp; peeled and deveined
- 1 garlic clove; finely chopped
- 5 dried red chilies
- 1 inch ginger; minced
- 1/4 cup coconut aminos
- A pinch of sea salt
- Black pepper to the taste
- 2 tbsp. coconut oil
- 2 tbsp. water
- 1 tbsp. lime juice
- 1 tsp. apple cider vinegar
- 1 tsp. raw honey
- A handful cilantro; finely chopped for serving

Instructions:

1. In a bowl; mix aminos with vinegar, honey, water and lime juice and whisk well.
2. Heat up a pan with the coconut oil over medium heat, add garlic and ginger, stir and cook for 2 minutes.
3. Add red chilies, onion, bell pepper, stir and cook for 4 minutes.
4. Add shrimp, a pinch of salt and pepper to the taste and the vinegar mix you've made, stir and cook for 5 minutes. Divide between plates and serve with cilantro sprinkled on top.

Nutrition: Calories: 157; Fat: 7g; Carbs: 11g; Fiber: 0g; Protein: 5g

222. Salmon Tartar Delight

Preparation Time: 15 minutes
Servings: 4

Ingredients:

- 7 oz. smoked salmon; minced
- 14 oz. salmon fillet; cut into very small cubes
- 3 tbsp. red onion; minced
- 2 tbsp. pickled cucumber; minced
- Zest and juice from 1 lemon
- 1 garlic clove; finely minced
- 2 tbsp. basil; minced
- 2 tsp. oregano; dried
- Black pepper to the taste
- 2 tbsp. mint leaves; minced
- 2 tbsp. Dijon mustard
- 5 tbsp. extra virgin olive oil
- Lime wedges for serving

Instructions:

1. In a bowl; mix onion with cucumber, garlic, lemon zest and juice, basil, mint, oregano, mustard, oil and pepper and stir well.
2. Add smoked and fresh salmon and stir well again. Divide tartar between plates and serve with lime wedges on the side.

Nutrition: Calories: 230; Fat: 16g; Carbs: 2.3g; Fiber: 0.4g; Protein: 17g

223. Salmon And Chili Sauce

Preparation Time: 25 minutes
Servings: 12

Ingredients:

- 1¼ cups coconut; shredded
- 1 lb. salmon; cut into medium cubes
- 1/3 cup coconut flour
- A pinch of sea salt
- Black pepper to the taste
- 1 egg
- 2 tbsp. coconut oil
- ¼ cup water
- 1/4 tsp. agar agar
- 4 red chilies; chopped
- 3 garlic cloves; minced
- 1/4 cup balsamic vinegar
- 1/2 cup honey

Instructions:

1. In a bowl; mix coconut flour with a pinch of salt and stir.
2. In another bowl; whisk the egg with black pepper.
3. Put coconut in a third bowl.
4. Dip salmon cubes in flour, egg and coconut and place them all on a working surface.
5. Heat up a pan with the oil over medium high heat, add salmon cubes, fry them for 3 minutes on each side, transfer them to paper towels, drain grease and divide them between plates.
6. Heat up a pan with the water over medium high heat.
7. Add chilies, cloves, vinegar, honey and agar agar, stir very well, bring to a gentle boil and simmer until all ingredients combine. Drizzle this over salmon cubes and serve.

Nutrition: Calories: 140; Fat: 1g; Fiber: 2g; Carbs: 4g; Protein: 15g

224. Salmon With Avocado Sauce

Preparation Time: 30 minutes
Servings: 5

Ingredients:

- 1 tsp. cumin
- 1 tsp. sweet paprika
- 1 tsp. chili powder
- 1 tsp. onion powder
- 1/2 tsp. garlic powder
- 2 lbs. salmon filets; cut into 4 pieces
- A pinch of sea salt
- Black pepper to the taste
- For the avocado sauce:
- 2 avocados; pitted, peeled and chopped
- 1 garlic clove; minced
- Juice from 1 lime
- 1 red onion; chopped
- 1 tbsp. extra virgin olive oil
- Black pepper to the taste

- 1 tbsp. cilantro; finely chopped

Instructions:
1. In a bowl; mix paprika with cumin, onion powder, garlic powder, chili powder, a pinch of sea salt and pepper to the taste.
2. Add salmon pieces, toss to coat and keep in the fridge for 20 minutes.
3. Put avocado in a bowl and mash well with a fork.
4. Add red onion, garlic clove, lime juice, olive oil, chopped cilantro and pepper to the taste and stir very well.
5. Take salmon out of the fridge, place it on preheated grill over medium high heat and cook it for 3 minutes.
6. Flip salmon, cook for 3 more minutes and divide on serving plates. Top each salmon piece with avocado sauce and serve.

Nutrition: Calories: 150; Fat: 12g; Carbs: 9g; Fiber: 6g; Protein: 24g

225. Roasted Trout

Preparation Time: 30 minutes
Servings: 4

Ingredients:
- 3 trout; cleaned and gutted
- 1 bunch dill
- 2 lemons; sliced
- 1 bunch rosemary
- 2 fennel bulbs; sliced
- A pinch of sea salt
- Black pepper to the taste
- 2 tbsp. extra virgin olive oil

Instructions:
1. Grease a baking dish with some oil, spread fennel slices on the bottom and add trout after you've seasoned them with a pinch of sea salt and pepper.
2. Fill each fish with lemon slices, dill and rosemary springs.
3. Top fish with the rest of the herbs and lemon slices, drizzle the rest of the oil, introduce everything in the oven at 500 °F and bake for 10 minutes.
4. Reduce heat to 425 °F and bake for 12 more minutes. Leave fish to cool down, divide between plates and serve.

Nutrition: Calories: 143; Fat: 2.3g; Carbs: 1g; Fiber: 0g; Protein: 6g

226. Fish Tacos

Preparation Time: 25 minutes
Servings: 4

Ingredients:
- 4 tilapia fillets; cut into medium pieces
- 1/4 cup coconut flour
- 2 eggs
- 3/4 cup tapioca starch
- 1/2 cup tapioca starch
- 1/4 cup sparkling water
- 2 cups cabbage; shredded
- 2 cups coconut oil
- A pinch of sea salt
- Black pepper to the taste
- Lime wedges for serving
- Cauliflower tortillas

For the Pico de Gallo:
- 2 tomatoes; chopped
- 2 tbsp. jalapeno; finely chopped
- 6 tbsp. yellow onion; finely chopped
- 2 tbsp. lime juice
- 1 tbsp. cilantro; finely chopped

For the mayo:
- 1 tbsp. Sriracha sauce
- 1/4 cup homemade mayonnaise
- 2 tsp. lime juice

Instructions:
1. In a bowl; mix tomatoes with tomatoes with onion, jalapeno, cilantro, 2 tbsp. lime juice and stir well, cover and keep in the fridge for now.
2. In another bowl; mix mayo with Sriracha and 2 tsp. lime juice, stir well, cover and also keep in the fridge.
3. In a bowl; mix 3/4 cup tapioca starch with coconut flour, sparkling water, a pinch of sea salt, pepper and eggs and whisk very well.
4. Put the rest of the tapioca starch in a separate bowl.

5. Pat dry tapioca pieces, coat with tapioca starch and dip each piece in eggs mix.
6. Heat up a pan with the coconut oil over medium high heat, transfer fish fillets to pan, cook for 1 minute, flip them, cook for 1 more minute, transfer to paper towels and drain excess fat.
7. Arrange tortillas on a working surface, divide cabbage on them, add a piece of fish on each, add some of the Pico de Gallo and top with mayo. Serve with lime wedges.

Nutrition: Calories: 230; Fat: 10g; Carbs: 12g; Fiber: 4g; Protein: 13g

It might seem like a very simple dish, but it's a delicious and fresh one!

227. Lobster And Sauce

Preparation Time: 18 minutes
Servings: 4

Ingredients:
- 2 tbsp. sriracha sauce
- 4 lobster tails; cut halfway through the center
- 1/4 cup ghee; melted
- 1 tbsp. chives; chopped
- 1 tbsp. parsley; chopped
- 1 tbsp. lime juice
- A pinch of sea salt
- Black pepper to the taste

Instructions:
1. In a bowl; mix ghee with a pinch of salt, black pepper, lime juice, chives and sriracha sauce and whisk well.
2. Fill lobster tails with half of this mix, place them on heated grill over medium high heat, cook for 5 minutes, flip, grill them for 3 minutes more and divide between plates.
3. Top lobster tails with the rest of the Sriracha sauce and parsley.

Nutrition: Calories: 223; Fat: 12g; Fiber: 0g; Carbs: 2g; Protein: 6g

228. Tuna Dish

Preparation Time: 25 minutes
Servings: 4

Ingredients:
- 1 tsp. fennel seeds
- 1 tsp. mustard seeds
- 4 medium tuna steaks
- 1/4 tsp. black peppercorns
- A pinch of sea salt
- Black pepper to the taste
- 4 tbsp. sesame seeds
- 3 tbsp. coconut oil

Instructions:
1. In your grinder, mix peppercorns with fennel and mustard seeds and grind well.
2. Add sesame seeds, a pinch of sea salt and pepper to the taste and grind again well.
3. Spread this mix on a plate, add tuna steaks and toss to coat.
4. Heat up a pan with the oil over medium high heat, add tuna steaks and cook for 3 minutes on each side. Divide between plates and serve with a side salad.

Nutrition: Calories: 240; Fat: 2g; Carbs: 0g; Fiber: 0g; Protein: 53

229. Salmon And Lemon Relish

Preparation Time: 1 hour 10 minutes
Servings: 2

Ingredients:
- 1 big salmon fillet; cut in halves
- Black pepper to the taste
- A drizzle of olive oil
- A pinch of sea salt
- For the relish:
- 1 tbsp. lemon juice
- 1 shallot; chopped
- 1 Meyer lemon; cut in wedges and then thinly sliced
- 2 tbsp. parsley; chopped
- 1/4 cup olive oil
- Black pepper to the taste

Instructions:
1. Put some water in a dish and place it in

the oven.
2. Put the salmon on a lined baking dish, drizzle some olive oil, season with a pinch of sea salt and black pepper, rub well, place in the oven at 370 °F and bake for 1 hour.
3. Meanwhile; in a bowl, mix shallot with the lemon juice, a pinch of salt and black pepper, stir and leave aside for 10 minutes.
4. In another bowl; mix marinated shallot with lemon slices, some salt, pepper, parsley and 1/4 cup oil and whisk well. Cut salmon in chunks, divide on plates and top with lemon relish.

Nutrition: Calories: 200; Fat: 3g; Fiber: 3g; Carbs: 6g; Protein: 20g

230. Salmon And Spicy Slaw

Preparation Time: 16 minutes
Servings: 4

Ingredients:

- 3 cups cold water
- 3 scallions; chopped
- 2 tsp. sriracha sauce
- 4 tsp. honey
- 3 tsp. avocado oil
- 4 tsp. cider vinegar
- 2 tsp. flax seed oil
- 4 medium salmon fillets; skinless and boneless
- A pinch of sea salt
- 1½ tsp. jerk seasoning
- 2 cups cabbage; chopped
- 4 cups baby arugula
- 2 cups radish; julienne cut
- 1/4 cup pepitas; toasted

Instructions:

1. Put scallions in a bowl; add cold water to them and leave aside.
2. In a bowl; mix Sriracha with honey and stir well.
3. In another bowl; combine 2 tsp. of the honey mix with 2 tsp. avocado oil, vinegar, a pinch of sea salt and black pepper and stir well.
4. Sprinkle salmon fillets with a pinch of sea salt, black pepper and jerk seasoning and rub well.
5. Heat up a pan with the rest of the avocado oil over medium high heat, add salmon, cook for 6 minutes, flip, take off heat, cover pan and leave aside for a few more minutes.
6. In a salad bowl; mix cabbage with arugula, radish, pepitas, a pinch of salt, black pepper, the honey and vinegar salad dressing and flax seed oil and toss to coat well.
7. Divide salmon on plates, drizzle the rest of the Sriracha sauce, add cabbage salad next to them and top with drained scallions.

Nutrition: Calories: 180; Fat: 3g; Fiber: 3g; Carbs: 4g; Protein: 8g

231. Grilled Salmon With Peaches

Preparation Time: 25 minutes
Servings: 4

Ingredients:

2 red onions; cut into wedges
- 3 peaches; cut in wedges
- 4 salmon steaks
- 1 tsp. thyme; chopped
- 1 tbsp. ginger; grated
- A pinch of sea salt
- Black pepper to the taste
- 1 tbsp. white wine vinegar
- 3 tbsp. extra virgin olive oil

Instructions:

1. In a bowl; mix wine with ginger, vinegar, thyme, a pinch of sea salt, pepper and olive oil and whisk very well.
2. In a bowl; mix peaches with onion, salt and pepper and toss to coat.
3. Heat up your kitchen grill over medium high heat, add salmon steaks after you've seasoned them with pepper to the taste, grill for 6 minutes on each side and divide between plates.
4. Add peaches and onions to grill, cook for 4 minutes on each side and transfer next

to salmon on plates. Drizzle the vinaigrette you've made all over salmon, onions and peaches and serve right away.

Nutrition: Calories: 448; Fat: 26g; Carbs: 13g; Fiber: 2; Sugar: 8g; Protein: 40

232. Wrapped Scallops

Preparation Time: 10 minutes
Cooking time: 6 minutes
Servings: 4

Ingredients:
- 12 oz scallops
- 7 oz bacon, sliced
- ½ teaspoon ground coriander
- 1 teaspoon lemon juice
- ½ teaspoon salt
- 1 teaspoon white pepper
- ½ teaspoon dried rosemary

Directions:
1. Mix up together ground coriander, salt, white pepper, and dried rosemary.
2. Rub the scallops with the spice mixture and sprinkle with lemon juice.
3. After this, wrap every scallop in the bacon slices and string into the skewers.
4. Preheat grill to 375F.
5. Place the scallop skewers in the grill and cook them for 3 minutes from each side.
6. Remove the cooked seafood from the skewers and transfer on the serving plates.

Nutrition value/serving: calories 345, fat 21.4, fiber 0.2, carbs 3.2, protein 32.7

233. Tuna Cups

Preparation Time: 10 minutes
Servings: 6

Ingredients:
- 6 lettuce leaves
- 8 oz tuna, canned
- 1 tablespoon mayonnaise
- ½ white onion, diced
- 1 tablespoon fresh parsley, chopped
- ½ teaspoon ground nutmeg
- ½ teaspoon chives, chopped

Directions:
1. Chop the tuna and mix it up with mayonnaise, diced onion, chopped parsley, and ground nutmeg. Add chopped chives.
2. Mix up the mixture until homogenous.
3. Fill the lettuce leaves with the tuna mixture.

Nutrition value/serving: calories 85, fat 4, fiber 0.3, carbs 1.7, protein 10.2

234. Tuna Skewers in Marinara Sauce

Preparation Time: 20 minutes
Cooking time: 7 minutes
Servings: 4

Ingredients:
- 1-pound tuna fillet
- 1 tablespoon marinara sauce
- 1 teaspoon olive oil
- 1 teaspoon sriracha
- ½ teaspoon ground black pepper

Directions:
1. Make a sauce: mix up together marinara sauce, olive oil, sriracha, and ground black pepper.
2. Tub the tuna fillet with the sauce and leave for 15 minutes to marinate.
3. Then chop the fish into medium size cubes.
4. String the fish into the skewers.
5. Preheat oven to 365F.
6. Place the tuna skewers on the tray and sprinkle with remaining sauce.
7. Bake the tuna skewers for 7 minutes.

Nutrition value/serving: calories 378, fat 32.3, fiber 0.2, carbs 1, protein 21.1

235. Piri-Piri Cod

Preparation Time: 15 minutes
Cooking time: 8 minutes
Servings: 2

Ingredients:
- 1-pound cod fillet
- 1 tablespoon piri piri sauce

- 1 teaspoon dried dill
- 1 tablespoon apple cider vinegar
- ½ teaspoon salt
- ½ teaspoon minced garlic
- 1 tablespoon butter

Directions:
1. Cut cod fillet into 2 servings.
2. Then sprinkle it with piri piri sauce and apple cider vinegar.
3. Add salt and dried dill. Massage the fish well and leave it for 10 minutes to marinate.
4. Meanwhile, toss the butter in the skillet and melt it.
5. Add minced garlic and cook it for 1 minute.
6. After this, add cod fillets and cook them for 3 minutes from each side over the medium heat.
7. When the fish is cooked, sprinkle it with the melted garlic butter mixture and transfer in the serving plates.

Nutrition value/serving: calories 296, fat 9.3, fiber 0.6, carbs 7.1, protein 45.3

236. Steamed Salmon with Lemon

Preparation Time: 10 minutes
Cooking time: 15 minutes
Servings:4

Ingredients:
- 4 salmon fillets
- ½ lemon
- 1 rosemary, fresh
- 1 oz scallions, chopped
- ½ cup heavy cream
- 1 teaspoon ground black pepper
- ½ teaspoon salt

Directions:
1. Pour heavy cream in the saucepan.
2. Add fresh rosemary, chopped scallions, ground black pepper, and salt.
3. Slice the lemon and add it in the cream liquid.
4. Bring heavy cream to boil and add salmon fillet.
5. Close the lid and steam the fish for 10 minutes.
6. Then remove salmon from the saucepan and cut into 4 pieces.
7. Sprinkle salmon with the remaining heavy cream sauce before serving.

Nutrition value/serving: calories 293, fat 16.6, fiber 0.6, carbs 2.1, protein 35.1

237. Tilapia Stew

Preparation Time: 10 minutes
Cooking time: 25 minutes
Servings:4

Ingredients:
- 9 oz tilapia fillet, chopped
- 1 carrot, chopped
- 1 white onion, chopped
- ½ cup of water
- 3 tablespoons cream cheese
- 1 teaspoon salt
- 1 tablespoon butter
- ½ teaspoon chili pepper

Directions:
1. Toss the butter in the saucepan and melt it.
2. Add chopped tilapia and sprinkle it with salt and chili pepper.
3. Mix up the fish and cook it for 5 minutes.
4. Add carrot, white onion, and cream cheese. Mix up the ingredients well.
5. After this, add water and close the lid.
6. Saute the stew for 20 minutes over the medium-low heat.
7. When the vegetables are tender, the stew is cooked.

Nutrition value/serving: calories 122, fat 6.1, fiber 1, carbs 4.3, protein 12.9

238. Grilled Hake

Preparation Time: 10 minutes
Cooking time: 8 minutes
Servings:4

Ingredients:
- 4 hake fillets

- 1 teaspoon salt
- ½ teaspoon ground nutmeg
- 1 tablespoon butter, melted
- ½ teaspoon cayenne pepper

Directions:
1. In the mixing bowl, mix up together salt, ground nutmeg, and cayenne pepper.
2. Rub the hake fillets with the spice mixture and brush with the melted butter.
3. Preheat the grill to 375F.
4. Place the fish on the grill and cook it for 4 minutes from each side.

Nutrition value/serving: calories 142, fat 4.3, fiber 0.1, carbs 1.5, protein 25.5

239. Glazed Salmon Fillet

Preparation Time: 10 minutes
Cooking time: 10 minutes
Servings:2

Ingredients:
- 2 salmon fillets
- 1 tablespoon Erythritol
- 1 teaspoon lemon juice
- 1 tablespoon butter
- 1 teaspoon sage
- 1 garlic clove, peeled
- 1 teaspoon canola oil

Directions:
1. Pour canola oil in the skillet and add garlic clove and sage.
2. Bring the mixture to boil.
3. Add salmon fillets and cook them for 4 minutes from each side over the medium-high heat.
4. Then remove the fish from the skillet.
5. Add Erythritol in the skillet and wait until it is dissolved.
6. Then add lemon juice and butter. Mix up the mixture.
7. Return the fish back in the skillet and coat in the sweet mixture. Cook it for 1 minute and transfer in the serving plates.

Nutrition value/serving: calories 311, fat 19.2, fiber 0.2, carbs 0.8, protein 34.8

240. Curry Fish

Preparation Time: 10 minutes
Cooking time: 20 minutes
Servings:6

Ingredients:
- 1-pound tilapia
- 1 tablespoon curry paste
- ½ teaspoon curry powder
- ½ teaspoon dried cilantro
- 1 teaspoon dried dill
- 1 teaspoon paprika
- 1 teaspoon chili flakes
- 1 cup of coconut milk
- 2 bell peppers, chopped
- 1 teaspoon butter
- 1 teaspoon tomato paste

Directions:
1. Chop tilapia roughly and place in the pan.
2. Add butter and cook the ingredients for 2 minutes over the medium heat.
3. Then sprinkle fish with dried cilantro, dill, paprika, chili flakes, and bell peppers.
4. Add curry powder and curry paste.
5. Then add coconut milk and tomato paste.
6. Mix up the ingredients carefully until you get a light red color.
7. Close the lid and cook curry fish for 15 minutes over the medium-low heat.

Nutrition value/serving: calories 192, fat 12.5, fiber 1.7, carbs 6.5, protein 15.7

241. Tagine

Preparation Time: 10 minutes
Cooking time: 30 minutes
Servings:4

Ingredients:
- 10 oz sea eel
- 1 teaspoon turmeric
- ¼ teaspoon fresh ginger, grated
- 1 teaspoon salt
- ½ teaspoon smoked paprika
- ½ teaspoon chili flakes
- 1 tomato, chopped
- 2 oz celery stalk, chopped

- 3 oz turnip, chopped
- 1 white onion, peeled, chopped
- ½ teaspoon ground black pepper
- 4 kalamata olives
- 2 tablespoons butter

Directions:
1. Chop the sea eel roughly and place in the casserole dish (or use tagine.
2. Sprinkle it with turmeric, fresh ginger, salt, smoked paprika, chili flakes, and ground black pepper. Mix up gently.
3. Add chopped tomato, celery stalk, turnip, onion, and kalamata olives.
4. Add butter and cover the casserole dish with foil. Secure the edges.
5. Preheat the oven to 375F.
6. Place the meal in the oven and cook it for 30 minutes.
7. When the time is over, remove tagine from the oven and discard the foil.
8. Mix up the meal gently.

Nutrition value/serving: calories 167, fat 12.4, fiber 1.8, carbs 8, protein 7

242. Thyme Seabass

Preparation Time: 10 minutes
Cooking time: 20 minutes
Servings:4

Ingredients:
- 2-pound seabass
- 1 tablespoon fresh thyme
- ¼ teaspoon fresh rosemary
- ½ teaspoon ground black pepper
- 1 teaspoon salt
- 1 tablespoon butter
- 1 teaspoon lemon juice

Directions:
1. Peel and trim the seabass.
2. Then rub the fish with ground black pepper and salt. Fill it with fresh thyme, fresh rosemary, and butter.
3. Sprinkle fish with lemon juice.
4. Preheat the grill to 380F.
5. Wrap the fish in the foil and place in the preheated grill.
6. Cook the seabass for 20 minutes. Flip it from time to time.
7. When the time is over, transfer the cooked seabass on the plate and remove the foil.

Nutrition value/serving: calories 234, fat 9, fiber 0.4, carbs 3.7, protein 0.1

243. Fish Chowder

Preparation Time: 15 minutes
Cooking time: 25 minutes
Servings:5

Ingredients:
- 7 oz cod fillet, chopped
- 5 oz shrimps, peeled
- 6 oz bacon, chopped
- 1 white onion, diced
- ½ teaspoon minced garlic
- 1 tablespoon butter
- 1 teaspoon ground coriander
- 1 carrot, peeled, chopped
- 5 oz celery stalk, chopped
- 1 teaspoon salt
- ½ cup coconut cream
- ½ teaspoon paprika
- 3 cups of water

Directions:
1. Place bacon in the skillet and roast it for 5 minutes over the medium-high heat. Stir it from time to time.
2. Then transfer the cooked bacon in the saucepan.
3. Put diced onion and minced garlic in the skillet. Add butter.
4. Roast the ingredients for 2 minutes and transfer in the saucepan too. Add cod fillet.
5. Sprinkle the saucepan mixture with ground coriander and paprika.
6. Add coconut cream, shrimp, water, and chopped celery stalk. Mix up gently with the help of the spoon.
7. Close the lid and simmer the chowder for 15 minutes over the medium heat.
8. Then remove the chowder from the heat and let it rest with the closed lid for 10

minutes.

Nutrition value/serving: calories 345, fat 23.2, fiber 2.4, carbs 6.6, protein 27.3

244. Coconut Pollock

Preparation Time: 10 minutes
Cooking time: 15 minutes
Servings: 3

Ingredients:

- 11 oz pollock fillet
- 1 bell pepper, chopped
- 1 teaspoon smoked paprika
- ½ teaspoon salt
- 6 oz Cheddar cheese, shredded
- 1 tablespoon butter
- ½ cup of coconut milk
- ½ teaspoon turmeric

Directions:

1. Put the butter in the saucepan and melt it.
2. Add chopped bell pepper. Cook it for 3 minutes.
3. Chop the pollock fillet roughly.
4. Add it in the melted butter mixture.
5. Sprinkle the fish with smoked paprika, salt, and turmeric. Mix up it gently.
6. Simmer the fish for 5 minutes.
7. In the separated saucepan pour coconut milk. Bring it to boil.
8. Switch off the heat and add Cheddar cheese.
9. Mix up the liquid carefully until cheese is dissolved.
10. Pour coconut milk mixture over the pollock and bring it to boil.
11. Then remove the meal from the heat and let it rest for 5 minutes.

Nutrition value/serving: calories 463, fat 33.3, fiber 1.8, carbs 6.6, protein 36

245. Spicy Paella

Preparation Time: 15 minutes
Cooking time: 20 minutes
Servings: 3

Ingredients:

- 1 cup cauliflower, shredded
- 3 oz shrimps, peeled
- 3 oz clams
- 1 garlic clove, peeled
- 1 teaspoon sage
- ½ teaspoon saffron
- 1 teaspoon turmeric
- ½ teaspoon ground coriander
- 1 teaspoon salt
- 1 tablespoon butter
- 4 oz chicken fillet, chopped
- ½ teaspoon chili flakes
- 1 teaspoon oregano
- 2 cup of water
- ½ cup heavy cream

Directions:

1. Mix up together sage, saffron, turmeric, ground coriander, salt, chili flakes, and oregano.
2. Place the butter in the pan and melt it.
3. Add shrimps and clams.
4. Sprinkle the seafood with the spice mixture and mix up well.
5. Then add chopped chicken fillet, garlic clove, and heavy cream. Mix up the ingredients well and cook for 5 minutes.
6. Add water and shredded cauliflower.
7. Close the lid and saute paella for 10 minutes.
8. Remove it from the heat and leave for 10 minutes to rest.
9. Serve paella only hot or warm.

Nutrition value/serving: calories 237, fat 14.8, fiber 1.4, carbs 7.2, protein 18.9

246. Fennel Seabass with Peppercorns

Preparation Time: 10 minutes
Cooking time: 30 minutes
Servings: 4

Ingredients:

- 1-pound seabass
- 8 oz fennel bulb
- 1 onion, sliced
- 1 teaspoon peppercorns
- 1 tablespoon butter

- 1 teaspoon ground black pepper
- ½ teaspoon ground nutmeg
- 1 teaspoon lemon juice
- ½ teaspoon apple cider vinegar
- 1 teaspoon coriander
- 1 tablespoon canola oil
- 1 teaspoon cumin seeds

Directions:
1. Rub the seabass with ground black pepper, nutmeg, and coriander.
2. Then sprinkle the fish with canola oil, apple cider vinegar, and transfer in the tray.
3. Slice the fennel bulb and arrange it near the seabass.
4. Sprinkle the fennel with the lemon juice, peppercorns, and cumin seeds. Add sliced onion.
5. Cover the tray with foil and transfer in the preheated to the 370F oven.
6. Cook the fish for 30 minutes.

Nutrition value/serving: calories 193, fat 9.8, fiber 2.6, carbs 9, protein 1.2

247. Tuna Pie

Preparation Time: 15 minutes
Cooking time: 40 minutes
Servings: 6

Ingredients:
- 1 cup cauliflower, chopped
- 3 eggs, boiled
- 1 white onion, sliced
- 1 bell pepper, chopped
- 1 cup heavy cream
- 7 oz Monterey Jack cheese, shredded
- 1 tablespoon butter
- 1 teaspoon ground black pepper
- ½ teaspoon sage
- 1 teaspoon salt
- 12 oz tuna, chopped
- 1 tablespoon chives, chopped
- 1 teaspoon dried dill

Directions:
1. Place the cauliflower in the tray and bake it in the preheated to the 365F oven for 15 minutes.
2. Meanwhile, mix up together chopped tuna, dried dill, salt, sage, ground black pepper, and transfer the mixture in the skillet.
3. Roast it for 5 minutes over the medium heat. Stir it from time to time.
4. After this, transfer the mixture in the pie mold.
5. Add the layer of the white onion and bell pepper.
6. Then add heavy cream.
7. Remove the cooked cauliflower from the oven and transfer in the food processor.
8. Blend it until you get a smooth texture.
9. Peel the boiled eggs and cut them into the halves.
10. Spread the smooth cauliflower mixture over the tuna mixture.
11. Then add the layer of the halved boiled eggs and top the pie with the shredded cheese.
12. Place the pie in the preheated to 365F oven and bake for 20 minutes.
13. When the pie is cooked, chill it to the room temperature and cut into the servings.

Nutrition value/serving: calories 366, fat 26.2, fiber 1.2, carbs 5.4, protein 27.2

248. Fish Cakes with Greens

Preparation Time: 10 minutes
Cooking time: 5 minutes
Servings: 4

Ingredients:
- 8 oz salmon fillet
- 4 oz cod fillet
- 1 tablespoon chives, chopped
- 1 tablespoon fresh parsley, chopped
- 1 teaspoon ground coriander
- 2 eggs, beaten
- 2 tablespoons almond flour
- 1 teaspoon salt
- 1 tablespoon avocado oil

Directions:

1. Chop the cod and salmon fillets into the tiny pieces and transfer in the mixing bowl.
2. Add eggs, chives, fresh parsley, ground coriander, almond flour, and salt.
3. Mix up the fish mixture with the help of the spoon.
4. Make the medium size cakes from the mixture with the help of the fingertips.
5. Pour avocado oil in the skillet.
6. Add the prepared fish cakes and roast them for 2.5 minutes from each side.
7. Dry the cooked fish cakes with the paper towel if needed and transfer in the serving plate.

Nutrition value/serving: calories 214, fat 13.4, fiber 1.7, carbs 3.5, protein 21.9

249. Fish Bars

Preparation Time: 10 minutes
Cooking time: 15 minutes
Servings: 6

Ingredients:

- 10 oz tilapia fillet
- ½ cup coconut flour
- 2 eggs, whisked
- 1 teaspoon salt
- ½ teaspoon ground black pepper
- 3 oz Parmesan, grated
- 1 teaspoon butter

Directions:

1. Mince the tilapia fillet and place it in the mixing bowl.
2. Add coconut flour, whisked eggs, salt, ground black pepper, and grated cheese.
3. Mix up the mixture with the help of the spoon until homogenous.
4. Spread the casserole mold with the butter generously.
5. Place the fish mixture in the mold and flatten it well. Cut the mixture into the bars with the help of the knife.
6. Preheat the oven to 360F.
7. Place the casserole mold in the oven and cook the fish bars for 15 minutes or until the fish bars get the golden brown surface.
8. Chill the cooked meal well and only after this, transfer it in the serving plates.

Nutrition value/serving: calories 128, fat 5.8, fiber 0.5, carbs 1.4, protein 17.6

250. Pan-fried Cod

Preparation Time: 5 minutes
Cooking time: 10 minutes
Servings: 2

Ingredients:

- 12 oz cod fillet
- 1 tablespoon scallions, chopped
- 1 tablespoon butter
- 1 tablespoon coconut oil
- 1 teaspoon garlic, diced
- 1 teaspoon cumin seeds
- 1 teaspoon coriander seeds
- 1 teaspoon salt

Directions:

- Place butter and coconut oil in the skillet and melt them.
- Add garlic, cumin and coriander seeds.
- Rub the fish fillet with salt and place it in the skillet.
- Fry the fish for 2 minutes from each side or until it is light brown.
- Transfer the cooked cod fillet in the plate and cut into 2 servings.

Nutrition value/serving: calories 253, fat 14.3, fiber 0.2, carbs 1.2, protein 30.8

251. Crab Fat Bombs

Preparation Time: 10 minutes
Cooking time: 5 minutes
Servings: 4

Ingredients:

- 4 tablespoons cream cheese
- 1 tablespoon minced garlic
- 8 oz crab meat, canned
- 4 oz bacon, chopped
- 4 oz Parmesan, grated
- ½ teaspoon ground black pepper

Directions:

1. Place the chopped bacon in the skillet and roast it for 5 minutes or until it is crispy.
2. Meanwhile, finely chop the crab meat and mix it up with the minced garlic, cream cheese, ground black pepper, and grated Parmesan.
3. When the mixture is homogenous, make the balls with the help of 2 spoons.
4. Chill the bacon well.
5. Coat the crab bombs into the crispy bacon.

Nutrition value/serving: calories 334, fat 22.4, fiber 0.1, carbs 3.6, protein 27.6

252. Stuffed Salmon Fillets

Preparation Time: 30 minutes
Servings: 2

Ingredients:

- 2 medium salmon fillets; boneless
- 5 oz. tiger shrimp; peeled, deveined and chopped
- 6 mushrooms; chopped
- 3 green onions; chopped
- 2 cups spinach; chopped
- 1/4 cup macadamia nuts; toasted and chopped
- A pinch of sea salt
- Black pepper to the taste
- A pinch of nutmeg; ground
- 1/4 cup Paleo mayonnaise
- Bacon fat for cooking

Instructions:

1. Heat up a pan with some bacon fat over medium heat, add onions and mushrooms, a pinch of salt and black pepper, stir and cook for 4 minutes.
2. Add nuts, stir and cook for 2 minutes more.
3. Add spinach, stir and cook for 1 minute.
4. Add shrimp, stir and cook for another minute.
5. Take this mix off heat, leave it aside to cool down a bit, add Paleo mayo and nutmeg and stir everything.
6. Make an incision lengthwise in each salmon fillet, season with some black pepper and stuff with the shrimp mix.
7. Heat up a pan with some bacon fat over high heat, add salmon fillets and cook skin side down for 1 minute.
8. Cover the pan, reduce temperature to medium-low and cook for 8 minutes more.
9. Introduce pan in preheated broiler and broil for 2 minutes. Divide stuffed salmon fillets on plates and serve.

Nutrition: Calories: 450; **Fat:** 6g; **Fiber:** 4g; **Carbs:** 7g; **Protein:** 40

253. Shrimp Burgers

Preparation Time: 30 minutes
Servings: 4

Ingredients:

- 2 tbsp. cilantro; chopped
- 1½ lbs. shrimp; peeled and deveined
- 2 tbsp. chives; chopped
- Black pepper to the taste
- 1 garlic clove; minced
- 1/4 cup radishes; minced
- 1 tsp. lemon zest
- 1/4 cup celery; minced
- 1 egg; whisked
- 1 tbsp. lemon juice
- 1/4 cup almond meal

For the salsa:

- 1 avocado; pitted, peeled and chopped
- 1 cup pineapple; chopped
- 2 tbsp. red onion; chopped
- 1/4 cup bell peppers; chopped
- 1 tbsp. lime juice
- 1 tbsp. cilantro; finely chopped
- A pinch of sea salt
- Black pepper to the taste

Instructions:

1. In a bowl; mix pineapple with avocado, bell peppers, 2 tbsp. red onion, 1 tbsp. lime juice, pepper to the taste and 1 tbsp. cilantro, stir well and keep in the fridge for now.
2. In your food processor, mix shrimp with

2 tbsp. cilantro, chives and garlic and blend well.
3. Transfer to a bowl and mix with radishes, celery, lemon zest, lemon juice, egg, almond meal, a pinch of sea salt and pepper to the taste and stir well.
4. Shape 4 burgers, place them on preheated grill over medium high heat and cook for 5 minutes on each side. Divide shrimp burgers between plates and serve with the salsa you've made earlier on the side.

Nutrition: Calories: 238; Fat: 12g; Carbs: 13.2g; Fiber: 3g; Protein: 15.4

254. Salmon Delight

Preparation Time: 37 minutes
Servings: 4

Ingredients:

- 10 oz. spinach; chopped
- 5 sun-dried tomatoes; chopped
- 1/4 tsp. red pepper flakes
- 4 medium salmon fillets
- A pinch of sea salt
- Black pepper to the taste
- 1 tbsp. coconut oil
- 1/4 cup shallots; chopped
- 4 garlic cloves

Instructions:

1. Heat up a pan with the oil over medium high heat, add shallots, stir and cook for 3 minutes.
2. Add garlic, stir and cook for 1 minute. Add tomatoes, pepper flakes and spinach, stir and cook for 3 minutes.
3. Season with a pinch of salt and black pepper to the taste, stir; take off heat and leave aside for now.
4. Arrange salmon fillets on a lined baking sheet, season with a pinch of salt and some black pepper, top with the spinach mix, place in the oven at 350 °F and bake for 20 minutes.
5. Divide between plates and serve right away.

Nutrition: Calories: 140; Fat: 2g; Fiber: 2g; Carbs: 3g; Protein: 10g

255. Scallops Tartar

Preparation Time: 15 minutes
Servings: 2

Ingredients:

- 6 scallops; diced
- A pinch of sea salt
- Black pepper to the taste
- 3 strawberries; chopped
- 1 tbsp. extra virgin olive oil
- 1 tbsp. green onions; minced
- Juice from 1/2 lemon
- 1/2 tbsp. basil leaves; finely chopped

Instructions:

1. In a bowl; mix strawberries with scallops, basil and onions and stir well.
2. Add olive oil, a pinch of salt, pepper to the taste and lemon juice and stir well again. Keep in the fridge until you serve.

Nutrition: Calories: 180; Fat: 27g; Carbs: 3g; Fiber: 0g; Protein: 24g

256. Shrimp Skewers

Preparation Time: 20 minutes
Servings: 4

Ingredients:

- 1/2 lb. sausages; chopped and already cooked
- 1/2 lb. shrimp; peeled and deveined
- 2 tbsp. extra virgin olive oil
- 2 zucchinis; cubed
- A pinch of sea salt
- Black pepper to the taste
- *For the Creole seasoning:*
- 1/2 tbsp. garlic powder
- 2 tbsp. paprika
- 1/2 tbsp. onion powder
- 1/4 tbsp. oregano; dried
- 1/2 tbsp. chili powder
- 1/4 tbsp. thyme; dried

Instructions:

1. In a bowl; mix paprika with garlic powder, onion one, chili powder, oregano and

thyme and stir well.
2. In another bowl; mix shrimp with sausage, zucchini and oil and toss to coat.
3. Pour paprika mix over shrimp mix and stir well.
4. Arrange sausage, shrimp and zucchini on skewers alternating pieces, season with a pinch of sea salt and black pepper, place them on preheated grill over medium high heat and cook for 8 minutes, flipping skewers from time to time. Arrange on a platter and serve.

Nutrition: Calories: 360; Fat: 32g; Carbs: 4.3g; Fiber: 0.8; Sugar: 1g; Protein: 18.1

257. Infused Clams

Preparation Time: 22 minutes
Servings: 2

Ingredients:

- 1 tbsp. olive oil
- 3 oz. pancetta
- 3 tbsp. ghee
- 2 lb. little clams; scrubbed
- 1 shallot; minced
- 2 garlic cloves; minced
- 1 bottle infused cider
- 1 apple; cored and chopped
- Juice of 1/2 lemon

Instructions:

1. Heat up a pan with the oil over medium high heat, add pancetta and brown for 3 minutes.
2. Add ghee, shallot and garlic, stir and cook for 3 minutes.
3. Add cider, stir well and cook for 1 minute.
4. Add clams and thyme, cover and simmer for 5 minutes. Add apple and lemon juice, stir; divide everything into bowls and serve.

Nutrition: Calories: 120; Fat: 1g; Fiber: 2g; Carbs: 4g; Protein: 10g

258. Halibut And Tasty Salsa

Preparation Time: 25 minutes
Servings: 4

Ingredients:

- 4 medium halibut fillets
- 2 tsp. olive oil
- 4 tsp. lemon juice
- 1 garlic clove; minced
- 1 tsp. sweet paprika
- A pinch of sea salt
- Black pepper to the taste

For the salsa:
- 1/4 cup green onions; chopped
- 1 cup red bell pepper; chopped
- 4 tsp. oregano; chopped
- 1 small habanero pepper; chopped
- 1 garlic clove; minced
- 1/4 cup lemon juice

Instructions:

1. In a bowl; mix red bell pepper with habanero, green onion, 1/4 cup lemon juice, 1 garlic clove, oregano, a pinch of sea salt and black pepper, stir well and keep in the fridge for now.
2. In a large bowl; mix paprika, olive oil, 1 garlic clove and 4 tsp. lemon juice and stir well.
3. Add fish, rub well, cover bowl and leave aside for 10 minutes.
4. Place marinated fish on preheated grill over medium high heat, season with a pinch of sea salt and black pepper, cook for 4 minutes on each side and divide between plates. Top fish with the salsa you've made earlier and serve.

Nutrition: Calories: 150; Fat: 3g; Fiber: 2g; Carbs: 3g; Protein: 12g

259. Shrimp With Mango And Avocado Mix

Preparation Time: 15 minutes
Servings: 2

Ingredients:

- 1 avocado; pitted, peeled and chopped
- 1 lb. shrimp; peeled and deveined
- 1 tomato; chopped

- 1 mango; peeled and chopped
- 1 jalapeno; chopped
- 1 tbsp. lime juice
- Bacon fat
- 1/4 cup green onions; chopped
- 4 garlic cloves; minced
- A pinch of sea salt
- Black pepper to the taste

Instructions:
1. In a bowl; mix lime juice with jalapeno, mango, tomato, avocado and green onions, stir well and leave aside.
2. Heat up a pan with some bacon fat over medium high heat, add garlic, stir and cook for 2 minutes.
3. Add shrimp, a pinch of sea salt and black pepper, stir and cook for 5 minutes. Divide shrimp on plates, add mango and avocado mix on the side.

Nutrition: Calories: 140; Fat: 2g; Fiber: 3g; Carbs: 3g; Protein: 8g

260. Grilled Oysters

Preparation Time: 17 minutes
Servings: 7

Ingredients:
- 1/4 cup red onion; chopped
- 2 tomatoes; chopped
- A handful cilantro; chopped
- 1 jalapeno; chopped
- A pinch of sea salt
- Black pepper to the taste
- Juice from 1 lime
- 2 limes; cut into wedges
- 24 oysters; scrubbed

Instructions:
1. In a bowl; tomatoes with onion, cilantro, jalapeno, a pinch of salt, black pepper and juice from 1 lime, stir well and leave aside.
2. Heat up your grill over medium high heat, add oysters, grill them for 7 minutes.
3. Open them completely and divide oysters between plates. Top with the tomatoes mix and serve with lime wedges on the side.

Nutrition: Calories: 140; Fat: 2g; Fiber: 2g; Carbs: 4g; Protein: 8g

261. Stuffed Calamari

Preparation Time: 1 hour 5 minutes
Servings: 4

Ingredients:
- 4 big calamari; tentacles separated and chopped
- 2 tbsp. parsley; chopped
- 5 oz. kale; chopped
- 2 garlic cloves; minced
- 1 red bell pepper; chopped
- 1 tsp. oregano; dried
- 14 oz. canned tomato puree
- Some bacon fat
- 1 onion; chopped
- A pinch of sea salt
- Black pepper to the taste

Instructions:
1. Heat up a pan with some bacon fat over medium heat, add onion and garlic, stir and cook for 2 minutes.
2. Add bell pepper, stir and cook for 3 minutes.
3. Add calamari tentacles, stir and cook for 6 minutes more.
4. Add kale, a pinch of sea salt and black pepper, stir; cook for a couple more minutes and take off heat.
5. Stuff calamari tubes with this mix and secure with toothpicks.
6. Heat up a pan with some bacon fat over medium high heat, add calamari, brown them for 2 minutes on each side and then mix with tomato puree.
7. Also add parsley, oregano and some black pepper to the pan, stir gently, cover, reduce heat to medium-low and simmer for 40 minutes. Divide stuffed calamari on plates and serve.

Nutrition: Calories: 222; Fat: 10g; Fiber: 1g; Carbs: 7g; Protein: 15g

262. Shrimp Cocktail

Preparation Time: 36 minutes
Servings: 4

Ingredients:

- 20 jumbo shrimp; deveined but shelled
- 2 cups ice
- A pinch of sea salt
- A drizzle of olive oil
- 1 cup water
- *For the cocktail sauce:*
- 1 cup tomato sauce
- 1/4 tsp. Worcestershire sauce
- Juice of 1 lemon
- Zest from 1 lemon
- 1 tbsp. prepared horseradish
- Chili sauce to the taste

Instructions:

1. In a bowl; mix water with ice, a pinch of sea salt and shrimp, stir; cover and keep in the fridge for 30 minutes.
2. Discard water from shrimp, rinse them, pat dry them, drizzle olive oil over them and rub well.
3. Arrange shrimp on a lined baking sheet, place in preheated broiler and broil them for 3 minutes.
4. Flip, broil for 2 minutes more and leave aside.
5. In a bowl; mix tomato sauce with Worcestershire sauce, lemon juice, lemon zest, chili sauce to the taste and horseradish and whisk well. Arrange shrimp on a platter and serve with the cocktail sauce on the side.

Nutrition: Calories: 160; Fat: 3g; Fiber: 2g; Carbs: 3g; Protein: 14g

263. Grilled Calamari

Preparation Time: 15 minutes
Servings: 4

Ingredients:

- 2 lbs. calamari tentacles and tubes cut into rings
- 2 tbsp. parsley; minced
- 1 lemon; sliced
- 1 lime; sliced
- 2 garlic cloves; minced
- 3 tbsp. lemon juice
- 1/4 cup olive oil
- A pinch of sea salt
- Black pepper to the taste

Instructions:

1. In a bowl; mix calamari with parsley, lime slices, lemon slices, garlic, lemon juice, a pinch of salt, black pepper and olive oil and stir well.
2. Place calamari rings on preheated grill over medium high heat, cook for 5 minutes and divide between plates. Serve with the lemon and lime slices and some of the marinade drizzled on top.

Nutrition: Calories: 130; Fat: 4g; Fiber: 1g; Carbs: 3g; Protein: 12g

264. Grilled Salmon And Avocado Sauce

Preparation Time: 25 minutes
Servings: 4

Ingredients:

- 1 avocado; pitted, peeled and chopped
- 4 salmon fillets
- 1/4 cup cilantro; chopped
- 1/3 cup coconut milk
- 1 tbsp. lime juice
- 1 tbsp. lime zest
- 1 tsp. onion powder
- 1 tsp. garlic powder
- A pinch of sea salt
- Black pepper to the taste

Instructions:

1. Season salmon fillets with a pinch of salt, black pepper and lime zest, rub well, place on heated grill over medium heat, cook for 15 minutes flipping once and divide between plates.
2. In your food processor, mix avocado with cilantro, garlic powder, onion powder, lime juice and coconut milk and blend well.

3. Add a pinch of sea salt and some black pepper, blend again and drizzle this over salmon fillets. Serve right away.

Nutrition: Calories: 170; Fat: 7g; Fiber: 2g; Carbs: 3g; Protein: 20g

265. Crusted Salmon

Preparation Time: 30 minutes
Servings: 4

Ingredients:
- 1 cup pistachios; chopped
- 4 salmon fillets
- 1/4 cup lemon juice
- 2 tbsp. honey
- 1 tsp. dill; chopped
- A pinch of sea salt
- Black pepper to the taste
- 1 tbsp. mustard

Instructions:
1. In a bowl; mix pistachios with mustard, honey, lemon juice, a pinch of salt, black pepper and dill and stir well.
2. Spread this over salmon fillets, press well, place them on a lined baking sheet, place in the oven at 375 °F and bake for 20 minutes. Divide salmon between plates and serve with a side salad.

Nutrition: Calories: 150; Fat: 3g; Fiber: 2g; Carbs: 5g; Protein: 12g

---

266. Tuna with Chimichurri Sauce

Preparation time: 10 minutes
Cooking time: 5 minutes
Servings: 4

Ingredients:
- 1 small red onion, chopped
- ½ cup cilantro, chopped
- 1/3 cup olive oil+ 2 tablespoons
- 1 jalapeno pepper, chopped
- 2 tablespoons basil, chopped
- 3 tablespoons vinegar
- 3 garlic cloves, minced
- 1 teaspoon red pepper flakes
- 1 teaspoon thyme, chopped
- A pinch of sea salt
- Black pepper to taste
- 1 pound sushi grade tuna
- 2 avocados, pitted, peeled and chopped
- 6 ounces arugula

Directions:
1. In a bowl, mix 1/3 cup oil with onion, jalapeno, cilantro, basil, vinegar, garlic, parsley, pepper flakes, thyme, a pinch of salt and black pepper and whisk well.
2. Heat up a pan with the rest of the oil over medium-high heat, add tuna, season salt and black pepper, cook for 2 minutes on each side, transfer to a cutting board, leave aside to cool down and slice.
3. In a bowl, mix arugula with half of the chimichurri sauce you've made earlier, toss to coat well and divide between plates.
4. Also divide tuna slices, and avocado pieces and drizzle the rest of the sauce on top.
5. Enjoy!

Nutrition: calories 938, fat 62,8, fiber 10, carbs 51,9, protein 43,8

267. Salmon and Chili Sauce

Preparation time: 10 minutes
Cooking time: 15 minutes
Servings: 12

Ingredients:
- 1 and ¼ cups coconut, shredded
- 1 pound salmon meat, cubed
- 1/3 cup coconut flour
- A pinch of sea salt
- Black pepper to taste
- 1 egg
- 2 tablespoons coconut oil
- ¼ cup water
- 4 red chilies, chopped
- 3 garlic cloves, minced
- ¼ cup balsamic vinegar
- ½ cup honey

Directions:

1. In a bowl, mix coconut flour with a pinch of salt and stir.
2. In another bowl, whisk the egg with black pepper.
3. Put coconut in a third bowl.
4. Dip salmon cubes in flour, egg and coconut and place them all on a working surface.
5. Heat up a pan with the oil over medium-high heat, add salmon cubes, fry them for 3 minutes on each side, transfer them to paper towels, drain grease and divide them between plates.
6. Heat up a pan with the water over medium-high heat.
7. Add chilies, cloves, vinegar, honey and agar agar, stir well, bring to a gentle boil and simmer until all ingredients combine.
8. Drizzle this over salmon cubes and serve.
9. Enjoy!

Nutrition: calories 180, fat 8,5, fiber 0,9, carbs 19,7, protein 7,7

268. Infused Clams

Preparation time: 10 minutes
Cooking time: 12 minutes
Servings: 2

Ingredients:

- 3 tablespoons ghee, melted
- 2 pound little clams, scrubbed
- 1 shallot, minced
- 2 garlic cloves, minced
- 1 cup cider
- 1 apple, cored and chopped
- Juice of ½ lemon

Directions:

1. Heat up a pan with the ghee over medium-high heat, add the shallot and garlic, stir and cook for 3 minutes.
2. Add cider, stir well and cook for 1 minute.
3. Add clams and thyme, cover and simmer for 5 minutes.
4. Add apple and lemon juice, stir, divide everything into bowls and serve.
5. Enjoy!

Nutrition: calories 610, fat 23,6, fiber 2,9, carbs 43,7, protein 55,1

269. Salmon and Apple Mix

Preparation time: 10 minutes
Cooking time: 30 minutes
Servings: 6

Ingredients:

- 2 tablespoons ghee, melted
- A pinch of sea salt
- Black pepper to taste
- 3 cups chicken stock
- ½ teaspoon fennel seeds
- 1 teaspoon mustard seeds
- 2 apples, cored, peeled and cubed
- 4 salmon fillets, skin on and bone in

Directions:

1. Put the stock in a pot, heat up over medium heat, add mustard seeds, a pinch of salt, black pepper and fennel seeds, stir and boil for 25 minutes.
2. Strain this into a bowl, add half of the ghee, stir well and leave aside for now.
3. Heat up a pan with the rest of the ghee over medium heat, add apple pieces, stir and cook for 6 minutes.
4. Brush salmon pieces with some of the stock mix, season with a pinch of salt and black pepper, place on a lined baking sheet, also add apple pieces, introduce everything in the oven at 350 degrees F and bake for 25 minutes.
5. Divide salmon between plates and serve with the rest of the stock drizzled on top.
6. Enjoy!

Nutrition: calories 241, fat 12,2, fiber 2, carbs 10,9, protein 23,7

270. Smoked Shrimp Mix

Preparation time: 10 minutes
Cooking time: 5 minutes
Servings: 4

Ingredients:

- 1 pound big shrimp, peeled and deveined
- 2 teaspoons olive oil
- 1 cup cilantro, chopped
- 1 cup parsley, chopped
- Juice from 2 limes
- ½ cup olive oil
- ¼ cup yellow onion, chopped
- A pinch of sea salt
- ½ teaspoon smoked paprika
- 2 garlic cloves, minced

Directions:
1. Heat up a pan with 2 teaspoons olive oil over medium heat, add shrimp, cook them for 5 minutes and reduce heat to low.
2. In a food processor, mix ½ cup oil with onion, sea salt, paprika, garlic, lime juice, parsley and cilantro and pulse well.
3. Divide shrimp on plates, top with the chimichurri and serve.
4. Enjoy!

Nutrition: calories 374, fat 26,9, fiber 1, carbs 4,3, protein 30,5

271. Scallops, Grapes and Spinach Bowls

Preparation time: 10 minutes
Cooking time: 13 minutes
Servings: 4

Ingredients:
- 1 shallot, minced
- 3 garlic cloves, minced
- 1 and ½ cups chicken stock
- ¼ cup walnuts, toasted and chopped
- 1 and ½ cups grapes, halved
- 2 cups spinach
- 1 tablespoon avocado oil
- 1 pound scallops
- A pinch of sea salt
- Black pepper to taste

Directions:
1. Heat up a pan with the oil over medium heat, add the shallot and the garlic, stir and cook for 2 minutes.
2. Add the walnuts, grapes, salt and pepper, stir and cook for 3 more minutes.
3. Add the scallops and cook them for 2 minutes on each side.
4. Add the spinach, toss, cook everything for 3 more minutes, divide everything into bowls and serve.
5. Enjoy!

Nutrition: calories 205, fat 7,4, fiber 1,5, carbs 17,5, protein 24,9

272. Crab Cakes and Red Pepper Sauce

Preparation time: 10 minutes
Cooking time: 7 minutes
Servings: 8

Ingredients:
- 1 cup crab meat
- 2 tablespoons parsley, chopped
- 2 tablespoons old bay seasoning
- 2 teaspoons Dijon mustard
- 1 egg, whisked
- 1 tablespoons lemon juice
- 2 tablespoons coconut oil
- 1 and ½ tablespoons coconut flour

For the sauce:
- 1 tablespoons olive oil
- ¼ cup roasted red peppers
- 1 tablespoon lemon juice
- ¼ cup avocado, peeled and chopped

Directions:
1. In a bowl, mix crabmeat with old bay seasoning, parsley, mustard, egg, 1 tablespoon lemon juice and coconut flour and stir everything very well.
2. Shape 8 patties from this mix and place them on a plate.
3. Heat up a pan with 2 tablespoons coconut oil over medium-high heat, add crab patties, cook for 3 minutes on each side and divide between plates.
4. In a food processor, mix olive oil with red peppers, avocado and 1 tablespoon lemon juice and blend well.
5. Spread this on the crab patties and serve.
6. Enjoy!

Nutrition: calories 69, fat 6,8, fiber 0,5, carbs

1,1, protein 1,4

273. Grilled Oysters

Preparation time: 10 minutes
Cooking time: 7 minutes
Servings: 4

Ingredients:

- ¼ cup red onion, chopped
- 2 tomatoes, chopped
- A handful cilantro, chopped
- 1 jalapeno, chopped
- A pinch of sea salt
- Black pepper to taste
- Juice from 1 lime
- 2 limes, cut into wedges
- 24 oysters, scrubbed

Directions:

1. In a bowl, tomatoes with onion, cilantro, jalapeno, a pinch of salt, black pepper and juice from 1 lime, stir well and leave aside.
2. Heat up your grill over medium-high heat, add oysters, grill them for 7 minutes.
3. Open them completely and divide oysters between plates.
4. Top with the tomatoes mix and serve with lime wedges on the side.
5. Enjoy!

Nutrition: calories 287, fat 8,9, fiber 2,1, carbs 21,7, protein 29,9

274. Squid and Guacamole

Preparation time: 10 minutes
Cooking time: 5 minutes
Servings: 2

Ingredients:

- 2 medium squid, cleaned, tentacles and tubes separated
- A pinch of sea salt
- Black pepper to taste
- 1 tablespoon olive oil
- Juice of ½ lime
- For the guacamole:
- 1 tablespoon coriander, chopped
- 2 red chilies, chopped
- 2 avocados, pitted, peeled and chopped
- 1 tomato, chopped
- 1 red onion, chopped
- Juice from 2 limes

Directions:

1. In a bowl, mix chilies with avocados, coriander, tomato, red onion and juice from 2 limes and stir well.
2. Heat up your grill over medium-high heat, add squid pieces after you've rubbed it with 1 tablespoon olive oil, season with salt and pepper to taste, grill for 3 minutes, flip and cook for 2 minutes on the other side.
3. Transfer squid to a cutting board, slice, drizzle juice of ½ lime. Toss to coat and divide between plates.
4. Serve with the guacamole on the side.
5. Enjoy!

Nutrition: calories 619, fat 48,1, fiber 15,2, carbs 28,9, protein 24,7

275. Shrimp and Cauliflower Rice

Preparation time: 10 minutes
Cooking time: 20 minutes
Servings: 4

Ingredients:

- 1 tablespoon ghee, melted
- 1 cauliflower head, florets separated
- ¼ cup coconut milk
- 1 pound shrimp, peeled and deveined
- 2 garlic cloves, minced
- 8 ounces mushrooms, sliced
- 3 small shallots, peeled, sliced
- A pinch of red pepper flakes
- A handful mixed parsley and chives, chopped
- ½ cup beef stock
- Black pepper to taste

Directions:

1. Heat up a pan over medium-high heat, add shallots slices, cook for 3 minutes on each side, drain grease on paper towels and leave aside.
2. Put cauliflower florets in a food

processor, blend until you obtain your "rice" and transfer to a heated pan over medium-high heat.
3. Cook cauliflower rice for 5 minutes stirring often.
4. Add coconut milk and 1 tablespoon ghee, stir and cook for a couple more minutes.
5. Blend everything using an immersion blender, add black pepper to taste, stir, reduce heat to low and cook for 3 more minutes
6. Heat up the pan where you cooked the shallots over medium-high heat, add the shrimp, cook for 2 minutes on each side and transfer to a plate.
7. Heat up the pan again over medium heat, add mushrooms, stir and cook for a few minutes.
8. Add garlic, pepper flakes and black pepper, stir and cook for 1 minute.
9. Add stock, return shrimp to pan, stir and cook for 4 minutes.
10. Divide cauliflower rice between plates, top with shrimp and mushrooms mix, top with crispy shallots and sprinkle parsley and chives on top.
11. Enjoy!

Nutrition: calories 241, fat 9,1, fiber 3,1, carbs 10,7, protein 30,4

276. Stuffed Salmon Fillets

Preparation time: 10 minutes
Cooking time: 20 minutes
Servings: 2

Ingredients:
- 2 medium salmon fillets, boneless
- 5 ounces tiger shrimp, peeled, deveined and chopped
- 6 mushrooms, chopped
- 3 green onions, chopped
- 2 cups spinach, chopped
- ¼ cup macadamia nuts, toasted and chopped
- A pinch of sea salt
- Black pepper to taste
- A pinch of nutmeg, ground
- ¼ cup avocado mayonnaise
- A drizzle of olive oil

Directions:
1. Heat up a pan with some over medium heat, add onions and mushrooms, salt and black pepper, stir and cook for 4 minutes.
2. Add nuts, stir and cook for 2 minutes more.
3. Add spinach, stir and cook for 1 minute.
4. Add shrimp, stir and cook for another minute.
5. Take this mix off heat, leave it aside to cool down a bit, add the mayo and nutmeg and stir everything.
6. Make an incision lengthwise in each salmon fillet, season with some black pepper and stuff with the shrimp mix.
7. Heat up a pan with some olive oil over high heat, add salmon fillets and cook them skin side down for 1 minute.
8. Cover the pan, reduce temperature to medium-low and cook for 8 minutes.
9. Place pan under preheated broiler and broil for 2 minutes over medium heat.
10. Divide stuffed salmon fillets between plates and serve.
11. Enjoy!

Nutrition: calories 702, fat 61,8, fiber 3,3, carbs 6,9, protein 53,7

277. Salmon and Coconut Sweet Potato Mash

Preparation time: 10 minutes
Cooking time: 40 minutes
Servings: 2

Ingredients:
- 2 salmon fillets, boneless
- 2 tablespoons mustard
- 1 tablespoon maple syrup
- A pinch of sea salt
- Black pepper to taste
- 2 sweet potatoes, peeled and chopped
- 2 teaspoons coconut oil
- ¼ cup coconut milk
- 3 garlic cloves, minced

Directions:

1. In a bowl, mix maple syrup with mustard and whisk well.
2. Season salmon fillets with a pinch of sea salt and black pepper to taste and brush them with half of the maple mix.
3. Heat up a pan with 1 teaspoon coconut oil over medium-high heat, add salmon, skin side down and cook for 4 minutes.
4. Transfer salmon to a baking dish, brush with the rest of the maple syrup mix, place in the oven at 425 degrees F and roast for 10 minutes.
5. Put sweet potatoes in a large saucepan, add water to cover, bring to a boil over medium heat, cover and cook for 20 minutes.
6. Heat up a pan with the rest of the oil over medium heat, add garlic, stir and cook for 1 minute.
7. Add sweet potatoes, stir well and then mash everything with a potato masher.
8. Add coconut milk, a pinch of salt and black pepper to taste and blend using an immersion blender.
9. Divide this mash between plates, add salmon on the side and serve.
10. Enjoy!

Nutrition: calories 606, fat 26,2, fiber 8,6, carbs 55,6, protein 40,6

278. Salmon and Spicy Slaw

Preparation time: 10 minutes
Cooking time: 6 minutes
Servings: 4

Ingredients:

- 3 cups cold water
- 3 scallions, chopped
- 2 teaspoons sriracha sauce
- 3 teaspoons avocado oil
- 4 teaspoons cider vinegar
- 2 teaspoons olive oil
- 4 medium salmon fillets, skinless and boneless
- A pinch of sea salt and black pepper
- 2 cups cabbage, chopped
- 4 cups baby arugula
- 2 cups radish, julienne cut
- ¼ cup pepitas, toasted

Directions:

1. In a bowl, combine 2 teaspoons avocado oil, vinegar, a pinch of sea salt and black pepper and whisk.
2. Sprinkle salmon fillets with salt, black pepper.
3. Heat up a pan with the rest of the avocado oil over medium-high heat, add salmon, cook for 6 minutes, flip, take off heat, cover pan and leave aside for a few more minutes.
4. In a salad bowl, mix cabbage with arugula, radish, pepitas, a pinch of salt, black pepper, the vinegar salad dressing and the olive oil and toss to coat well.
5. Divide salmon between plates, add cabbage salad on the side and top with scallions.
6. Enjoy!

Nutrition: calories 325, fat 17,5, fiber 2,8, carbs 6,3, protein 36,8

279. Spicy Shrimp

Preparation time: 10 minutes
Cooking time: 4 minutes
Servings: 2

Ingredients:

- 12 jumbo shrimp, peeled and deveined
- A pinch of sea salt
- Black pepper to taste
- 2 garlic cloves, minced
- 2 tablespoons olive oil
- ¼ teaspoon red pepper flakes
- 1 teaspoon steak seasoning
- 1 teaspoon lemon zest
- 1 tablespoon parsley, chopped
- 2 teaspoons lemon juice

Directions:

1. Heat up a pan with the oil over medium-high heat, add pepper flakes, garlic and shrimp, stir and cook for 4 minutes.
2. Season with a pinch of sea salt, black pepper, parsley, lemon juice and lemon zest, stir well, divide between plates and

serve.
3. Enjoy!

Nutrition: calories 368, fat 14,1, fiber 0,3, carbs 1,6, protein 60,4

280. Salmon and Lemon Relish

Preparation time: 10 minutes
Cooking time: 1 hour
Servings: 2

Ingredients:

- 1 big salmon fillet, cut in halves
- Black pepper to taste
- A drizzle of olive oil
- A pinch of sea salt
- For the relish:
- 1 tablespoon lemon juice
- 1 shallot, chopped
- 1 Meyer lemon, cut into wedges and then thinly sliced
- 2 tablespoons parsley, chopped
- ¼ cup olive oil
- Black pepper to taste

Directions:

1. Put some water in a dish and place it in the oven.
2. Put the salmon on a lined baking dish, drizzle some olive oil, season with a pinch of sea salt and black pepper, rub well, place in the oven at 370 degrees F and bake for 1 hour.
3. Meanwhile, in a bowl, mix shallot with the lemon juice, a pinch of salt and black pepper, stir and leave aside for 10 minutes.
4. In another bowl, mix marinated shallot with lemon slices, some salt, pepper, parsley and ¼ cup oil and whisk well.
5. Cut salmon into chunks, divide between plates and top with lemon relish.
6. Enjoy!

Nutrition: calories 549, fat 43,8, fiber 3,2, carbs 11,2, protein 35,8

281. Mussels Mix

Preparation time: 10 minutes
Cooking time: 15 minutes
Servings: 6

Ingredients:

- 3 garlic cloves, minced
- 1 yellow onion, chopped
- 1 tablespoon olive oil
- 1 handful parsley, chopped
- 1 teaspoon red pepper flakes
- 25 ounces fresh tomatoes, peeled, chopped
- 2 cups chicken stock
- 25 ounces fresh crushed tomatoes
- 2 pounds mussels, scrubbed

Directions:

1. Heat up a large saucepan with the oil over medium heat, add onions, garlic, parsley and pepper flakes, stir and cook for 2 minutes.
2. Add crushed and chopped tomatoes, black pepper and stock, stir, cover and bring to a boil.
3. Add mussels, stir, cover and cook until they open.
4. Ladle this into bowls and serve.
5. Enjoy!

Nutrition: calories 234, fat 6,3, fiber 5,8, carbs 22,5, protein 22,5

282. Mahi-Mahi and Cilantro Butter

Preparation time: 10 minutes
Cooking time: 10 minutes
Servings: 4

Ingredients:

- 4 mahi-mahi fillets, skinless, boneless
- ½ tablespoon sweet paprika
- ½ teaspoon garlic powder
- ½ teaspoon oregano, dried
- 1 tablespoon chili powder
- 2 tablespoons olive oil
- 2 tablespoons coconut oil
- ½ teaspoon onion powder
- A handful cilantro, chopped
- Lime wedges
- For the cilantro butter:

- Juice of 1 lemon
- 1 garlic clove, minced
- ¼ cup ghee, melted
- 2 tablespoons cilantro, chopped

Directions:

1. In a bowl, mix ¼ cup ghee with 1 garlic clove, juice from 1 lemon and 2 tablespoons cilantro, whisk very well and leave aside for now.
2. In another bowl, mix garlic powder with onion powder, chili powder, oregano and paprika and stir well.
3. Season mahi-mahi with this mix, drizzle the olive oil over them and rub well.
4. Heat up a pan with the coconut oil over medium-high heat, add fish fillets, cook for 4 minutes on each side and divide them between plates.
5. Add cilantro butter over fish and serve.
6. Enjoy!

Nutrition: calories 339, fat 27,1, fiber 1,7, carbs 5,4, protein 21,8

283. Herbed Shrimp Mix

Preparation time: 10 minutes
Cooking time: 8 minutes
Servings: 4

Ingredients:

- 2 tablespoons sriracha sauce
- 1 pound shrimp, peeled and deveined
- ¼ cup ghee, melted and heated up
- 1 tablespoon chives, chopped
- 1 tablespoon parsley, chopped
- 1 tablespoon lime juice
- A pinch of sea salt
- Black pepper to taste

Directions:

1. In a bowl, mix ghee with a pinch of salt, black pepper, lime juice, chives, parsley, sriracha sauce and whisk well.
2. Put the shrimp on heated grill over medium-high heat, cook for 3 minutes on each side and transfer them to a bowl.
3. Add melted ghee mix, toss well and serve.
4. Enjoy!

Nutrition: calories 298, fat 19,7, fiber 0,1, carbs 2,6, protein 25,9

284. Grilled Salmon and Lime Sauce

Preparation time: 10 minutes
Cooking time: 15 minutes
Servings: 4

Ingredients:

- 4 salmon fillets, boneless
- ¼ cup cilantro, chopped
- 1/3 cup coconut milk
- 1 tablespoon lime juice
- 1 tablespoon lime zest
- 1 teaspoon onion powder
- 1 teaspoon garlic powder
- A pinch of sea salt
- Black pepper to taste

Directions:

1. Season salmon fillets with a pinch of salt and black pepper, rub well, place on heated grill over medium heat, cook for 15 minutes flipping once and divide between plates.
2. In a food processor, mix cilantro, garlic powder, onion powder, lime juice, salt, pepper and coconut milk and blend well.
3. Drizzle this over salmon fillets and serve right away.
4. Enjoy!

Nutrition: calories 288, fat 15,8, fiber 0,8, carbs 2,7, protein 35,2

285. Shrimp Pan

Preparation time: 10 minutes
Cooking time: 8 minutes
Servings: 4

Ingredients:

- 1 pound shrimp, deveined
- 2 tablespoons parsley, minced
- 2 garlic cloves, minced
- 3 tablespoons lemon juice
- 2 tablespoons olive oil
- A pinch of sea salt
- Black pepper to taste

Directions:
1. Heat up a pan with the oil over medium heat, add the shrimp, and cook for 3 minutes on each side.
2. Add garlic, parsley, lemon juice, salt and pepper, toss, cook for 2 more minutes, divide into bowls and serve.
3. Enjoy!

Nutrition: calories 200, fat 9, fiber 0,1, carbs 2,6, protein 26,1

286. Shrimp and Cucumber Noodles

Preparation time: 10 minutes
Cooking time: 6 minutes
Servings: 2

Ingredients:
- 2 cucumbers, cut with a spiralizer
- 1 pound shrimp, peeled and deveined
- 4 garlic cloves, minced
- 2 tablespoons olive oil
- 2 tablespoons lemon juice
- 2 tablespoons chives, minced
- A pinch of sea salt
- Black pepper to taste

Directions:
1. Heat up a pan with the oil over medium heat, add garlic, stir and cook for 3 minutes.
2. Add the shrimp and the lemon juice, stir, cook for 4 minutes more and transfer to a bowl.
3. Add cucumber noodles, salt, pepper and the chives, toss and serve.
4. Enjoy!

Nutrition: calories 448, fat 18,3, fiber 1,8, carbs 16,8, protein 54,2

287. Walnut Crusted Salmon

Preparation time: 10 minutes
Cooking time: 20 minutes
Servings: 4

Ingredients:
- 1 cup walnuts, chopped
- 4 salmon fillets, boneless
- ¼ cup lemon juice
- 2 tablespoons stevia
- 1 teaspoon dill, chopped
- A pinch of sea salt
- Black pepper to taste
- 1 tablespoon mustard

Directions:
1. In a bowl, mix the walnuts with mustard, stevia, lemon juice, a pinch of salt, black pepper and dill and stir well.
2. Spread this over salmon fillets, press well, place them on a lined baking sheet, place in the oven at 375 degrees F and bake for 20 minutes.
3. Divide salmon between plates and serve with a side salad.
4. Enjoy!

Nutrition: calories 446, fat 30,4, fiber 2,6, carbs 4,5, protein 42,9

288. Stuffed Calamari

Preparation time: 15 minutes
Cooking time: 50 minutes
Servings: 4

Ingredients:
- 4 big calamari, tentacles separated and chopped
- 2 tablespoons parsley, chopped
- 5 ounces kale, chopped
- 2 garlic cloves, minced
- 1 red bell pepper, chopped
- 1 teaspoon oregano, dried
- 15 ounces homemade tomato puree
- Olive oil
- 1 yellow onion, chopped
- A pinch of sea salt
- Black pepper to taste

Directions:
1. Heat up a pan with some olive oil over medium heat, add onion and garlic, stir and cook for 2 minutes.
2. Add bell pepper, stir and cook for 3 minutes.
3. Add calamari tentacles, stir and cook for 6

minutes more.
4. Add kale, a pinch of sea salt and black pepper, stir, cook for a couple more minutes and take off heat.
5. Stuff calamari tubes with this mix and secure with toothpicks.
6. Heat up a pan with some olive oil over medium-high heat, add calamari, brown them for 2 minutes on each side and then mix with tomato puree.
7. Also add parsley, oregano and some black pepper to the pan, stir gently, cover, reduce heat to medium-low and simmer for 40 minutes.
8. Divide stuffed calamari on plates and serve.
9. Enjoy!

Nutrition: calories 637, fat 23,7, fiber 6,3, carbs 57,9, protein 42,9

289. Salmon and Chives

Preparation time: 10 minutes
Cooking time: 12 minutes
Servings: 4

Ingredients:
- 2 tablespoons dill, chopped
- 4 salmon fillets, boneless
- 2 tablespoons chives, chopped
- 1/3 cup maple syrup
- A drizzle of olive oil
- 3 tablespoons balsamic vinegar
- A pinch of sea salt
- Black pepper to taste
- Lime wedges for serving

Directions:
1. Heat up a pan with the oil over medium-high heat, add fish fillets, season them with a pinch of sea salt and black pepper, cook for 3 minutes, cover pan and cook for 6 minutes more.
2. Add balsamic vinegar and maple syrup and cook for 3 minutes basting fish with this mix.
3. Add dill and chives, cook for 1 minute, divide the fish between plates and serve with lime wedges on the side.
4. Enjoy!

Nutrition: calories 346, fat 14,7, fiber 0,7, carbs 20,4, protein 35

290. Shrimp Salsa

Preparation time: 10 minutes
Cooking time: 0 minutes
Servings: 4

Ingredients:
- 1 pound shrimp, peeled, deveined, and cooked
- 1 cup kalamata olives, pitted and sliced
- 1 cup cherry tomatoes, cubed
- ½ cup basil, chopped
- A pinch of salt and black pepper
- 2 tablespoons lime juice
- 2 teaspoons chili powder

Directions:
1. In a bowl, combine the shrimp with the kalamata, tomatoes and the other ingredients, toss well, divide into smaller bowls and serve.

Nutrition: calories 186, fat 5.8, fiber 2.1, carbs 6.4, protein 26.8

291. Salmon Bites

Preparation time: 10 minutes
Cooking time: 14 minutes
Servings: 4

Ingredients:
- 1 pound salmon fillets, boneless and cubed
- 2 tablespoons olive oil
- 1 teaspoon Italian seasoning
- 1 teaspoon garlic, minced
- ½ cup kalamata olives, pitted and chopped
- ¼ cup basil, chopped
- Salt and black pepper to the taste

Directions:
1. In a bowl, combine the salmon with the oil, the Italian seasoning and the other ingredients, toss, arrange on a baking

sheet lined with parchment paper and cook at 400 degrees F for 14 minutes.
2. Divide the salmon into bowls and serve.

Nutrition: calories 270, fat 7.5, fiber 2, carbs 7, protein 7

292. Avocado Salsa

Preparation time: 10 minutes
Cooking time: 0 minutes
Servings: 4

Ingredients:

- 2 avocados, peeled, pitted and roughly cubed
- 2 tablespoons olive oil
- 1 cup kalamata olives, pitted and halved
- ½ cup cherry tomatoes, cubed
- Juice of 1 lime
- Salt and black pepper to the taste
- 1 tablespoon basil, chopped

Directions:

1. In a bowl, combine the avocados with the lime juice and the other ingredients, toss, divide into small bowls and serve as a snack.

Nutrition: calories 180, fat 3, fiber 5, carbs 8, protein 6

293. Mussels and Shrimp Bowls

Preparation time: 5 minutes
Cooking time: 10 minutes
Servings: 4

Ingredients:

- 1 pound mussels, debearded and scrubbed
- ½ pound shrimp, peeled and deveined
- 4 scallions, chopped
- 2 garlic cloves, minced
- 1 tablespoon olive oil
- 1 tablespoon lemon juice

Directions:

1. Heat up a pan with the oil over medium heat, add the scallions and the garlic and sauté for 2 minutes.
2. Add the rest of the ingredients, toss, cook over medium heat for 8 minutes more, divide into bowls and serve.

Nutrition: calories 90, fat 4, fiber 5, carbs 5, protein 2

294. Calamari Bowls

Preparation time: 10 minutes
Cooking time: 20 minutes
Servings: 4

Ingredients:

- 1 pound calamari rings
- 2 tablespoons olive oil
- ½ cup chicken stock
- A pinch of cayenne pepper
- A pinch of salt and black pepper
- 1 tablespoons lemon juice
- 1 teaspoon chili powder
- 1 teaspoon cumin, ground
- 1 tablespoon chives, chopped

Directions:

1. Heat up a pan with the oil over medium heat, add the calamari, the stock and the other ingredients, toss, cook for 20 minutes, divide into small bowls and serve.

Nutrition: calories 155, fat 8, fiber 3, carbs 3, protein 7

295. Seafood Platter

Preparation time: 10 minutes
Cooking time: 12 minutes
Servings: 4

Ingredients:

- 1 cup calamari rings
- 1 cup clams, scrubbed
- 1 pound shrimp, peeled and deveined
- 1 tablespoon avocado oil
- 1 teaspoon lemon juice
- ½ teaspoon rosemary, dried
- 1 teaspoon chili powder
- ½ cup chicken stock
- Salt and black pepper to the taste

- ½ teaspoon turmeric powder

Directions:
1. Heat up a pan with the oil over medium heat, add the shrimp, the calamari rings, the clams and the other ingredients, toss, cook for 12 minutes, arrange on a platter and serve.

Nutrition: calories 238, fat 8, fiber 3, carbs 10, protein 8

296. Celery Dip

Preparation time: 10 minutes
Cooking time: 15 minutes
Servings: 4

Ingredients:
- 4 celery stalks
- 3 scallions, chopped
- 1 tablespoon olive oil
- 1 tablespoon lime juice
- ½ teaspoon chili powder
- 1 cup coconut cream
- Salt and black pepper to the taste
- 2 tablespoons parsley, chopped

Directions:
1. Heat up a pan with the oil over medium heat, add the scallions and sauté for 2 minutes.
2. Add the celery and the other ingredients, toss, cook over medium heat for 13 minutes more, blend using an immersion blender, divide into bowls and serve s a snack.

Nutrition: calories 140, fat 10, fiber 3, carbs 6, protein 13

297. Creamy Shrimp Bowls

Preparation time: 5 minutes
Cooking time: 10 minutes
Servings: 4

Ingredients:
- 1 pound shrimp, peeled and deveined
- 2 shallots, chopped
- 1 tablespoon olive oil
- Salt and black pepper to the taste
- 1 teaspoon rosemary, dried
- 2 cups coconut cream
- 1 cup cilantro, chopped

Directions:
1. Heat up a pan with the oil over medium heat, add the shallots and sauté for 2 minutes.
2. Add the shrimp and the other ingredients, toss, cook over medium heat for 8 minutes, divide into bowls and serve.

Nutrition: calories 220, fat 8, fiber 0, carbs 5, protein 12

298. Herbed Fennel Salsa

Preparation time: 10 minutes
Cooking time: 0 minutes
Servings: 4

Ingredients:
- 2 tablespoons olive oil
- 2 fennel bulbs, shredded
- 1 cup kalamata olives, pitted and halved
- 1 tablespoon balsamic vinegar
- A pinch of salt and black pepper
- 2 tablespoons lime juice
- 2 tablespoons parsley, chopped
- 2 tablespoons mint, chopped

Directions:
1. In a bowl, mix the fennel with the oil and the other ingredients, toss well, keep in the fridge for 10 minutes, divide into bowls and serve.

Nutrition: calories 160, fat 7, fiber 2, carbs 7, protein 8

299. Orange and Mango Salsa

Preparation time: 10 minutes
Cooking time: 0 minutes
Servings: 4

Ingredients:
- 2 mangoes, peeled and cubed
- 2 oranges, peeled and cut into segments
- ½ cup kalamata olives, pitted and halved

- Juice of 1 orange
- Zest of 1 orange, grated
- Juice of 1 lime
- 2 red chili peppers, chopped
- ½ teaspoon ginger, grated
- A pinch of salt and black pepper
- 1 tablespoon avocado oil
- ¼ cup cilantro, chopped

Directions:
1. In a bowl, mix the mangoes with the oranges and the other ingredients, toss, divide into smaller bowls and serve.

Nutrition: calories 170, fat 3, fiber 5.7, carbs 37.6, protein 2.5

300. Smoked Salmon Rolls

Preparation time: 10 minutes
Cooking time: 0 minutes
Servings: 4

Ingredients:
- 6 ounces smoked salmon, skinless and thinly sliced
- 1 red bell pepper, cut into strips
- 1 cucumber, cut into strips
- 2 tablespoons coconut cream

Directions:
1. Place the smoked salmon slices on a working surface, spread the coconut cream on each, divide the cucumber and the bell pepper strips on each slide, roll and serve as a snack.

Nutrition: calories 120, fat 6, fiber 6, carbs 12, protein 6

301. Hot Mussels Bowls

Preparation time: 10 minutes
Cooking time: 12 minutes
Servings: 4

Ingredients:
- 1 pound mussels, scrubbed
- 2 cups quinoa, cooked
- ½ cup chicken soup
- 1 teaspoon red pepper flakes, crushed
- 1 teaspoon hot paprika
- 2 garlic cloves, minced
- 2 tablespoons parsley, chopped
- 2 tablespoons avocado oil
- 1 yellow onion, chopped
- A pinch of salt and black pepper

Directions:
1. Heat up a pan with the oil over medium heat, add the onion and the garlic and sauté for 2 minutes.
2. Add the mussels, quinoa and the other ingredients, toss, cook over medium heat for 10 minutes more, divide into small bowls and serve.

Nutrition: calories 150, fat 3, fiber 3, carbs 6, protein 8

302. Tuna and Shrimp Bites

Preparation time: 10 minutes
Cooking time: 10 minutes
Servings: 4

Ingredients:
- 1 pound tuna fillets, boneless, skinless and cubed
- 1 pound shrimp, peeled and deveined
- 2 tablespoons olive oil
- 4 scallions, chopped
- Juice of 1 lime
- 1 teaspoon sweet paprika
- 1 teaspoon turmeric powder
- 2 tablespoons coconut aminos
- A pinch of salt and black pepper

Directions:
1. Heat up a pan with the oil over medium heat, add the scallions and sauté for 2 minutes.
2. Add the tuna bites and cook them for 2 minutes on each side.
3. Add the shrimp and the remaining ingredients, toss gently, cook everything for 4 minutes more, arrange everything on a platter and serve.

Nutrition: calories 210, fat 7, fiber 6, carbs 6, protein 7

303. Tomato and Berries Salsa

Preparation time: 10 minutes
Cooking time: 0 minutes
Servings: 4

Ingredients:

- 1 pound cherry tomatoes, cubed
- 1 cup blackberries
- ½ cup strawberries
- 2 tablespoons avocado oil
- 4 scallions, chopped
- 2 tablespoons garlic powder
- A pinch of salt and black pepper
- ½ tablespoon mint, chopped
- 1 tablespoon chives, chopped

Directions:

1. In a bowl, combine the tomatoes with the blackberries, strawberries and the other ingredients, toss, divide into small bowls and serve really cold.

Nutrition: calories 60, fat 3, fiber 2, carbs 6, protein 7

304. Tomato and Carrot Dip

Preparation time: 10 minutes
Cooking time: 12 minutes
Servings: 6

Ingredients:

- 1 pound tomatoes, chopped
- 2 carrots, grated
- 4 ounces coconut cream
- A pinch of salt and black pepper
- 1 teaspoon chili powder
- Cooking spray

Directions:

1. In a pan, combine the tomatoes with the carrots and the other ingredients, toss and cook over medium heat for 12 minutes.
2. Blend using an immersion blender, divide into small bowls and serve as a party dip.

Nutrition: calories 150, fat 4, fiber 6, carbs 14, protein 6

305. Cayenne Avocado and Shrimp Mix

Preparation time: 10 minutes
Cooking time: 0 minutes
Servings: 2

Ingredients:

- 2 avocados, halved, pitted and cubed
- ½ pound shrimp, cooked, peeled and deveined
- A pinch of salt and black pepper
- 1 tablespoon lemon juice
- 2 tablespoons olive oil
- 1 teaspoon cayenne pepper
- ½ teaspoon rosemary, dried
- ½ teaspoon oregano, dried
- 1 teaspoon sweet paprika

Directions:

1. In a bowl, combine the avocados with the shrimp, salt, pepper and the other ingredients, toss, divide into small bowls and serve.

Nutrition: calories 160, fat 10, fiber 7, carbs 12, protein 7

306. Radish Bites

Preparation time: 5 minutes
Cooking time: 25 minutes
Servings: 4

Ingredients:

- 1 pound radishes, cut into wedges
- 2 tablespoons olive oil
- ½ teaspoon garam masala
- ½ teaspoon oregano, dried
- ½ teaspoon basil, dried
- Salt and black pepper to the taste
- 1 tablespoon chives, chopped

Directions:

1. Spread the radishes on a baking sheet lined with parchment paper, add the oil, garam masala and the other ingredients, toss and bake at 420 degrees F for 25 minutes.
2. Divide the radish bites into bowls and serve as a snack.

Nutrition: calories 30, fat 1, fiber 2, carbs 7,

protein 1

307. Avocado and Radish Dip

Preparation time: 5 minutes
Cooking time: 0 minutes
Servings: 4

Ingredients:

- 2 avocados, pitted, peeled and chopped
- 1 cup radishes, chopped
- 1 cup coconut cream
- 4 spring onions, chopped
- 1 tablespoon lemon juice
- A pinch of salt and black pepper
- 1 tablespoon avocado oil

Directions:

1. In a blender, combine the avocados with the radishes and the other ingredients, pulse well, divide into bowls and serve as a party dip.

Nutrition: calories 162, fat 8, fiber 4, carbs 6, protein 6

308. Orange and Olives Salsa

Preparation time: 10 minutes
Cooking time: 0 minutes
Servings: 6

Ingredients:

- 1 teaspoon cumin seeds
- 1 tablespoon avocado oil
- 2 oranges, peeled and cut into segments
- 1 cup kalamata olives, pitted and halved
- 1 tablespoon oregano, chopped
- 1 tablespoon chives, chopped
- 1 tablespoon balsamic vinegar
- ½ tablespoon ginger, grated
- ½ teaspoon fennel seeds

Directions:

1. In a bowl, combine the oranges with the olives, cumin and the other ingredients, toss, keep in the fridge for 10 minutes, divide into small bowls and serve.

Nutrition: calories 120, fat 1, fiber 3, carbs 5, protein 9

309. Peppers and Radishes Salsa

Preparation time: 5 minutes
Cooking time: 0 minutes
Servings: 4

Ingredients:

- 1 tablespoon olive oil
- 2 red bell peppers, cut into thin strips
- 2 green bell peppers, cut into strips
- 1 cup radishes, cubed
- 2 tablespoons balsamic vinegar
- 1 tablespoon ginger, grated
- 1 teaspoon chili powder
- 1 tablespoon lemon juice
- A pinch of salt and black pepper
- 1 tablespoon basil, chopped

Directions:

1. In a bowl, combine the bell peppers with the radishes, the oil and the other ingredients, toss, divide into small bowls and serve as a party salsa.

Nutrition: calories 107, fat 4, fiber 2, carbs 6, protein 6

310. Beans Spread

Preparation time: 10 minutes
Cooking time: 20 minutes
Servings: 6

Ingredients:

- 2 cups canned red kidney beans, drained
- 2 tablespoons olive oil
- 1 yellow onion, chopped
- ½ cup chicken stock
- ½ cup coconut cream
- ¼ teaspoon oregano, dried
- ¼ teaspoon garlic powder
- ¼ teaspoon onion powder
- Salt and black pepper to the taste
- 1 tablespoon chives, chopped

Directions:

1. Heat up a pan with the oil over medium heat, add the onion and sauté for 5 minutes.
2. Add the stock, oregano and the other

ingredients except the cream and the chives, stir, and cook over medium heat for 15 minutes more.
3. Add the cream, blend the mix using an immersion blender, divide into bowls and serve with the chives sprinkled on top.

Nutrition: calories 302, fat 10.2, fiber 10.2, carbs 40.7, protein 14.6

311. Mint Avocado and Tomato Dip

Preparation time: 10 minutes
Cooking time: 0 minutes
Servings: 4

Ingredients:
- 2 avocados, pitted, peeled and chopped
- 1 cup cherry tomatoes, chopped
- 1 tablespoon lemon juice
- 2 tablespoons coconut oil
- 1 teaspoon chili powder
- ½ cup mint, chopped
- A pinch of salt and black pepper

Directions:
1. In a blender, mix the tomatoes with the avocado and the other ingredients, pulse well, divide into small bowls and serve as a party dip.

Nutrition: calories 150, fat 7, fiber 6, carbs 8.8, protein 6

312. Shrimp, Watermelon and Berries Mix

Preparation time: 10 minutes
Cooking time: 0 minutes
Servings: 4

Ingredients:
- 2 tablespoons avocado oil
- 4 scallions, chopped
- 1 pound shrimp, cooked, deveined and peeled
- 1 cup watermelon, peeled and cubed
- ½ cup strawberries
- 2 tablespoons lemon juice
- A pinch of cayenne pepper
- 1 tablespoon balsamic vinegar

Directions:
1. In a bowl, combine the shrimp with the watermelon, scallions and the other ingredients, toss, divide into smaller bowls and serve.

Nutrition: calories 205, fat 12, fiber 2, carbs 9, protein 8

313. Berries Dip

Preparation time: 10 minutes
Cooking time: 0 minutes
Servings: 4

Ingredients:
- 1 avocado, pitted, peeled and chopped
- 1 red chili pepper, minced
- 1 cup blackberries
- ½ cup blueberries
- A pinch of cayenne pepper
- 2 tablespoons lemon juice

Directions:
1. In a blender, combine the avocado with the berries and the other ingredients, pulse well, divide into small bowls and serve as a party dip.

Nutrition: calories 120, fat 2, fiber 2, carbs 7, protein 4

314. Cilantro Squares

Preparation time: 5 minutes
Cooking time: 25 minutes
Servings: 4

Ingredients:
- 1 cup coconut flour
- A pinch of salt and black pepper
- 1 cup cilantro, chopped
- 1 teaspoon lemon zest, grated
- 1 tablespoon lemon juice
- 2 eggs, whisked
- ½ teaspoon baking powder

Directions:
1. In a bowl, mix the flour with the eggs and

the other ingredients, and stir well.
2. Spread the mix on a baking sheet lined with parchment paper, cut into triangles and cook at 380 degrees F for 25 minutes.
3. Cool the squares down and serve them as a snack.

Nutrition: calories 49, fat 2.7, fiber 1.4, carbs 2.8, protein 3.4

315. Spicy Baked Shrimp

Serving: 4
Preparation Time: 10 minutes
Cook Time: 25 minutes + 2-4 hours

Ingredients:

- ½ ounce large shrimp, peeled and deveined
- Cooking spray as needed
- 1 teaspoon low sodium coconut aminos
- 1 teaspoon parsley
- ½ teaspoon olive oil
- ½ tablespoon honey
- 1 tablespoon lemon juice

Directions:

1. Pre-heat your oven to 450 degrees F.
2. Take a baking dish and grease it well.
3. Mix in all the ingredients and toss.
4. Transfer to oven and bake for 8 minutes until shrimp turns pink.
5. Serve and enjoy!

Nutrition:
Calories: 321
Fat: 9g
Carbohydrates: 44g
Protein: 22g

316. Shrimp and Cilantro Meal

Serving: 4
Preparation Time: 10 minutes
Cook Time: 5 minutes
SmartPoints: 0

Ingredients:

- 1 ¾ pounds shrimp, deveined and peeled
- 2 tablespoons fresh lime juice
- ¼ teaspoon cloves, minced
- ½ teaspoon ground cumin
- 1 tablespoon olive oil
- 1 ¼ cups fresh cilantro, chopped
- 1 teaspoon lime zest
- ½ teaspoon sunflower seeds
- ¼ teaspoon pepper

Direction

1. Take a large sized bowl and add shrimp, cumin, garlic, lime juice, ginger and toss well.
2. Take a large sized non-stick skillet and add oil, allow the oil to heat up over medium-high heat.
3. Add shrimp mixture and sauté for 4 minutes.
4. Remove the heat and add cilantro, lime zest, sunflower seeds, and pepper.
5. Mix well and serve hot!

Nutrition:
Calories: 177
Fat: 6g
Carbohydrates: 2g
Protein: 27g

317. The Original Dijon Fish

Serving: 2
Preparation Time: 3 minutes
Cook Time: 12 minutes
SmartPoints: 2

Ingredients:

- 1 perch, flounder or sole fish florets
- 1 tablespoon Dijon mustard
- 1 ½ teaspoons lemon juice
- 1 teaspoon low sodium Worcestershire sauce, low sodium
- 2 tablespoons Italian seasoned bread crumbs
- 1 almond butter flavored cooking spray

Directions:

1. Preheat your oven to 450 degrees F.
2. Take an 11 x 7-inch baking dish and arrange your fillets carefully.
3. Take a small sized bowl and add lemon juice, Worcestershire sauce, mustard and mix it well.

4. Pour the mix over your fillet.
5. Sprinkle a good amount of breadcrumbs.
6. Bake for 12 minutes until fish flakes off easily.
7. Cut the fillet in half portions and enjoy!

Nutrition:
Calories: 125
Fat: 2g
Carbohydrates: 6g
Protein: 21g

318. Lemony Garlic Shrimp

Serving: 4
Preparation Time: 5-10 minutes
Cook Time: 10-15 minutes

Ingredients:

- 1 ¼ pounds shrimp, boiled or steamed
- 3 tablespoons garlic, minced
- ¼ cup lemon juice
- 2 tablespoons olive oil
- ¼ cup parsley

Directions:

1. Take a small skillet and place over medium heat, add garlic and oil and stir-cook for 1 minute.
2. Add parsley, lemon juice and season with sunflower seeds and pepper accordingly.
3. Add shrimp in a large bowl and transfer the mixture from the skillet over the shrimp.
4. Chill and serve.
5. Enjoy!

Nutrition:
Calories: 130
Fat: 3g
Carbohydrates: 2g
Protein: 22g

319. Baked Zucchini Wrapped Fish

Serving: 2
Preparation Time: 15 minutes
Cook Time: 15 minutes
SmartPoints: 0

Ingredients:

- 24-ounce cod fillets, skin removed
- 1 tablespoon of blackening spices
- 2 zucchini, sliced lengthwise to form ribbon
- ½ tablespoon of olive oil

Directions:

1. Season the fish fillets with blackening spice.
2. Wrap each fish fillet with zucchini ribbons.
3. Place fish on a plate.
4. Take a skillet and place over medium heat.
5. Pour oil and allow the oil to heat up.
6. Add wrapped fish to the skillet and cook each side for 4 minutes.
7. Serve and enjoy!

Nutrition:
Calories: 397
Fat: 23g
Carbohydrates: 2g
Protein: 46g

320. Heart-Warming Medi Tilapia

Serving: 4
Preparation Time: 15 minutes
Cook Time: 15 minute

Ingredients:

- 3 tablespoons sun-dried tomatoes, packed in oil, drained and chopped
- 1 tablespoon capers, drained
- 2 tilapia fillets
- 1 tablespoon oil from sun-dried tomatoes
- 2 tablespoons kalamata olives, chopped and pitted

Directions:

1. Pre-heat your oven to 372 degrees F.
2. Take a small sized bowl and add sun-dried tomatoes, olives, capers and stir well.
3. Keep the mixture on the side.
4. Take a baking sheet and transfer the tilapia fillets and arrange them side by side.
5. Drizzle olive oil all over them.
6. Bake in your oven for 10-15 minutes.

7. After 10 minutes, check the fish for a "Flaky" texture.
8. Once cooked, top the fish with the tomato mixture and serve!

Nutrition:
Calories: 183
Fat: 8g
Carbohydrates: 18g
Protein:83g

321. Baked Salmon and Orange Juice

Serving: 2
Preparation Time: 10 minutes
Cook Time: 10 minutes

Ingredients:

- ½ pound salmon steak
- Juice of 1 orange
- Pinch ginger powder, black pepper, and sunflower seeds
- Juice of ½ lemon
- 1-ounce coconut almond milk

Directions:

1. Preheat oven to 350 degrees F.
2. Rub salmon steak with spices and let it sit for 15 minutes.
3. Take a bowl and squeeze an orange.
4. Squeeze lemon juice as well and mix.
5. Pour almond milk into the mixture and stir.
6. Take a baking dish and line with aluminum foil.
7. Place steak on it and pour the sauce over steak.
8. Cover with another sheet and bake for 10 minutes.
9. Serve and enjoy!

Nutrition:
Calories: 300
Fat: 3g
Carbohydrates: 1g
Protein: 7g

322. Lemon and Almond butter Cod

Serving: 2
Preparation Time: 5 minutes
Cook Time: 20 minutes

Ingredients:

- 4 tablespoons almond butter, divided
- 4 thyme sprigs, fresh and divided
- 4 teaspoons lemon juice, fresh and divided
- 4 cod fillets, 6 ounces each
- Sunflower seeds to taste

Directions:

1. Pre-heat your oven to 400 degrees F.
2. Season cod fillets with sunflower seeds on both sides.
3. Take four pieces of foil, each foil should be 3 times bigger than the fillets.
4. Divide fillets between the foil and top with almond butter, lemon juice, thyme.
5. Fold to form a pouch and transfer pouches to the baking sheet.
6. Bake for 20 minutes.
7. Open and let the steam out.
8. Serve and enjoy!

Nutrition:
Calories: 284
Fat: 18g
Carbohydrates: 2g
Protein: 32g

323. Shrimp Scampi

Serving: 4
Preparation Time: 25 minutes
Cook Time: Nil
SmartPoints: 1

Ingredients:

- 4 teaspoons olive oil
- 1 ¼ pounds medium shrimp
- 6-8 garlic cloves, minced
- ½ cup low sodium chicken broth
- ½ cup dry white wine
- ¼ cup fresh lemon juice
- ¼ cup fresh parsley + 1 tablespoon extra, minced
- ¼ teaspoon sunflower seeds
- ¼ teaspoon fresh ground pepper
- 4 slices lemon

Directions:

1. Take a large sized bowl and place it over medium-high heat.
2. Add oil and allow the oil to heat up.
3. Add shrimp and cook for 2-3 minutes.
4. Add garlic and cook for 30 seconds.
5. Take a slotted spoon and transfer the cooked shrimp to a serving platter.
6. Add broth, lemon juice, wine, ¼ cup of parsley, pepper, and sunflower seeds to the skillet.
7. Bring the whole mix to a boil.
8. Keep boiling until the sauce has been reduced to half.
9. Spoon the sauce over the cooked shrimp.
10. Garnish with parsley and lemon.
11. Serve and enjoy!

Nutrition:
Calories: 184
Fat: 6g
Carbohydrates: 6g
Protein: 15g

324. Lemon and Garlic Scallops

Serving: 4
Preparation Time: 10 minutes
Cook Time: 5 minutes
SmartPoints: 2

Ingredients:

- 1 tablespoon olive oil
- 1 ¼ pounds dried scallops
- 2 tablespoons all-purpose flour
- ¼ teaspoon sunflower seeds
- 4-5 garlic cloves, minced
- 1 scallion, chopped
- 1 pinch of ground sage
- 1 lemon juice
- 2 tablespoons parsley, chopped

Direction

1. Take a non-stick skillet and place over medium-high heat.
2. Add oil and allow the oil to heat up.
3. Take a medium sized bowl and add scallops alongside sunflower seeds and flour.
4. Place the scallops in the skillet and add scallions, garlic, and sage.
5. Sauté for 3-4 minutes until they show an opaque texture.
6. Stir in lemon juice and parsley.
7. Remove heat and serve hot!

Nutrition:
Calories: 151
Fat: 4g
Carbohydrates: 10g
Protein: 18g

325. Walnut Encrusted Salmon

Serving: 34
Preparation Time: 10 minutes
Cook Time: 14 minutes

Ingredients:

- ½ cup walnuts
- 2 tablespoons stevia
- ½ tablespoon Dijon mustard
- ¼ teaspoon dill
- 2 salmon fillets (3 ounces each
- 1 tablespoon olive oil
- Sunflower seeds and pepper to taste

Directions:

1. Pre-heat your oven to 350 degrees F.
2. Add walnuts, mustard, stevia to food processor and process until your desired consistency is achieved.
3. Take a frying pan and place it over medium heat.
4. Add oil and let it heat up.
5. Add salmon and sear for 3 minutes.
6. Add walnut mix and coat well.
7. Transfer coated salmon to baking sheet, bake in oven for 8 minutes.
8. Serve and enjoy!

Nutrition:
Calories: 373
Fat: 43g
Carbohydrates: 4g
Protein: 20g

326. Roasted Lemon Swordfish

Serving: 4
Preparation Time: 10 minutes
Cook Time: 70-80 minutes

Ingredients:

- ¼ cup parsley, chopped
- ½ teaspoon garlic, chopped
- ½ teaspoon canola oil
- 4 swordfish fillets, 6 ounces each
- ¼ teaspoon sunflower seeds
- 1 tablespoon sugar
- 2 lemons, quartered and seeds removed

Directions:

1. Preheat your oven to 375 degrees F.
2. Take a small-sized bowl and add sugar, sunflower seeds, lemon wedges.
3. Toss well to coat them.
4. Take a shallow baking dish and add lemons, cover with aluminum foil.
5. Roast for about 60 minutes until lemons are tender and browned (Slightly.
6. Heat your grill and place the rack about 4 inches away from the source of heat.
7. Take a baking pan and coat it with cooking spray.
8. Transfer fish fillets to the pan and brush with oil on top spread garlic on top.
9. Grill for about 5 minutes each side until fillet turns opaque.
10. Transfer fish to a serving platter, squeeze roasted lemon on top.
11. Sprinkle parsley, serve with a lemon wedge on the side.
12. Enjoy!

Nutrition:
Calories: 280
Fat: 12g
Net Carbohydrates: 4g
Protein: 34g

327. Especial Glazed Salmon

Serving: 4
Preparation Time: 45 minutes
Cook Time: 10 minutes

Ingredients:

- 4 pieces salmon fillets, 5 ounces each
- 4 tablespoons coconut aminos
- 4 teaspoon olive oil
- 2 teaspoons ginger, minced
- 4 teaspoons garlic, minced
- 2 tablespoons sugar-free ketchup
- 4 tablespoons dry white wine
- 2 tablespoons red boat fish sauce, low sodium

Directions:

1. Take a bowl and mix in coconut aminos, garlic, ginger, fish sauce and mix.
2. Add salmon and let it marinate for 15-20 minutes.
3. Take a skillet/pan and place it over medium heat.
4. Add oil and let it heat up.
5. Add salmon fillets and cook on high heat for 3-4 minutes per side.
6. Remove dish once crispy.
7. Add sauce and wine.
8. Simmer for 5 minutes on low heat.
9. Return salmon to the glaze and flip until both sides are glazed.
10. Serve and enjoy!

Nutrition:
Calories: 372
Fat: 24g
Carbohydrates: 3g
Protein: 35g

328. Generous Stuffed Salmon Avocado

Serving: 2
Preparation Time: 10 minutes
Cook Time: 30 minutes

Ingredients:

- 1 ripe organic avocado
- 2 ounces wild caught smoked salmon
- 1 ounce cashew cheese
- 2 tablespoons extra virgin olive oil
- Sunflower seeds as needed

Directions:

1. Cut avocado in half and deseed.
2. Add the rest of the ingredients to a food processor and process until coarsely chopped.
3. Place mixture into avocado.
4. Serve and enjoy!

Nutrition:

Calories: 525
Fat: 48g
Carbohydrates: 4g
Protein: 19g

329. Spanish Mussels

Serving: 4
Preparation Time: 10 minutes
Cook Time: 23 minutes

Ingredients:

- 3 tablespoons olive oil
- 2 pounds mussels, scrubbed
- Pepper to taste
- 3 cups canned tomatoes, crushed
- 1 shallot, chopped
- 2 garlic cloves, minced
- 2 cups low sodium vegetable stock
- 1/3 cup cilantro, chopped

Directions:

1. Take a pan and place it over medium-high heat, add shallot and stir-cook for 3 minutes.
2. Add garlic, stock, tomatoes, pepper, stir and reduce heat, simmer for 10 minutes.
3. Add mussels, cilantro, and toss.
4. Cover and cook for 10 minutes more.
5. Serve and enjoy!

Nutrition:

Calories: 210
Fat: 2g
Carbohydrates: 5g
Protein: 8g

330. Tilapia Broccoli Platter

[MOU9]
Serving: 2
Preparation Time: 4 minutes
Cook Time: 14 minutes

Ingredients:

- 6 ounce tilapia, frozen
- 1 tablespoon almond butter
- 1 tablespoon garlic, minced
- 1 teaspoon lemon pepper seasoning
- 1 cup broccoli florets, fresh

Directions:

1. Pre-heat your oven to 350 degrees F.
2. Add fish in aluminum foil packets.
3. Arrange broccoli around fish.
4. Sprinkle lemon pepper on top.
5. Close the packets and seal.
6. Bake for 14 minutes.
7. Take a bowl and add garlic and almond butter, mix well and keep the mixture on the side.
8. Remove the packet from oven and transfer to platter.
9. Place almond butter on top of the fish and broccoli, serve and enjoy!

Nutrition:

Calories: 362
Fat: 25g
Carbohydrates: 2g
Protein: 29g

331. Salmon with Peas and Parsley Dressing

Serving: 4
Preparation Time: 15 minutes
Cook Time: 15 minutes

Ingredients:

- 16 ounces salmon fillets, boneless and skin-on
- 1 tablespoon parsley, chopped
- 10 ounces peas
- 9 ounces vegetable stock, low sodium
- 2 cups water
- ½ teaspoon oregano, dried
- ½ teaspoon sweet paprika
- 2 garlic cloves, minced
- A pinch of black pepper

Directions:

1. Add garlic, parsley, paprika, oregano and stock to a food processor and blend.
2. Add water to your Instant Pot.
3. Add steam basket.
4. Add fish fillets inside the steamer basket.
5. Season with pepper.
6. Lock the lid and cook on HIGH pressure for 10 minutes.

7. Release the pressure naturally over 10 minutes .
8. Divide the fish amongst plates.
9. Add peas to the steamer basket and lock the lid again, cook on HIGH pressure for 5 minutes.
10. Quick release the pressure.
11. Divide the peas next to your fillets and serve with the parsley dressing drizzled on top
12. Enjoy!

Nutrition:
Calories: 315
Fat: 5g
Carbohydrates: 14g
Protein: 16g

332. Mackerel and Orange Medley

Serving: 4
Preparation Time: 10 minutes
Cook Time: 10 minutes

Ingredients:
- 4 mackerel fillets, skinless and boneless
- 4 spring onion, chopped
- 1 teaspoon olive oil
- 1-inch ginger piece, grated
- Black pepper as needed
- Juice and zest of 1 whole orange
- 1 cup low sodium fish stock

Directions:
1. Season the fillets with black pepper and rub olive oil.
2. Add stock, orange juice, ginger, orange zest and onion to Instant Pot.
3. Place a steamer basket and add the fillets.
4. Lock the lid and cook on HIGH pressure for 10 minutes.
5. Release the pressure naturally over 10 minutes.
6. Divide the fillets amongst plates and drizzle the orange sauce from the pot over the fish.
7. Enjoy!

Nutrition:
Calories: 200
Fat: 4g
Carbohydrates: 19g
Protein: 14g

333. Spicy Chili Salmon

Serving: 4
Preparation Time: 10 minutes
Cook Time: 7 minutes

Ingredients:
- 4 salmon fillets, boneless and skin-on
- 2 tablespoons assorted chili peppers, chopped
- Juice of 1 lemon
- 1 lemon, sliced
- 1 cup water
- Black pepper

Directions:
1. Add water to the Instant Pot.
2. Add steamer basket and add salmon fillets, season the fillets with salt and pepper.
3. Drizzle lemon juice on top.
4. Top with lemon slices.
5. Lock the lid and cook on HIGH pressure for 7 minutes.
6. Release the pressure naturally over 10 minutes.
7. Divide the salmon and lemon slices between serving plates.
8. Enjoy!

Nutrition:
Calories: 281
Fats: 8g
Carbs: 19g
Protein:7g

334. Simple One Pot Mussels

Serving: 4
Preparation Time: 10 minutes
Cook Time: 5 minutes

Ingredients:
- 2 tablespoons butter
- 2 chopped shallots
- 4 minced garlic cloves
- ½ cup broth

- ½ cup white wine
- 2 pounds cleaned mussels
- Lemon and parsley for serving

Directions:
1. Clean the mussels and remove the beard.
2. Discard any mussels that do not close when tapped against a hard surface.
3. Set your pot to Sauté mode and add chopped onion and butter.
4. Stir and sauté onions.
5. Add garlic and cook for 1 minute.
6. Add broth and wine.
7. Lock the lid and cook for 5 minutes on HIGH pressure.
8. Release the pressure naturally over 10 minutes.
9. Serve with a sprinkle of parsley and enjoy!

Nutrition:
Calories: 286
Fats: 14g
Carbs: 12g
Protein: 28g

335. Lemon Pepper and Salmon

Serving: 3
Preparation Time: 5 minute
Cook Time: 6 minutes

Ingredients:
- ¾ cup water
- Few sprigs of parsley, basil, tarragon, basil
- 1 pound of salmon, skin on
- 3 teaspoons ghee
- ¼ teaspoon salt
- ½ teaspoon pepper
- ½ lemon, thinly sliced
- 1 whole carrot, julienned

Directions:
1. Set your pot to Sauté mode and water and herbs.
2. Place a steamer rack inside your pot and place salmon.
3. Drizzle the ghee on top of the salmon and season with salt and pepper.
4. Cover lemon slices.
5. Lock the lid and cook on HIGH pressure for 3 minutes.
6. Release the pressure naturally over 10 minutes.
7. Transfer the salmon to a serving platter.
8. Set your pot to Sauté mode and add vegetables.
9. Cook for 1-2 minutes.
10. Serve with vegetables and salmon.
11. Enjoy!

Nutrition:
Calories: 464
Fat: 34g
Carbohydrates: 3g
Protein: 34g

336. Simple Sautéed Garlic and Parsley Scallops

Serving: 4
Preparation Time: 5 minutes
Cook Time: 25 minutes

Ingredients:
- 8 tablespoons almond butter
- 2 garlic cloves, minced
- 16 large sea scallops
- Sunflower seeds and pepper to taste
- 1 ½ tablespoons olive oil

Directions:
1. Seasons scallops with sunflower seeds and pepper.
2. Take a skillet, place it over medium heat, add oil and let it heat up.
3. Sauté scallops for 2 minutes per side, repeat until all scallops are cooked.
4. Add almond butter to the skillet and let it melt.
5. Stir in garlic and cook for 15 minutes.
6. Return scallops to skillet and stir to coat.
7. Serve and enjoy!

Nutrition:
Calories: 417
Fat: 31g
Net Carbohydrates: 5g
Protein: 29g

337. Salmon and Cucumber Platter

Serving: 4
Preparation Time: 10 minutes
Cook Time: nil

Ingredients:

- 2 cucumbers, cubed
- 2 teaspoons fresh squeezed lemon juice
- 4 ounces non-fat yogurt
- 1 teaspoon lemon zest, grated
- Pepper to taste
- 2 teaspoons dill, chopped
- 8 ounces smoked salmon, flaked

Directions:

1. Take a bowl and add cucumbers, lemon juice, lemon zest, pepper, dill, salmon, yogurt and toss well.
2. Serve cold.
3. Enjoy!

Nutrition:

Calories: 242
Fat: 3g
Carbohydrates: 3g
Protein: 3g

338. Tuna Paté

Serving: 4
Preparation Time: 10 minutes
Cook Time: nil

Ingredients:

- 6 ounces canned tuna, drained and flaked
- 3 teaspoons fresh lemon juice
- 1 teaspoon onion, minced
- 8 ounces low-fat cream cheese
- ¼ cup parsley, chopped

Directions:

1. Take a bowl and mix in tuna, cream cheese, lemon juice, parsley, onion and stir well.
2. Serve cold and enjoy!

Nutrition:

Calories: 172
Fat: 2g
Carbohydrates: 8g
Protein: 4g

339. Cinnamon Salmon

Serving: 4
Preparation Time: 10 minutes
Cook Time: 10 minutes

Ingredients:

- 2 salmon fillets, boneless and skin on
- Pepper to taste
- 1 tablespoon cinnamon powder
- 1 tablespoon organic olive oil

Directions:

1. Take a pan and place it over medium heat, add oil and let it heat up.
2. Add pepper, cinnamon and stir.
3. Add salmon, skin side up and cook for 5 minutes on both sides.
4. Divide between plates and serve.
5. Enjoy!

Nutrition:

Calories: 220
Fat: 8g
Carbohydrates: 11g
Protein: 8g

340. Scallop and Strawberry Mix

Serving: 4
Preparation Time: 10 minutes
Cook Time: 6 minutes

Ingredients:

- 4 ounces scallops
- ½ cup Pico De Gallo
- ½ cup strawberries, chopped
- 1 tablespoon lime juice
- Pepper to taste

Directions:

1. Take a pan and place it over medium heat, add scallops and cook for 3 minutes on both sides.
2. Remove heat.
3. Take a bowl and add strawberries, lime juice, Pico De Gallo, scallops, pepper and toss well.
4. Serve and enjoy!

Nutrition:

Calories: 169
Fat: 2g
Carbohydrates: 8g
Protein: 13g

341. Salmon and Orange Dish

Serving: 4
Preparation Time: 10 minute
Cook Time: 15 minutes

Ingredients:

- 4 salmon fillets
- 1 cup orange juice
- 2 tablespoons arrowroot and water mixture
- 1 teaspoon orange peel, grated
- 1 teaspoon black pepper

Directions:

1. Add the listed ingredients to your pot.
2. Lock the lid and cook on HIGH pressure for 12 minutes.
3. Release the pressure naturally.
4. Serve and enjoy!

Nutrition:

Calories: 583
Fat: 20g
Carbohydrates: 71g
Protein: 33g

342. Mesmerizing Coconut Haddock

Serving: 3
Preparation Time: 10 minutes
Cook Time: 12 minutes

Ingredients:

- 4 haddock fillets, 5 ounces each, boneless
- 2 tablespoons coconut oil, melted
- 1 cup coconut, shredded and unsweetened
- ¼ cup hazelnuts, ground
- Sunflower seeds to taste

Directions:

1. Pre-heat your oven to 400 degrees F.
2. Line a baking sheet with parchment paper.
3. Keep it on the side.
4. Pat fish fillets with paper towel and season with sunflower seeds.
5. Take a bowl and stir in hazelnuts and shredded coconut.
6. Drag fish fillets through the coconut mix until both sides are coated well.
7. Transfer to baking dish.
8. Brush with coconut oil.
9. Bake for about 12 minutes until flaky.
10. Serve and enjoy!

Nutrition:

Calories: 299
Fat: 24g
Carbohydrates: 1g
Protein: 20g

343. Asparagus and Lemon Salmon Dish

Serving: 3
Preparation Time: 5 minutes
Cook Time: 15 minutes

Ingredients:

- 2 salmon fillets, 6 ounces each, skin on
- Sunflower seeds to taste
- 1 pound asparagus, trimmed
- 2 cloves garlic, minced
- 3 tablespoons almond butter
- ¼ cup cashew cheese

Directions:

1. Pre-heat your oven to 400 degrees F.
2. Line a baking sheet with oil.
3. Take a kitchen towel and pat your salmon dry, season as needed.
4. Put salmon onto the baking sheet and arrange asparagus around it.
5. Place a pan over medium heat and melt almond butter.
6. Add garlic and cook for 3 minutes until garlic browns slightly.
7. Drizzle sauce over salmon.
8. Sprinkle salmon with cheese and bake for 12 minutes until salmon looks cooked all the way and is flaky.
9. Serve and enjoy!

Nutrition:

Calories: 434
Fat: 26g

Carbohydrates: 6g
Protein: 42g

344. Ecstatic "Foiled" Fish

Serving: 4
Preparation Time: 20 minutes
Cook Time: 40 minutes

Ingredients:

- 2 rainbow trout fillets
- 1 tablespoon olive oil
- 2 teaspoon garlic salt
- 1 teaspoon ground black pepper
- 1 fresh jalapeno pepper, sliced
- 1 lemon, sliced

Directions:

1. Pre-heat your oven to 400 degrees F.
2. Rinse your fish and pat them dry.
3. Rub the fillets with olive oil, season with some garlic salt and black pepper.
4. Place each of your seasoned fillets on a large sized sheet of aluminum foil.
5. Top it with some jalapeno slices and squeeze the juice from your lemons over your fish.
6. Arrange the lemon slices on top of your fillets.
7. Carefully seal up the edges of your foil and form a nice enclosed packet.
8. Place your packets on your baking sheet.
9. Bake them for about 20 minutes.
10. Once the flakes start to flake off with a fork, the fish is ready!

Nutrition:
Calories: 213
Fat: 10g
Carbohydrates: 8g
Protein: 24g

345. Brazilian Shrimp Stew

Serving: 4
Preparation Time: 20 minutes
Cook Time: 25 minutes

Ingredients:

- 4 tablespoons lime juice
- 1 ½ tablespoons cumin, ground
- 1 ½ tablespoons paprika
- 2 ½ teaspoons garlic, minced
- 1 ½ teaspoons pepper
- 2 pounds tilapia fillets, cut into bits
- 1 large onion, chopped
- 3 large bell peppers, cut into strips
- 1 can (14 ounces tomato, drained
- 1 can (14 ounces coconut milk
- Handful of cilantro, chopped

Directions:

1. Take a large sized bowl and add lime juice, cumin, paprika, garlic, pepper and mix well.
2. Add tilapia and coat it up.
3. Cover and allow to marinate for 20 minutes.
4. Set your Instant Pot to Saute mode(HIGH [MOU10][F11]and add olive oil.
5. Add onions and cook for 3 minutes until tender.
6. Add pepper strips, tilapia, and tomatoes to a skillet.
7. Pour coconut milk and cover, simmer for 20 minutes.
8. Add cilantro during the final few minutes.
9. Serve and enjoy!

Nutrition:
Calories: 471
Fat: 44g
Carbohydrates: 13g
Protein: 12g

346. Inspiring Cajun Snow Crab

Serving: 2
Preparation Time: 10 minutes
Cook Time: 10 minutes

Ingredients:

- 1 lemon, fresh and quartered
- 3 tablespoons Cajun seasoning
- 2 bay leaves
- 4 snow crab legs, precooked and defrosted
- Golden ghee

Directions:

1. Take a large pot and fill it about halfway with sunflower seeds and water.
2. Bring the water to a boil.
3. Squeeze lemon juice into the pot and toss in remaining lemon quarters.
4. Add bay leaves and Cajun seasoning.
5. Season for 1 minute.
6. Add crab legs and boil for 8 minutes (make sure to keep them submerged the whole time.
7. Melt ghee in microwave and use as dipping sauce, enjoy!

Nutrition:

Calories: 643
Fat: 51g
Carbohydrates: 3g
Protein: 41g

347. Grilled Lime Shrimp

Serving: 8
Preparation Time: 25 minutes
Cook Time: 5 minutes

Ingredients:

- 1 pound medium shrimp, peeled and deveined
- 1 lime, juiced
- ½ cup olive oil
- 3 tablespoons Cajun seasoning

Directions:

1. Take a re-sealable zip bag and add lime juice, Cajun seasoning, olive oil.
2. Add shrimp and shake it well, let it marinate for 20 minutes.
3. Pre-heat your outdoor grill to medium heat.
4. Lightly grease the grate.
5. Remove shrimp from marinade and cook for 2 minutes per side.
6. Serve and enjoy!

Nutrition:

Calories: 188
Fat: 3g
Net Carbohydrates: 1.2g
Protein: 13g

348. Calamari Citrus

Serving: 4
Preparation Time: 10 minutes
Cook Time: 5 minutes

Ingredients:

- 1 lime, sliced
- 1 lemon, sliced
- 2 pounds calamari tubes and tentacles, sliced
- Pepper to taste
- ¼ cup olive oil
- 2 garlic cloves, minced
- 3 tablespoons lemon juice
- 1 orange, peeled and cut into segments
- 2 tablespoons cilantro, chopped

Directions:

1. Take a bowl and add calamari, pepper, lime slices, lemon slices, orange slices, garlic, oil, cilantro, lemon juice and toss well.
2. Take a pan and place it over medium-high heat.
3. Add calamari mix and cook for 5 minutes.
4. Divide into bowls and serve.
5. Enjoy!

Nutrition:

Calories: 190
Fat: 2g
Net Carbohydrates: 11g
Protein: 14g

349. Spiced Up Salmon

Serving: 4
Preparation Time: 10 minutes
Cook Time: 10 minutes

Ingredients:

- 4 salmon fillets
- 2 tablespoons olive oil
- 1 teaspoon cumin, ground
- 1 teaspoon sweet paprika
- 1 teaspoon chili powder
- ½ teaspoon garlic powder
- Pinch of pepper

Directions:

1. Take a bowl and add cumin, paprika, onion, chili powder, garlic powder, pepper and toss well.
2. Rub the salmon in the mixture.
3. Take a pan and place it over medium heat, add oil and let it heat up.
4. Add salmon and cook for 5 minutes, both sides.
5. Divide between plates and serve.
6. Enjoy!

Nutrition:

Calories: 220
Fat: 10g
Net Carbohydrates: 8g
Protein: 10g

350. Coconut Cream Shrimp

Serving: 4
Preparation Time: 10 minutes
Cook Time: nil

Ingredients:

- 1 pound shrimp, cooked, peeled and deveined
- 1 tablespoon coconut cream
- ¼ teaspoon jalapeno, chopped
- ½ teaspoon lime juice
- 1 tablespoon parsley, chopped
- Pinch of pepper

Directions:

1. Take a bowl and add shrimp, cream, jalapeno, lime juice, parsley, pepper.
2. Toss well and divide into small bowls.
3. Serve and enjoy!

Nutrition:

Calories: 183
Fat: 5g
Net Carbohydrates: 12g
Protein: 8g

351. Shrimp and Avocado Platter

Serving: 8
Preparation Time: 10 minutes
Cook Time: nil

Ingredients:

- 2 green onions, chopped
- 2 avocados, pitted, peeled and cut into chunks
- 2 tablespoons cilantro, chopped
- 1 cup shrimp, cooked, peeled and deveined
- Pinch of pepper

Directions:

1. Take a bowl and add cooked shrimp, avocado, green onions, cilantro, pepper.
2. Toss well and serve.
3. Enjoy!

Nutrition:

Calories: 160
Fat: 2g
Net Carbohydrates: 5g
Protein: 6g

352. Calamari

Serving: 4
Preparation Time: 10 minutes +1 hour marinating
Cook Time: 8 minutes

Ingredients:

- 2 tablespoons extra virgin olive oil
- 1 teaspoon chili powder
- ½ teaspoon ground cumin
- Zest of 1 lime
- Juice of 1 lime
- Dash of sea sunflower seeds
- 1 ½ pounds squid, cleaned and split open, with tentacles cut into ½ inch rounds
- 2 tablespoons cilantro, chopped
- 2 tablespoons red bell pepper, minced

Directions:

1. Take a medium bowl and stir in olive oil, chili powder, cumin, lime zest, sea sunflower seeds, lime juice and pepper.
2. Add squid and let it marinade and stir to coat, coat and let it refrigerate for 1 hour
3. Pre-heat your oven to broil.
4. Arrange squid on a baking sheet, broil for 8 minutes turn once until tender.
5. Garnish the broiled calamari with cilantro and red bell pepper.
6. Serve and enjoy!

Nutrition:

Calories: 159
Fat: 13g
Carbohydrates: 12g
Protein: 3g

353. Hearty Deep Fried Prawn and Rice Croquettes

Serving: 8
Preparation Time: 25 minute
Cook Time: 13 minutes

Ingredients:

- 2 tablespoons almond butter
- ½ onion, chopped
- 4 ounces shrimp, peeled and chopped
- 2 tablespoons all-purpose flour
- 1 tablespoon white wine
- ½ cup almond milk
- 2 tablespoons almond milk
- 2 cups cooked rice
- 1 tablespoon parmesan, grated
- 1 teaspoon fresh dill, chopped
- 1 teaspoon sunflower seeds
- Ground pepper as needed
- Vegetable oil for frying
- 3 tablespoons all-purpose flour
- 1 whole egg
- ½ cup breadcrumbs

Directions:

1. Take a large skillet and place it over medium heat, add almond butter and let it melt.
2. Add onion, cook and stir for 5 minutes.
3. Add shrimp and cook for 1-2 minutes.
4. Stir in 2 tablespoons flour, white wine, pour in almond milk gradually and cook for 3-5 minutes until the sauce thickens.
5. Remove white sauce from heat and stir in rice, mix evenly.
6. Add parmesan, cheese, dill, sunflower seeds, pepper and let it cool for 15 minutes.
7. Heat oil in large saucepan and bring it to 350 degrees F.
8. Take a bowl and whisk in egg, spread breadcrumbs on a plate.
9. Form rice mixture into 8 balls and roll 1 ball in flour, dip in egg and coat with crumbs, repeat with all balls.
10. Deep fry balls for 3 minutes.
11. Enjoy!

Nutrition:

Calories: 182
Fat: 7g
Carbohydrates: 21g
Protein: 7g

354. Easy Garlic Almond butter Shrimp

Serving: 4
Preparation Time: 15 minutes
Cook Time: 30 minutes

Ingredients:

- 4 pounds shrimp
- 1-2 tablespoons garlic, minced
- ½ cup almond butter
- 1 tablespoon lemon pepper seasoning
- ½ teaspoon garlic powder

Directions:

1. Pre-heat your oven to 300 degrees F.
2. Take a bowl and mix in garlic and almond butter.
3. Place shrimp in a pan and dot with almond butter garlic mix.
4. Sprinkle garlic powder and lemon pepper.
5. Bake for 30 minutes.
6. Enjoy!

Nutrition:

Calories: 749
Fat: 30g
Net Carbohydrates: 7g
Protein: 74g

355. Blackened Tilapia

Serving: 2
Preparation Time: 9 minutes
Cook Time: 9 minutes

Ingredients:

- 1 cup cauliflower, chopped
- 1 teaspoon red pepper flakes

- 1 tablespoon Italian seasoning
- 1 tablespoon garlic, minced
- 6 ounces tilapia
- 1 cup English cucumber, chopped with peel
- 2 tablespoons olive oil
- 1 sprig dill, chopped
- 1 teaspoon stevia
- 3 tablespoons lime juice
- 2 tablespoons Cajun blackened seasoning

Directions:
1. Take a bowl and add the seasoning ingredients (except Cajun.
2. Add a tablespoon of oil and whip.
3. Pour dressing over cauliflower and cucumber.
4. Brush the fish with olive oil on both sides.
5. Take a skillet and grease it well with 1 tablespoon of olive oil.
6. Press Cajun seasoning on both sides of fish.
7. Cook fish for 3 minutes per side.
8. Serve with vegetables and enjoy!

Nutrition:
Calories: 530
Fat: 33g
Net Carbohydrates: 4g
Protein: 32g

356. Light Lobster Bisque

Serving: 4
Preparation Time: 10 minutes
400 Cook Time: 6 minutes

Ingredients:
- 1 cup diced carrots
- 1 cup diced celery
- 29 ounces diced tomatoes
- 2 minced whole shallots
- 1 clove of minced garlic
- 1 tablespoon butter
- 32 ounce chicken broth, low-sodium
- 1 teaspoon dill, dried
- 1 teaspoon freshly ground black pepper
- ½ teaspoon paprika
- 4 lobster tails
- 1 pint heavy whipping cream

Directions:
1. Add butter, garlic and minced shallots to a microwave safe bowl.
2. Microwave for 2-3 minutes on HIGH.
3. Add tomatoes, celery, carrot, minced shallots, garlic to your Instant Pot.
4. Add chicken broth and spices to the Pot.
5. Use a knife to cut the lobster tails if you prefer and add them to the Instant Pot.
6. Lock the lid and cook on HIGH pressure for 4 minutes.
7. Release the pressure naturally over 10 minutes.
8. Use an immersion blender to puree to your desired chunkiness.
9. Serve and enjoy!

Nutrition:
Calories: 437
Fats: 17g
Carbs: 21g
Protein: 38g

357. Herbal Shrimp Risotto

Serving: 4
Preparation Time: 10 minutes
Cook Time: 8 minutes

Ingredients:
- 2 pounds shrimp with their tails removed
- 1 cup instant rice
- 2 cups vegetable broth
- 1 chopped up onion
- 1 cup chicken breast cut into fine strips
- ¼ cup lemon juice
- 1 teaspoon crushed red pepper
- ¼ cup parsley
- ¼ cup fresh dill
- 6 pieces chopped up garlic cloves
- 1 tablespoon black pepper
- ½ cup parmesan
- 1 cup mozzarella cheese

Directions:
1. Add the listed ingredients to your Instant

Pot and stir.
2. Lock the lid and cook on HIGH pressure for 8 minutes.
3. Release the pressure naturally over 10 minutes.
4. Open lid and top with cheese.
5. Serve hot and enjoy!

Nutrition:

Calories: 463
Fat: 8g
Carbohydrates: 63g
Protein: 29g

358. Thai Pumpkin Seafood Stew

Serving: 4
Preparation Time: 5 minutes
Cook Time: 35 minutes

Ingredients:

- 1 ½ tablespoons fresh galangal, chopped
- 1 teaspoon lime zest
- 1 small kabocha squash
- 32 medium sized mussels, fresh
- 1 pound shrimp
- 16 thai leaves
- 1 can coconut milk
- 1 tablespoon lemongrass, minced
- 4 garlic cloves, roughly chopped
- 32 medium clams, fresh
- 1 ½ pounds fresh salmon
- 2 tablespoons coconut oil
- Pepper to taste

Directions:

1. Add coconut milk, lemongrass, galangal, garlic, lime leaves in a small-sized saucepan, bring to a boil.
2. Let it simmer for 25 minutes.
3. Strain mixture through a fine sieve into the large soup pot and bring to a simmer.
4. Add oil to a pan and heat up, add Kabocha squash.
5. Season with salt and pepper, sauté for 5 minutes.
6. Add mix to coconut mix.
7. Heat oil in a pan and add fish shrimp, season with salt and pepper, cook for 4 minutes.
8. Add mixture to coconut milk, mix alongside clams and mussels.
9. Simmer for 8 minutes, garnish with basil and enjoy!

Nutrition:

Calories: 370
Fat: 16g
Net Carbohydrates: 10g
Protein: 16g

359. Pistachio Sole Fish

Serving: 4
Preparation Time: 5 minutes
Cook Time: 10 minutes

Ingredients:

- 4 (5 ounces boneless sole fillets
- Sunflower seeds and pepper as needed
- ½ cup pistachios, finely chopped
- Juice of 1 lemon
- 1 teaspoon extra virgin olive oil

Directions:

1. Pre-heat your oven to 350 degrees F.
2. Line a baking sheet with parchment paper and keep it on the side.
3. Pat fish dry with kitchen towels and lightly season with sunflower seeds and pepper.
4. Take a small bowl and stir in pistachios.
5. Place sole on the prepared baking sheet and press 2 tablespoons of pistachio mixture on top of each fillet.
6. Drizzle fish with lemon juice and olive oil.
7. Bake for 10 minutes until the top is golden and fish flakes with a fork.
8. Serve and enjoy!

Nutrition:

Calories: 166
Fat: 6g
Carbohydrates: 2g

Poultry

360. Chicken with Tomato Rice

Preparation time: 10 minutes
Cooking time: 30 minutes
Servings: 4

Ingredients:
- 1 yellow onion, chopped
- 2 tablespoons olive oil
- 1 pound chicken breast, skinless, boneless and cubed
- 1 tablespoon lemon zest, grated
- 2 tablespoons lemon juice
- 3 garlic cloves, minced
- 1 cup brown rice
- 2 cups chicken stock
- ½ cup grape tomatoes, halved
- 1 tablespoon parsley, chopped

Directions:
1. Heat up a pan with the oil over medium heat, add the onion and sauté for 5 minutes.
2. Add the meat and brown for 5 minutes.
3. Add the rest of the ingredients, toss, cook everything for 20 minutes more, divide between plates and serve.

Nutrition: calories 288, fat 6, fiber 5, carbs 14, protein 20

361. Turkey with Tomato Asparagus

Preparation time: 10 minutes
Cooking time: 30 minutes
Servings: 4

Ingredients:
- 1 pound turkey breast, skinless, boneless and sliced
- 2 tablespoons olive oil
- 4 scallions, chopped
- A pinch of salt and black pepper
- 1 cup chicken stock
- ¼ cup tomato sauce
- 1 bunch asparagus, sliced
- 2 teaspoons lemon juice
- 2 garlic cloves, minced
- 1 tablespoon coriander, chopped

Directions:
1. Heat up a pan with the oil over medium-high heat, add the scallions and the garlic and sauté for 5 minutes.
2. Add the meat and brown for 5 minutes more.
3. Add the rest of the ingredients, toss, cook over medium heat for 20 minutes more, divide between plates and serve.

Nutrition: calories 271, fat 6, fiber 7, carbs 8, protein 16

362. Chicken Wings and Potatoes

Preparation time: 10 minutes
Cooking time: 50 minutes
Servings: 4

Ingredients:
- 2 tablespoons olive oil
- 1 yellow onion, chopped
- 2 tablespoons olive oil
- A pinch of salt and black pepper
- 2 pounds chicken wings
- ½ pound sweet potatoes, peeled and cut into wedges
- ½ cup coconut cream
- 1 and ½ tablespoons tarragon, chopped

Directions:
1. Heat up a pan with the oil over medium-high heat, add the onion and sauté for 5 minutes.
2. Add the meat and cook for 5 minutes more.
3. Add the rest of the ingredients, toss, introduce in the oven and bake at 360 degrees F for 40 minutes.
4. Divide the mix between plates and serve.

Nutrition: calories 698, fat 38.1, fiber 3.6, carbs 20.1, protein 67.5

363. Walnuts Chicken Mix

Preparation time: 10 minutes
Cooking time: 45 minutes
Servings: 4

Ingredients:
- 1 yellow onion, chopped
- 2 tablespoons olive oil
- 3 garlic cloves, minced
- 1 pound chicken thighs, skinless, boneless
- ½ cup chicken stock
- 2 bay leaves
- 3 tablespoons walnuts, chopped
- A pinch of salt and black pepper
- 2 tablespoons chives, chopped

Directions:
1. Heat up a pan with the oil over medium-high heat, add the onion and the garlic and sauté for 5 minutes.
2. Add the chicken and brown for 5 minutes more.
3. Add the rest of the ingredients, stir, cook over medium heat for 30 minutes more, divide between plates and serve.

Nutrition: calories 229, fat 7, fiber 7, carbs 15, protein 18

364. Chicken with Kidney Beans

Preparation time: 5 minutes
Cooking time: 8 hours
Servings: 4

Ingredients:
- 1 yellow onion, chopped
- 2 carrots, sliced
- 2 garlic cloves, minced
- 2 pounds chicken breast, skinless, boneless and cubed
- 10 ounces canned kidney beans, drained and rinsed
- 1 teaspoon cumin, ground
- ½ teaspoon basil, dried
- A pinch of salt and black pepper
- 1 tablespoon oregano, chopped

Directions:
1. In a slow cooker, combine chicken with the onion, the carrots, the garlic and the other ingredients, toss, put the lid on and cook on Low for 8 hours.
2. Divide the mix between plates and serve.

Nutrition: calories 299, fat 3, fiber 7, carbs 13, protein 19

365. Chicken Thighs and Green Beans Mix

Preparation time: 5 minutes
Cooking time: 30 minutes
Servings: 4

Ingredients:
- 1 cup chicken stock
- 2 tablespoons olive oil
- 1 pound chicken thighs, bone-in and skin-on
- A pinch of salt and black pepper
- 1 yellow onion, chopped
- 2 cups green beans, trimmed and halved
- ¼ cup basil, chopped
- 2 tablespoons capers
- 1 tablespoon lemon juice

Directions:
1. Heat up a pan with the oil over medium-high heat, add the onion and the chicken and sauté for 5 minutes.
2. Add the rest of the ingredients, toss, cook over medium heat for 25 minutes more, divide between plates and serve.

Nutrition: calories 300, fat 5, fiber 7, carbs 11, protein 16

366. Chicken with Sprouts and Beets

Preparation time: 10 minutes
Cooking time: 40 minutes
Servings: 4

Ingredients:
- 1 pound chicken breast, skinless, boneless and sliced
- A pinch of salt and black pepper
- 1 teaspoon sweet paprika
- 1 yellow onion, chopped

- 1 teaspoon coriander, ground
- 2 tablespoons avocado oil
- Juice of 1 lemon
- 4 garlic cloves, minced
- 1 cup Brussels sprouts, trimmed and halved
- 2 beets, peeled and cubed
- 1 tablespoon rosemary, chopped

Directions:
1. Heat up a pan with the oil over medium-high heat, add the onion and the garlic and sauté for 5 minutes.
2. Add the meat and brown for 5 minutes more.
3. Add the rest of the ingredients, toss, cook over medium heat for 30 minutes more, divide between plates and serve.

Nutrition: calories 297, fat 7, fiber 6, carbs 11, protein 19

367. Chicken with Grapes

Preparation time: 10 minutes
Cooking time: 40 minutes
Servings: 4

Ingredients:
- 1 cup grapes, halved
- 2 pounds chicken breast, skinless, boneless and cubed
- 2 teaspoons curry powder
- 2 tablespoons avocado oil
- 4 scallions, chopped
- A pinch of salt and black pepper
- 1 tablespoon chives, chopped

Directions:
1. Heat up a pan with the oil over medium-high heat, add the scallions and sauté for 5 minutes.
2. Add the chicken and brown for 5 minutes more.
3. Add the rest of the ingredients, toss, cook over medium heat for 30 minutes more, divide between plates and serve.

Nutrition: calories 222, fat 5, fiber 7, carbs 14, protein 17

368. Chicken with Bok Choy

Preparation time: 10 minutes
Cooking time: 40 minutes
Servings: 4

Ingredients:
- 2 pounds chicken breast, skinless, boneless and cubed
- 1 cup bok choy, torn
- 2 tablespoons olive oil
- 4 garlic cloves, minced
- A pinch of salt and black pepper
- Cooking spray
- ½ cup pecans, roasted
- 1 tablespoon chives, chopped

Directions:
1. Heat up a pan with the oil over medium-high heat, add the garlic and sauté for 2 minutes.
2. Add the meat and brown for 5 minutes more.
3. Add the rest of the ingredients, toss, cook over medium heat for 33 minutes more, divide between plates and serve.

Nutrition: calories 300, fat 12, fiber 7, carbs 15, protein 18

369. Tarragon Turkey and Tomatoes

Preparation time: 10 minutes
Cooking time: 40 minutes
Servings: 4

Ingredients:
- 1 yellow onion, chopped
- 2 garlic cloves, minced
- 1 pound turkey breast, skinless, boneless and cut into strips
- 1 cup tomatoes, roughly cubed
- 2 tablespoons olive oil
- 1 tablespoon tarragon, chopped
- A pinch of salt and black pepper
- 1 teaspoon smoked paprika

Directions:
1. Heat up a pan with the oil over medium-high heat, add the onion and the garlic and sauté for 5 minutes.

2. Add the meat and brown for 5 minutes more.
3. Add the remaining ingredients, toss, cook over medium for 30 minutes more, divide between plates and serve.

Nutrition: calories 298, fat 8, fiber 4, carbs 14, protein 15

370. Chicken and Thyme Mushrooms

Preparation time: 10 minutes
Cooking time: 40 minutes
Servings: 4

Ingredients:
- 2 tablespoons olive oil
- 1 yellow onion, chopped
- ½ pounds Bella mushrooms, sliced
- 2 pounds chicken thighs, boneless and skinless
- 3 carrots, sliced
- 2 celery stalks, chopped
- ½ cup coconut cream
- 1 tablespoon thyme, chopped
- 1 tablespoon cilantro, chopped

Directions:
1. Heat up a pan with the oil over medium heat, add the onion, carrots and the celery and sauté for 5 minutes.
2. Add the mushrooms and the meat and brown for 5 minutes more.
3. Add the rest of the ingredients, toss, cook over medium heat for 30 minutes more, divide between plates and serve.

Nutrition: calories 300, fat 6, fiber 7, carbs 15, protein 16

371. Chicken with Plums

Preparation time: 10 minutes
Cooking time: 45 minutes
Servings: 4

Ingredients:
- 2 pounds chicken breast, skinless, boneless and cubed
- 4 scallions, chopped
- 2 tablespoons olive oil
- A pinch of salt and black pepper
- 1 teaspoon ginger, grated
- 4 garlic cloves, minced
- 2 cups plums, pitted and halved
- 1 tablespoon balsamic vinegar
- 2 tablespoons cilantro, chopped

Directions:
1. Heat up a pan with the oil over medium heat, add the scallions, ginger and the garlic and sauté for 5 minutes.
2. Add the chicken and brown for 5 minutes more.
3. Add the plums and the rest of the ingredients, toss, cook over medium heat for 35 minutes more, divide between plates and serve.

Nutrition: calories 280, fat 8, fiber 4, carbs 12, protein 17

372. Turkey with Apples and Peaches

Preparation time: 10 minutes
Cooking time: 45 minutes
Servings: 4

Ingredients:
- 2 pound turkey breast, skinless, boneless and sliced
- 1 green apple, cored and cut into wedges
- 1 cup peaches, pitted and cubed
- 1 tablespoon olive oil
- 2 green chilies, chopped
- A pinch of black pepper
- 1 teaspoon chili powder
- 1 tablespoon lime juice

Directions:
1. In a roasting pan, combine the turkey with the apple, peaches and the other ingredients, toss and bake at 390 degrees F for 45 minutes.
2. Divide everything between plates and serve.

Nutrition: calories 314, fat 7.6, fiber 3.3, carbs 22.1, protein 39.3

373. Chicken with Green Onions Quinoa

Preparation time: 10 minutes
Cooking time: 40 minutes
Servings: 4

Ingredients:

- 2 tablespoons avocado oil
- 1 pound chicken breast, skinless, boneless and cubed
- A pinch of salt and black pepper
- 1 cup quinoa
- ½ teaspoon chili powder
- ½ teaspoon cumin, ground
- 3 cups chicken stock
- 4 green onions, chopped
- 1 tablespoon sesame seeds, toasted

Directions:

1. Heat up a pan with the oil over medium heat, add the green onions and the chicken and brown for 5 minutes.
2. Add the rest of the ingredients, toss, bring to a simmer and cook over medium heat for 35 minutes more.
3. Divide everything between plates and serve.

Nutrition: calories 322, fat 8, fiber 4.1, carbs 30.2, protein 31.4

374. Chicken with Blackberry Sauce

Preparation time: 10 minutes
Cooking time: 35 minutes
Servings: 4

Ingredients:

- 4 scallions, chopped
- 2 tablespoons avocado oil
- 2 pounds chicken breasts, skinless, boneless and sliced
- 2 tablespoons balsamic vinegar
- 1 cup chicken stock
- 2 cups raspberries
- A pinch of salt and black pepper
- 1 tablespoon cilantro, chopped

Directions:

1. Heat up a pan with the oil over medium-high heat, add the scallions and the meat and brown for 5 minutes.
2. Add the rest of the ingredients, toss, cook over medium heat for 30 minutes more, divide between plates and serve.

Nutrition: calories 481, fat 18.3, fiber 4.7, carbs 9.1, protein 66.9

375. Turkey Curry

Preparation time: 10 minutes
Cooking time: 40 minutes
Servings: 4

Ingredients:

- 1 pound turkey breast, boneless, skinless and cubed
- 1 yellow onion, chopped
- 1 red bell pepper, chopped
- 2 tablespoons avocado oil
- 1 cup coconut cream
- 1 cup chicken stock
- ½ teaspoon chili powder
- 1 teaspoon coriander, ground
- 3 tablespoons curry powder
- 2 tablespoons cilantro, chopped
- A pinch of salt and black pepper

Directions:

1. Heat up a pan with the oil over medium-high heat, add the onion and the turkey meat and brown for 5 minutes.
2. Add the bell pepper and the other ingredients, toss, cook over medium heat for 35 minutes more, divide into bowls and serve.

Nutrition: calories 280, fat 13, fiber 7, carbs 8, protein 15

376. Chicken and Avocado

Preparation time: 10 minutes
Cooking time: 35 minutes
Servings: 4

Ingredients:

- 4 garlic cloves, minced
- 4 scallions, chopped
- 2 pounds chicken thighs, skinless and boneless
- 2 tablespoons olive oil

- 1 avocado, peeled, pitted and sliced
- 1 teaspoon turmeric powder
- A pinch of salt and black pepper
- 1 teaspoon red chili flakes

Directions:
1. Heat up a pan with the oil over medium-high heat, add the scallions and the garlic and sauté for 5 minutes.
2. Add the meat and brown for 5 minutes more.
3. Add the rest of the ingredients, toss, cook over medium heat for 25 minutes more, divide between plates and serve.

Nutrition: calories 200, fat 10, fiber 1, carbs 12, protein 24

377. Ginger Chicken Thighs with Potatoes

Preparation time: 5 minutes
Cooking time: 40 minutes
Servings: 4

Ingredients:
- 2 pounds chicken thighs, boneless, skinless
- 2 tablespoons olive oil
- 4 scallions, chopped
- 2 sweet potatoes, peeled and cut into wedges
- 1 tablespoon lemon juice
- 1 teaspoon coriander, ground
- A pinch of salt and black pepper
- 1 tablespoon ginger, minced
- 1 tablespoon rosemary, chopped

Directions:
1. Heat up a pan with the oil over medium-high heat, add the scallions, ginger and the meat and brown for 10 minutes stirring often.
2. Add the rest of the ingredients, toss, cook over medium heat for 30 minutes more, divide between plates and serve.

Nutrition: calories 210, fat 8, fiber 4, carbs 12, protein 17

378. Chili Turkey and Peppers

Preparation time: 10 minutes
Cooking time: 1 hour
Servings: 4

Ingredients:
- 2 tablespoons avocado oil
- 2 pounds turkey breast, skinless, boneless and cubed
- 1 green bell pepper, chopped
- 1 orange bell pepper, chopped
- 2 garlic cloves, minced
- 3 scallions, chopped
- 1 red chili, chopped
- ½ teaspoon chili flakes, crushed
- 1 tablespoon chili powder
- 15 ounces canned tomatoes, chopped
- 1 cup veggie stock
- A pinch of salt and black pepper

Directions:
1. Heat up a pan with the oil over medium heat, add the scallions and the garlic and sauté for 5 minutes.
2. Add the meat and brown for 5 minutes more.
3. Add the bell peppers and the other ingredients, toss, cook over medium heat for 50 minutes more, divide into bowls and serve.

Nutrition: calories 220, fat 8, fiber 4, carbs 14, protein 13

379. Chicken with Turmeric Mushrooms

Preparation time: 10 minutes
Cooking time: 40 minutes
Servings: 4

Ingredients:
- 1 yellow onion, chopped
- 1 pound chicken breast, skinless, boneless and roughly cubed
- 2 tablespoons olive oil
- 1 cup white mushrooms, sliced
- 1 teaspoon turmeric powder
- 1 cup chicken stock
- 2 garlic cloves, minced

- 2 teaspoons rosemary, chopped
- Salt and black pepper to the tastes
- 1 tablespoon balsamic vinegar
- 1 tablespoon cilantro, chopped

Directions:
1. Heat up a pan with the oil over medium heat, add the onion and the mushrooms and sauté for 10 minutes.
2. Add the meat and brown for 5 minutes more.
3. Add the garlic and the other ingredients, toss, cook over medium heat for 25 minutes more, divide between plates and serve.

Nutrition: calories 210, fat 5, fiber 8, carbs 15, protein 11

380. Baked Turkey

Preparation time: 10 minutes
Cooking time: 1 hour
Servings: 4

Ingredients:
- 2 pounds turkey breast, skinless, boneless and sliced
- 2 tablespoons avocado oil
- 1 yellow onion, sliced
- 2 spring onions, chopped
- A pinch of salt and black pepper
- 1 cup chicken stock
- 2 teaspoons lemon juice
- 1 teaspoon coriander, ground

Directions:
1. In a roasting pan, combine the turkey with the oil, the onion and the other ingredients, toss and bake at 390 degrees F for 1 hour.
2. Divide the mix between plates and serve.

Nutrition: calories 300, fat 4, fiber 4, carbs 15, protein 27

381. Maple Chicken Wings

Preparation time: 10 minutes
Cooking time: 1 hour
Servings: 4

Ingredients:
- 2 pounds chicken wings, halved
- 2 tablespoons maple syrup
- A pinch of sea salt and black pepper
- 1 tablespoon apple cider vinegar
- ½ teaspoon thyme, dried
- ½ teaspoon chili powder

Directions:
1. In a roasting pan, combine the chicken wings with the maple syrup and the other ingredients, toss and bake at 390 degrees F for 1 hour.
2. Divide the mix between plates and serve.

Nutrition: calories 274, fat 6, fiber 8, carbs 14, protein 12

382. Hot Chicken Wings with Artichokes

Preparation time: 10 minutes
Cooking time: 40 minutes
Servings: 4

Ingredients:
- 2 pounds chicken wings, halved
- 2 tablespoons olive oil
- 1 cup canned artichoke hearts, drained and quartered
- 1 bunch green onions, chopped
- ½ cup chili sauce
- A pinch of salt and black pepper

Directions:
1. Spread the chicken wings on a baking sheet lined with parchment paper, add the oil and the other ingredients, toss and bake at 420 degrees F for 40 minutes.
2. Divide the mix between plates and serve.

Nutrition: calories 260, fat 4, fiber 2, carbs 12, protein 14

383. Chicken and Cilantro Sauce

Preparation time: 10 minutes
Cooking time: 40 minutes
Servings: 4

Ingredients:
- 1 cup cilantro, chopped

- 1 tablespoon pine nuts, toasted
- ½ cup olive oil
- 1 cup chicken stock
- 4 garlic cloves, minced
- 2 pounds chicken breast, skinless, boneless and sliced
- A pinch of salt and black pepper

Directions:
1. In a blender, combine the cilantro with the pine nuts, the oil and the garlic and pulse well.
2. In a roasting pan, combine the chicken with the cilantro sauce and the remaining ingredients, toss and bake at 390 degrees F for 40 minutes.
3. Divide everything between plates and serve.

Nutrition: calories 254, fat 3, fiber 3, carbs 7, protein 12

384. Greek Style Chicken

Preparation Time: 10 minutes
Cooking time: 20 minutes
Servings: 3

Ingredients:
- 1-pound chicken breast, skinless, boneless
- 2 tablespoons lemon juice
- 1 teaspoon lemon zest, grated
- ½ teaspoon ground black pepper
- 1 teaspoon chili flakes
- ½ cup sour cream
- 1 tablespoon butter
- 1 teaspoon olive oil
- 1 garlic clove, diced
- ½ teaspoon dried oregano

Directions:
1. Chop the chicken breast roughly and place in the saucepan.
2. Sprinkle the chicken with lemon juice, lemon zest, ground black pepper, chili flakes, and diced garlic. Add oregano.
3. Add olive oil and roast it for 3-4 minutes. Stir it from time to time.
4. After this, add butter, sour cream, and mix up the chicken well.
5. Close the lid and cook the meal with the closed lid for 15 minutes over the medium-high heat. Stir the chicken from time to time.

Nutrition value/serving: calories 308, fat 17.3, fiber 0.3, carbs 2.7, protein 33.5

385. Classic Whole Chicken with Herbs

Preparation Time: 15 minutes
Cooking time: 60 minutes
Servings: 7

Ingredients:
- 3-pound whole chicken
- 1 tablespoon rosemary
- 1 teaspoon thyme
- 4 garlic cloves, peeled, crushed
- 1 tablespoon ground paprika
- 1 tablespoon olive oil
- 1 white onion, chopped
- 1 teaspoon ground black pepper
- 1 teaspoon salt
- ½ teaspoon dried cilantro
- ¼ teaspoon cayenne pepper

Directions:
1. Trim the chicken if needed.
2. In the shallow bowl, mix up together thyme, rosemary, crushed garlic, ground paprika, olive oil, ground black pepper, salt, dried cilantro, and cayenne pepper.
3. Then rub the chicken with the mixture from inside and outside.
4. Fill the chicken with the chopped onion and transfer in the baking tray.
5. Add the remaining spice mixture and bake the chicken for 60 minutes at 365F.
6. Then check if the chicken is cooked and sprinkle it with "chicken juice" from the tray.

Nutrition value/serving: calories 401, fat 16.7, fiber 1.1, carbs 3.2, protein 56.7

386. Chicken Jalapeno Quesadillas

Preparation Time: 15 minutes
Cooking time: 10 minutes

Servings: 4

Ingredients:

- ½ cup almond flour
- 1 egg, beaten
- 3 teaspoons butter, softened
- 1 teaspoon ground paprika
- 1 tablespoon olive oil
- 2 jalapeno peppers, minced
- 8 oz chicken fillet, boiled
- 1 tablespoon mayonnaise
- ½ teaspoon tomato paste
- 5 oz Cheddar cheese, shredded
- 1 tablespoon fresh parsley, chopped

Directions:

1. Make the tortillas: mix up together almond flour, beaten egg, and butter.
2. Knead the soft dough.
3. Cut the dough into 2 parts and roll up 2 tortillas.
4. After this, mix up together ground paprika, minced jalapeno peppers, mayonnaise, tomato paste, and chopped parsley.
5. Chop the boiled fillet.
6. Pour the olive oil in the skillet.
7. Add the first tortilla and spread it with the jalapeno mixture. Add chopped chicken fillet and shredded Cheddar cheese.
8. Cover the cheese with the second tortilla.
9. Cook the quesadillas for 3 minutes and then flip onto another side.
10. The quesadillas are cooked when it has a golden brown color.
11. Slice it into servings.

Nutrition value/serving: calories 361, fat 26.6, fiber 0.9, carbs 3.2, protein 27.7

387. Aromatic Tuscan Chicken

Preparation Time: 10 minutes
Cooking time: 20 minutes
Servings: 2

Ingredients:

- 8 oz chicken fillet
- 1 teaspoon butter
- ½ teaspoon ground black pepper
- ½ cup fresh spinach, chopped
- 4 oz Parmesan, grated
- ½ teaspoon chili flakes
- 1/3 cup coconut cream

Directions:

1. Cut the chicken fillet into 2 parts.
2. Then place the fillets in the skillet.
3. Add butter and roast them for 4 minutes from each side.
4. After this, remove the chicken from the skillet.
5. Add coconut cream in the skillet.
6. Then add chili flakes, grated Parmesan, spinach, and ground black pepper.
7. Mix up the liquid and cook it until cheese is melted.
8. Then add cooked chicken fillets and coat them in the cream mixture well.
9. Close the lid and cook the meal for 10 minutes over the medium heat.

Nutrition value/serving: calories 510, fat 32.1, fiber 1.2, carbs 4.9, protein 52.3

388. Baked Paprika Chicken Breast

Preparation Time: 10 minutes
Cooking time: 40 minutes
Servings: 5

Ingredients:

- 14 oz chicken breast, skinless, boneless
- 1 tablespoon ground paprika
- ½ teaspoon ground black pepper
- 1 teaspoon salt
- 1 teaspoon butter, melted
- 1 tablespoon heavy cream
- 1 tablespoon cream cheese
- 2 tablespoons water

Directions:

1. Rub the chicken breast with ground paprika, black pepper, and salt.
2. Place the chicken in the baking dish.
3. Add butter, cream cheese, and heavy cream.
4. Then add water and cover the dish with the foil.
5. Bake the chicken breast in the preheated

to 370F oven and cook it for 40 minutes.
6. Serve the chicken breast with the hot creamy sauce from it.

Nutrition value/serving: calories 119, fat 4.7, fiber 0.6, carbs 1, protein 17.3

389. Stuffed Chicken Fillets

Preparation Time: 15 minutes
Cooking time: 40 minutes
Servings: 4

Ingredients:

- 10 oz chicken fillet
- ¼ cup mushrooms, chopped
- 1 shallot, diced
- 1 teaspoon olive oil
- 2 oz Parmesan, grated
- ½ teaspoon ground black pepper
- 2 oz bacon, chopped
- ½ teaspoon cayenne pepper
- ¾ cup coconut cream

Directions:

1. In the skillet, mix up together chopped mushrooms, bacon, diced shallot, and olive oil.
2. Saute the mushroom mixture for 10 minutes.
3. Meanwhile, beat the chicken fillets with the help of the chicken hammer well.
4. Sprinkle the chicken fillets with cayenne pepper and ground black pepper.
5. Then add cooked mushroom mixture and roll the chicken fillets.
6. Secure them with the help of the toothpicks. And transfer in the baking tray.
7. Sprinkle the chicken fillets with the coconut cream and grated Parmesan.
8. Bake the chicken fillets for 30 minutes at 365F.
9. When the meal is cooked, let it chill little and slice roughly.

Nutrition value/serving: calories 373, fat 26.2, fiber 1.2, carbs 3.7, protein 31.5

390. Grilled Chicken

Preparation Time: 20 minutes
Cooking time: 10 minutes
Servings: 4

Ingredients:

- 1 teaspoon lemon juice
- 1 teaspoon apple cider vinegar
- 1 tablespoon olive oil
- 1 teaspoon chili flakes
- 1 teaspoon chili powder
- ½ onion, diced
- 1 teaspoon salt
- 4 chicken thighs, skinless, boneless

Directions:

1. Sprinkle the chicken thighs with the apple cider vinegar, lemon juice, olive oil, chili flakes, chili powder, salt, and diced onion.
2. Mix up the chicken thighs well and let them marinate for at least 15 minutes.
3. Meanwhile, preheat the grill till 380F.
4. Place the marinated chicken thighs in the grill and cook for 4 minutes from each side.
5. If you want to get a crunchy crust, grill the chicken thighs for 4 minutes more.

Nutrition value/serving: calories 228, fat 13.9, fiber 0.5, carbs 1.7, protein 28

391. Cajun Chicken

Preparation Time: 10 minutes
Cooking time: 20 minutes
Servings: 2

Ingredients:

- 9 oz chicken breast, skinless, boneless
- 1 tablespoon Cajun seasoning
- ½ teaspoon salt
- 1 tablespoon lime juice
- 1 tablespoon olive oil
- ½ teaspoon garlic, minced

Directions:

1. Cut the chicken breast into 2 servings and rub with Cajun seasonings, salt, lime juice, and minced garlic.
2. Massage the chicken breast carefully.
3. Pour olive in the skillet and make it hot.
4. Place the marinated chicken breast in the

hot oil and roast them for 8 minutes from each side over the medium heat.

Nutrition value/serving: calories 208, fat 10.2, fiber 0, carbs 0.8, protein 27.2

392. Hasselback Chicken Breast

Preparation Time: 15 minutes
Cooking time: 40 minutes
Servings: 3

Ingredients:

- 1-pound chicken breast, skinless, boneless
- 5 oz Mozzarella, sliced
- 1 teaspoon white pepper
- 1 teaspoon salt
- ½ teaspoon chili flakes
- 1 tablespoon lemon juice
- ½ teaspoon paprika
- ¾ teaspoon turmeric
- 1 white onion, sliced
- 1 teaspoon olive oil
- ¾ cup heavy cream

Directions:

1. Rub the chicken breast with the white pepper, salt, chili flakes, lemon juice, paprika, and turmeric.
2. Then make the cuts in the chicken breast in the shape o the Hasselback.
3. Fill the Hasselback cuts with sliced Mozzarella and onion.
4. Transfer the chicken breast in the baking dish.
5. Pour it over with the olive oil and heavy cream.
6. Bake the Hasselback chicken breast for 40 minutes or until it is light brown.

Nutrition value/serving: calories 443, fat 25, fiber 1.3, carbs 7.1, protein 46.6

393. Chicken Tenders

Preparation Time: 15 minutes
Cooking time: 10 minutes
Servings: 6

Ingredients:

- 14 oz chicken fillet
- ½ cup coconut flour
- 4 oz Cheddar cheese, shredded
- 2 eggs, whisked
- ¾ cup heavy cream
- 1 tablespoon canola oil
- 1 teaspoon salt
- 1 teaspoon chili flakes

Directions:

1. Cut the chicken filet into the tenders and sprinkle them with the salt and chili flakes.
2. Mix up together shredded Cheddar cheese and coconut flour.
3. In the separated bowl, mix up together heavy cream and whisked eggs.
4. Dip the chicken tenders in the egg mixture.
5. Then coat them in the cheese mixture.
6. Pour canola oil in the skillet.
7. Arrange the chicken tenders in one layer and cook them for 3 minutes from each side or until light brown.

Nutrition value/serving: calories 335, fat 21.8, fiber 3.3, carbs 6.1, protein 27.3

394. Chicken Balls with Coconut Sauce

Preparation Time: 10 minutes
Cooking time: 10 minutes
Servings: 2

Ingredients:

- ½ cup ground chicken
- ¼ teaspoon chili powder
- ¾ teaspoon turmeric
- ¼ teaspoon salt
- 1 egg, whisked
- 1 tablespoon coconut flour
- 1/3 cup coconut cream
- 1 teaspoon butter
- ½ teaspoon minced garlic
- 1 teaspoon olive oil
- ½ teaspoon ground paprika

Directions:

1. In the mixing bowl, mix up together ground chicken, chili powder, turmeric,

salt, egg, coconut flour, ground paprika, and minced garlic.
2. Make the balls from the mixture.
3. Pour olive oil in the saucepan.
4. Add butter and melt the mixture.
5. Then add the prepared chicken balls and roast them for 4 minutes over the medium heat.
6. Then flip them onto another side and cook for 3 minutes more.
7. Add coconut cream and simmer for chicken balls for 3 minutes.
8. Serve the chicken balls with the coconut cream mixture (sauce.

Nutrition value/serving: calories 263, fat 19.8, fiber 3.9, carbs 7.6, protein 15.1

395. Butter Chicken

Preparation Time: 10 minutes
Cooking time: 25 minutes
Servings:4

Ingredients:

- 10 oz chicken fillets, sliced
- ½ cup cherry tomatoes, chopped
- 1 teaspoon chili powder
- 1 teaspoon chili flakes
- 1 tablespoon butter
- ¾ cup heavy cream
- 1 white onion, diced
- 1 teaspoon olive oil
- 1 teaspoon minced garlic
- 1 teaspoon minced ginger
- ½ teaspoon turmeric
- 1 teaspoon ground paprika

Directions:

1. Toss the butter in the saucepan.
2. Melt it over the low heat.
3. Meanwhile, mix up together chicken fillets, chili powder, and chili flakes.
4. Place the diced onion in the saucepan.
5. Add olive oil, minced ginger, minced garlic, turmeric, and ground paprika.
6. Saute the ingredients for 5 minutes.
7. Then add chopped cherry tomatoes, heavy cream, and mix up.
8. Simmer the ingredients for 5 minutes.
9. Then transfer the cooked mixture in the blender and blend well.
10. Add the chicken in the skillet and roast it for 5 minutes.
11. Add the blended tomato mixture and mix up well.
12. Close the lid and saute the butter chicken for 10 minutes over the medium heat.

Nutrition value/serving: calories 270, fat 18, fiber 1.4, carbs 5.5, protein 21.8

396. Hot Chicken Chowder

Preparation Time: 7 minutes
Cooking time: 30 minutes
Servings:4

Ingredients:

- 1 cup heavy cream
- 2 cups of water
- 1 teaspoon ground black pepper
- 1 tablespoon cream cheese
- 4 chicken thighs
- ½ teaspoon salt
- 1 teaspoon cayenne pepper
- 1 teaspoon chili flakes
- 1 teaspoon ground coriander
- 1 cup mushrooms, chopped
- 1 teaspoon olive oil
- ½ white onion, diced

Directions:

1. Pour olive oil in the skillet and add diced onion.
2. Roast the onion for 3 minutes over the medium heat.
3. Then add chopped mushrooms, ground coriander, chili flakes, salt, and cayenne pepper.
4. Cook the ingredients with the closed lid for 10 minutes.
5. Meanwhile, pour heavy cream and water in the saucepan.
6. Bring the liquid to boil and add ground black pepper and cream cheese.
7. Add chicken thighs and boil the soup for 10 minutes.
8. After this, add mushroom mixture and stir well.

9. Close the lid and simmer chowder for 2 minutes.
10. Then let it rest with the closed lid for 10 minutes before serving.

Nutrition value/serving: calories 412, fat 24.1, fiber 0.7, carbs 3.4, protein 43.9

397. Coconut Chicken Tenders

Preparation Time: 10 minutes
Cooking time: 5 minutes
Servings: 2

Ingredients:

- 6 oz chicken fillet
- 1 teaspoon salt
- 1 teaspoon ground black pepper
- 1 egg, whisked
- 1 tablespoon heavy cream
- 1/3 cup coconut flakes
- 1 tablespoon butter

Directions:

1. Cut the chicken fillet into the tenders and sprinkle with the salt and ground black pepper.
2. Then mix up together heavy cream and whisked the egg.
3. Place the chicken tenders in the egg mixture and stir well.
4. Then coat every chicken tender in the coconut flakes.
5. Toss the butter in the skillet and melt it.
6. Add the chicken tenders and roast them over the high heat for 2.5 minutes from each side.

Nutrition value/serving: calories 320, fat 21.5, fiber 1.5, carbs 3.1, protein 28.1

398. Chicken Loaf

Preparation Time: 15 minutes
Cooking time: 45 minutes
Servings: 6

Ingredients:

- 2 ½ cup ground chicken
- ¼ cup white onion, minced
- 1 teaspoon garlic powder
- 2 tablespoons coconut flour
- 1 teaspoon salt
- 1 teaspoon dried oregano
- 1 teaspoon olive oil
- 1 teaspoon ground paprika

Directions:

1. In the mixing bowl, mix up together ground chicken, minced white onion, garlic powder, coconut flour, salt, dried oregano, and ground paprika.
2. Stir the mixture well with the help of the fingertips.
3. After this, brush the loaf mold with the olive oil and transfer the ground chicken mixture inside it.
4. Flatten it gently to get the shape of the loaf. Cover the chicken loaf with the foil and secure the edges.
5. Bake the chicken loaf in the preheated to the 365F oven for 45 minutes.
6. Then chill the loaf till the room temperature and remove it from the mold.
7. Slice it.

Nutrition value/serving: calories 143, fat 5.8, fiber 2.1, carbs 3.8, protein 17.8

399. Chicken Bulgogi

Preparation Time: 10 minutes
Cooking time: 20 minutes
Servings: 4

Ingredients:

- 11 oz chicken fillet
- 1 tablespoon apple cider vinegar
- 1 teaspoon minced garlic
- ½ teaspoon minced ginger
- ½ teaspoon salt
- 1 teaspoon lemon juice
- ½ teaspoon ground black pepper
- ½ teaspoon white pepper
- 1 tablespoon olive oil
- ¾ teaspoon marjoram

Directions:

1. Put olive oil in the saucepan and preheat it.

2. Then slice the chicken fillet and place it in the hot oil.
3. Sprinkle the poultry with apple cider vinegar, minced garlic, minced ginger, salt, lemon juice, ground black pepper and white pepper, and marjoram.
4. Mix up the chicken bulgogi well and cook it for 15 minutes over the medium-high heat.
5. Stir the meal from time to time during cooking.

Nutrition value/serving: calories 182, fat 9.3, fiber 0.2, carbs 0.7, protein 22.7

400. Mustard Chicken

Preparation Time: 10 minutes
Cooking time: 15 minutes
Servings:2

Ingredients:

- 1 tablespoon mustard
- 1 tablespoon apple cider vinegar
- 2 chicken thighs, boneless, skinless
- ½ teaspoon ground black pepper
- 1 tablespoon sesame oil

Directions:

1. Mix up together mustard, apple cider vinegar, ground black pepper, and sesame oil.
2. Brush the chicken thighs in the mustard mixture and massage well.
3. Then preheat grill to 380F.
4. Place the chicken thighs in the grill and cook for 6 minutes from each side.

Nutrition value/serving: calories 367, fat 19.3, fiber 1, carbs 2.4, protein 43.7

401. Fajitas

Preparation Time: 15 minutes
Cooking time: 15 minutes
Servings:4

Ingredients:

- 9 oz chicken fillet
- 4 keto tortillas
- 1 bell pepper
- 1 white onion, sliced
- 1 teaspoon ground paprika
- 1 teaspoon salt
- 1 tablespoon ghee
- ¼ teaspoon Taco seasoning

Directions:

1. Slice the chicken.
2. Cut the bell pepper into the wedges.
3. Put ghee in the skillet and melt it.
4. Add chicken and sprinkle it with Taco seasoning. Stir well.
5. Cook the chicken for 10 minutes. Stir it from time to time.
6. After this, add sliced onion and bell pepper. Mix up well.
7. Roast the ingredients for 5 minutes more.
8. Fill the keto tortillas with the chicken mixture and fold them.

Nutrition value/serving: calories 324, fat 16.1, fiber 5.2, carbs 13.6, protein 31.2

402. Glazed Duck Breast

Preparation Time: 10 minutes
Cooking time: 40 minutes
Servings:6

Ingredients:

- 2-pound duck breast, skinless, boneless
- 2 tablespoons Erythritol
- 1 tablespoon butter
- 1 tablespoon lemon juice
- 1 tablespoon ground black pepper
- 1 teaspoon salt
- 1 teaspoon olive oil
- 1 teaspoon ground paprika
- ½ teaspoon chili flakes
- 2 tablespoons cream cheese

Directions:

1. Put olive oil in the skillet.
2. Sprinkle the duck breast with lemon juice, ground black pepper, salt, chili flakes, and ground paprika.
3. Put the duck breast in the skillet and roast it on the high heat for 7 minutes from each side.
4. After this, transfer the chicken breast in

the oven and cook for 15 minutes at 375F.
5. Meanwhile, toss the butter in the skillet, add Erythritol and melt the mixture.
6. When the duck breast is cooked, transfer it in the melted sweet mixture and stir well to coat all breast with sweet liquid.
7. Roast the duck breast for 3-4 minutes over the high heat.
8. Slice the cooked duck breast and sprinkle with the sweet liquid.

Nutrition value/serving: calories 235, fat 10, fiber 0.4, carbs 1, protein 33.7

403. Duck Confit

Preparation Time: 15 minutes
Cooking time: 25 minutes
Servings: 2

Ingredients:

- ¼ teaspoon cumin seeds
- 1/3 teaspoon coriander
- 1 teaspoon of sea salt
- 2 duck legs
- 1 tablespoon duck fat
- 1 teaspoon minced garlic
- 1 oz blackberries

Directions:

1. Blend the blackberries with minced garlic, sea salt, coriander, and cumin seeds.
2. When the mixture is smooth, transfer it in the mixing bowl.
3. Add duck legs and coat them well.
4. Let the duck legs stay for 10 minutes to marinate.
5. Meanwhile, line the baking tray with the parchment.
6. Transfer the marinated duck legs in the baking tray and sprinkle with the remaining blackberries marinade.
7. Bake the duck in the preheated to 375F oven for 25 minutes.
8. Check if the duck meat is tender and transfer the meal in the serving plates.

Nutrition value/serving: calories 199, fat 11, fiber 0.8, carbs 1.9, protein 22.2

404. Duck Drumsticks with Blackberry Sauce

Preparation Time: 10 minutes
Cooking time: 25 minutes
Servings: 4

Ingredients:

- 1/3 cup blackberries
- 1 teaspoon ground paprika
- 1 tablespoon butter
- 3 tablespoons water
- 1 teaspoon Erythritol
- 4 duck drumsticks
- 1 teaspoon olive oil
- 1 teaspoon ground thyme
- ½ teaspoon turmeric
- ¾ cup of coconut milk

Directions:

1. Sprinkle the duck drumsticks with the ground paprika, ground thyme, and turmeric.
2. Place the olive oil in the skillet.
3. Add duck drumsticks and roast them for 15 minutes over the medium heat.
4. Meanwhile, make the blackberry sauce: blend together blackberries, water, Erythritol, butter, and coconut milk.
5. When the mixture is smooth, it is cooked.
6. Pour the sauce over the roasted duck drumsticks. Mix up well with the help of the spatula.
7. Close the lid and cook the meal for 10 minutes more over the low heat.
8. Serve the cooked duck drumsticks with the hot sauce.

Nutrition value/serving: calories 358, fat 27, fiber 2, carbs 5.4, protein 24.4

405. Oregano Roasted Duck

Preparation Time: 15 minutes
Cooking time: 2 hours
Servings: 6

Ingredients:

- 2-pound whole duck
- 1 tablespoon dried oregano

- 1 teaspoon cumin seeds
- 1 tablespoon butter
- 1 teaspoon orange zest, grated
- 1 teaspoon ground black pepper
- 1 teaspoon salt
- 1 teaspoon chili flakes
- ½ teaspoon garlic powder
- 1 tablespoon olive oil

Directions:
1. In the shallow bowl, mix up together dried oregano, cumin seeds, butter, orange zest, ground black pepper, salt, chili flakes, garlic powder, and olive oil.
2. Then rub the duck with this mixture well.
3. Put all the remaining spice mixture inside the duck.
4. Wrap the duck in foil and place in the baking tray.
5. Bake the duck for 2 hours at 365F.
6. When the duck is cooked, switch off the oven and let it rest for 20 minutes. Then discard the foil and slice the duck into the servings.

Nutrition value/serving: calories 243, fat 13.4, fiber 0.5, carbs 1.1, protein 27.9

406. Crispy Duck Skin

Preparation Time: 10 minutes
Cooking time: 10 minutes
Servings: 4

Ingredients:
- 8 oz duck skin
- 1 teaspoon ground paprika
- ¾ teaspoon ground turmeric
- ½ teaspoon salt
- 1 tablespoon ghee

Directions:
1. Cut the duck skin into the servings.
2. Mix up together duck skin, ground paprika, ground turmeric, and salt.
3. Toss ghee in the skillet and melt it.
4. Then add prepared duck skin and roast it for approximately 10 minutes or until it is crunchy. Stir the duck skin from time to time.

Nutrition value/serving: calories 288, fat 26.4, fiber 0.3, carbs 0.6, protein 11.7

407. Keto Duck de Marietta

Preparation Time: 15 minutes
Cooking time: 2.5 hours
Servings: 4

Ingredients:
- 1 duck (12 oz
- ¼ cup strawberries
- ¾ cup blackberries
- 1 tablespoon lemon juice
- ½ teaspoon ground paprika
- 1 teaspoon of sea salt

Directions:
1. Fill the duck with strawberries and blackberries.
2. Then secure the duck hole with toothpicks.
3. Rub the duck with the ground paprika and sea salt, and sprinkle with lemon juice.
4. Bake the duck in the preheated to the 375F oven for 2.5 hours.
5. When the duck is cooked, cut it into the pieces and grill for 10 minutes more.

Nutrition value/serving: calories 127, fat 6.4, fiber 1.7, carbs 3.5, protein 13.5

408. Duck Pate

Preparation Time: 15 minutes
Cooking time: 15 minutes
Servings: 6

Ingredients:
- 11 oz duck liver
- 3 tablespoons butter
- 1 teaspoon coconut oil
- ½ white onion, diced
- 1 teaspoon salt
- ½ teaspoon chili powder
- 1 cup water, for cooking
- 1 bay leaf

Directions:

Boil the duck liver in the water with the bay leaf for 15 minutes. When the duck liver is soft, it is cooked.
Drain the water and discard the bay leaf.
Transfer the hot duck liver in the blender.
Add butter, chili powder, and salt. Blend the mixture until smooth.
After this, fry the diced onion in the coconut oil until it is translucent.
Add the onion in the liver mixture and pulse it for 10 seconds.
Transfer the cooked pate in the bowl and flatten the surface well.
Let the cooked pate chill well before serving.

Nutrition value/serving: calories 133, fat 9, fiber 0.3, carbs 2.8, protein 9.9

409. Soft Chicken Pate

Preparation Time: 15 minutes
Cooking time: 15 minutes
Servings: 6

Ingredients:

- 1-pound chicken breast, skinless, boneless
- 1 tablespoon butter
- ¾ cup heavy cream
- 1 tablespoon cream cheese
- 1 teaspoon salt
- 1 teaspoon ground paprika
- ¾ teaspoon white pepper
- 1 cup of water

Directions:

1. Boil chicken breast in the water for 15 minutes or until it is soft.
2. Meanwhile, toss the butter in the saucepan and melt it.
3. Add heavy cream, cream cheese, salt, ground paprika, and white pepper.
4. Bring the mixture to boil and remove it from the heat.
5. When the chicken breast is cooked, drain the water.
6. Blend the chicken breast until it is smooth.
7. Then add cream cheese mixture and blend the pate for 30 seconds more.
8. Transfer the cooked pate in the serving bowl.

Nutrition value/serving: calories 162, fat 10, fiber 0.2, carbs 0.8, protein 16.6

410. Cardamom Chicken Breast

Preparation Time: 10 minutes
Cooking time: 30 minutes
Servings: 2

Ingredients:

- 1 teaspoon ground cardamom
- 1 teaspoon chili flakes
- 10 oz chicken breast, skinless, boneless
- ½ teaspoon ground cinnamon
- 1 tablespoon coconut oil

Directions:

1. Rub the chicken breast with the ground cardamom, chili flakes, and ground cinnamon.
2. Then sprinkle the chicken breast with the coconut oil and transfer in the skillet.
3. Cook the chicken breast for 30 minutes at 365F.
4. The cooked chicken breast should have a light brown color.

Nutrition value/serving: calories 225, fat 10.4, fiber 0.6, carbs 1.2, protein 30.2

411. Balsamic Chicken Thighs

Preparation Time: 10 minutes
Cooking time: 25 minutes
Servings: 5

Ingredients:

- 5 chicken thighs, boneless, skinless
- 4 tablespoon balsamic vinegar
- ½ cup of water
- 1 tablespoon olive oil
- ½ teaspoon chili powder
- 2 garlic cloves, peeled
- ½ teaspoon salt
- 1 green pepper, chopped

Directions:

1. Place the chicken thighs in the saucepan.
2. Add balsamic vinegar, water, olive oil,

chili powder, peeled garlic cloves, salt, and chopped green pepper. Stir it gently and leave overnight to marinate.
3. Then cook the chicken thighs mixture with the closed lid for 25 minutes.
4. Serve the cooked meal with the remaining balsamic vinegar liquid from the saucepan.

Nutrition value/serving: calories 159, fat 9.9, fiber 0.1, carbs 0.7, protein 19.1

Meat

412. Sausage Casserole

Preparation Time: 60 minutes
Servings: 6

Ingredients:

- 6 sausage
- 2 green bell peppers; chopped
- 3 sweet potatoes; chopped
- 1-pint grape tomatoes; chopped
- A pinch of sea salt
- Black pepper to the taste
- 2 garlic cloves; minced
- 1 red onion; chopped
- A few thyme springs

Instructions:

1. In a baking dish, mix potatoes with tomatoes, onion, bell pepper, garlic, a pinch of sea salt and pepper and stir gently.
2. Heat up a pan over high heat, add sausages, brown them for 2 minutes on each side and transfer on top of veggies in the baking dish.
3. Add thyme, introduce in the oven at 400 °F and bake for 45 minutes. Divide between plates and serve hot.

Nutrition: Calories: 355; Fat: 10g; Carbs: 25g; Fiber: 2g; Protein: 16g

413. Mexican Steaks

Preparation Time: 25 minutes
Servings: 4

Ingredients:

- 2 tbsp. chili powder
- 4 medium sirloin steaks
- 1 tsp. cumin; ground
- 1/2 tbsp. sweet paprika
- 1 tsp. onion powder
- 1 tsp. garlic powder
- A pinch of sea salt and black pepper to the taste

For the Pico de gallo:

- 1 small red onion; chopped
- 2 tomatoes; chopped
- 2 garlic cloves; minced
- 2 tbsp. lime juice
- 1 small green bell pepper; chopped
- 1 jalapeno; chopped
- 1/4 cup cilantro; chopped
- 1/4 tsp. cumin; ground
- Black pepper to the taste

Instructions:

1. In a bowl; mix chili powder with a pinch of salt, black pepper, onion powder, garlic powder, paprika and 1 tsp. cumin and stir well.
2. Season steaks with this mix, rub well and place them on preheated grill over medium high heat.
3. Cook steaks for 5 minutes on each side and divide them between plates.
4. In a bowl; mix red onion with tomatoes, garlic, lime juice, bell pepper, jalapeno, cilantro, black pepper to the taste and 1/4 tsp. cumin and stir well. Top steaks with this mix and serve.

Nutrition: Calories: 200; Fat: 12g; Fiber: 4g; Carbs: 5g; Protein: 12g

414. Beef Tenderloin With Special Sauce

Preparation Time: 50 minutes
Servings: 4

Ingredients:

- 3 tbsp. Dijon mustard
- 3 lbs. beef tenderloin
- A pinch of sea salt
- Black pepper to the taste
- 1 tbsp. coconut oil
- 3 tbsp. balsamic vinegar
- For the sauce:
- 3 tbsp. basil leaves; chopped
- 1/2 cup parsley leaves; chopped
- Zest from 1 lemon

- 2 garlic cloves; finely chopped
- A pinch of sea salt
- Black pepper to the taste
- 1/4 cup extra virgin olive oil

Instructions:

1. In a bowl; mix mustard with vinegar, stir very well and leave aside.
2. Season beef with a pinch of sea salt and pepper to the taste put in a pan heated with the coconut oil over medium-high heat and cook for 2 minutes on each side.
3. Transfer beef to a baking pan, cover with the mustard mix, introduce in the oven at 475 °F and bake for 25 minutes.
4. Meanwhile; in a bowl, mix parsley with basil, lemon zest, garlic, olive oil, a pinch of sea salt and pepper to the taste and whisk very well.
5. Take beef tenderloin out if the oven, leave aside for a few minutes to cool down, slice and divide between plates. Serve with herbs sauce on the side.

Nutrition: Calories: 180; Fat: 13g; Carbs: 2g; Fiber: 2g; Protein: 7g

415. Roasted Duck Dish

Preparation Time: 2 hours 10 minutes
Servings: 4

Ingredients:

- 2 tsp. allspice; ground
- 4 duck legs
- 4 thyme springs
- 1 lemon; sliced
- 1 orange; sliced
- 1 cup chicken broth
- A pinch of sea salt
- Black pepper to the taste
- 1/2 cup orange juice

Instructions:

1. Heat up a pan over medium high heat, add duck legs, season with a pinch of salt and pepper to the taste and brown them for 3 minutes on each side.
2. Arrange half of lemon and orange slices on the bottom of a baking dish, place duck legs, top with the rest of the orange and lemon slices and thyme springs.
3. Add chicken stock, orange juice, sprinkle allspice, introduce in the oven at 350 °F and bake for 2 hours. Divide between plates and serve hot.

Nutrition: 255; Fat: 17g; Carbs: 6g; Protein: 33g; Fiber: 1

416. Steaks And Scallops

Preparation Time: 30 minutes
Servings: 2

Ingredients:

- 10 sea scallops
- 4 garlic cloves; minced
- 2 beef steaks
- 1 shallot; chopped
- 2 tbsp. lemon juice
- 2 tbsp. parsley; chopped
- 2 tbsp. basil; chopped
- 1 tsp. lemon zest
- 1/4 cup ghee
- 1/4 cup veggie stock
- Some bacon fat
- A pinch of sea salt
- Black pepper to the taste

Instructions:

1. Heat up a pan with some bacon fat over medium high heat, add steaks, season them with a pinch of salt and black pepper to the taste and cook for 4 minutes on each side.
2. Add shallot and garlic, stir and cook for 2 minutes more.
3. Add ghee and stir everything.
4. Add stock, basil, lemon juice, parsley and lemon zest and stir.
5. Add scallops, season them with some black pepper as well and cook for a couple more minutes. Divide steaks and scallops between plates and serve with pan juices.

Nutrition: Calories: 150; Fat: 2g; Fiber: 2g; Carbs: 4g; Protein: 14g

417. Beef Stir Fry

Preparation Time: 30 minutes
Servings: 4

Ingredients:

- 10 oz. mushrooms; sliced
- 10 oz. asparagus; sliced
- 1½ lbs. beef steak; thinly sliced
- 2 tbsp. honey
- 1/3 cup coconut amino
- 2 tsp. apple cider vinegar
- 1/2 tsp. ginger; minced
- 6 garlic cloves; minced
- 1 chili; sliced
- 1 tbsp. coconut oil
- Black pepper to the taste

Instructions:

1. In a bowl; mix garlic with coconut amino, honey, ginger and vinegar and whisk well.
2. Put some water in a pan, heat up over medium high heat, add asparagus and black pepper, cook for 3 minutes, transfer to a bowl filled with ice water, drain and leave aside.
3. Heat up a pan with the oil over medium-high heat, add mushrooms, cook for 2 minutes on each side, transfer to a bowl and also leave aside.
4. Heat up the same pan over high heat, add meat, brown for a few minutes and mix with chili pepper.
5. Cook for 2 more minutes and mix with asparagus, mushrooms and vinegar sauce you've made at the beginning. Stir well, cook for 3 minutes, take off heat, divide between plates and serve.

Nutrition: Calories: 165; Fat: 7.2g; Carbs: 6.33g; Fiber: 1.3; Sugar: 3g; Protein: 18.4

418. Pork With Pear Salsa

Preparation Time: 55 minutes
Servings: 4

Ingredients:

- 1 yellow onion; chopped
- 1 organic pork tenderloin
- 2 pears; chopped
- 2 garlic cloves; minced
- 1 tbsp. chives; chopped
- 1/4 cup walnuts; chopped
- 3 tbsp. balsamic vinegar
- Black pepper to the taste
- 1/2 cup chicken stock
- 1 tbsp. coconut oil
- 1 tbsp. lemon juice

Instructions:

1. In a bowl; mix walnuts with pear, chives, pepper and lemon juice and stir well.
2. Heat up a pan with the oil over medium high heat, add tenderloin and brown for 3 minutes on each side.
3. Reduce heat, add onion and garlic, stir and cook for 2 minutes. Add balsamic vinegar, stock, pear mix, stir; introduce in the oven at 400 °F and bake for 20 minutes.
4. Take pork out of the oven, leave aside for 4 minutes, slice, divide between plates and serve with pear salsa on top.

Nutrition: Calories: 170; Fat: 3g; Carbs: 19g; Fiber: 4.4; Sugar: 10g; Protein: 12g

419. Pork Tenderloin with Carrot Puree

Preparation Time: 55 minutes
Servings: 4

Ingredients:

- 2 sausages; casings removed
- A handful arugula
- Black pepper to the taste
- 1 grass fed pork tenderloin
- 1 tbsp. coconut oil
- For the puree:
- 1 sweet potato; chopped
- 3 carrots; chopped
- A pinch of sea salt
- Black pepper to the taste
- 1 tbsp. curry paste
- For the sauce:
- 2 tbsp. balsamic vinegar
- 1 tsp. mustard

- 2 shallots; finely chopped
- Black pepper to the taste
- 4 tbsp. extra virgin olive oil

Instructions:
1. Slice pork tenderloin in half horizontally but not all the way and open it up.
2. Use a meat tenderizer to even it up.
3. Place sausage in the middle, roll pork around it, tie with twine, season pepper to the taste and leave aside.
4. Heat up an oven proof pan with the coconut oil over medium high heat, add pork roll, cook for 3 minutes on each side, introduce in the oven at 350 °F and bake for 25 minutes.
5. Meanwhile; put potatoes and carrots in a pot, add water to cover, bring to a boil over medium high heat, cook for 20 minutes, drain and transfer to your food processor.
6. Pulse a few times until you obtain a puree, add a pinch of sea salt and pepper to the taste, blend again, transfer to a bowl and leave aside.
7. Take pork roll out of the oven, slice and divide between plates.
8. Heat up a pan with the olive oil over medium high heat, add shallots, stir and cook for 10 minutes.
9. Add balsamic vinegar, mustard, pepper, stir well and take off heat. Divide carrots puree next to pork slices, drizzle vinegar sauce on to and serve with arugula on the side.

Nutrition: Calories: 250; Fat: 34g; Carbs: 19g; Fiber: 2g; Protein: 53

420. Pork with Strawberry Sauce

Preparation Time: 45 minutes
Servings: 4

Ingredients:
- 4 lbs. pork tenderloin
- 1 cup strawberries; sliced
- 10 bacon slices
- A pinch of sea salt
- Black pepper to the taste
- 4 garlic cloves; minced
- 1/2 cup balsamic vinegar
- 2 tbsp. extra virgin olive oil

Instructions:
1. Wrap bacon slices around tenderloin, secure with toothpicks and season with salt and pepper.
2. Heat up your grill over indirect medium high heat, put tenderloin on it and cook for 30 minutes.
3. Heat up a pan with the oil over medium high heat, add garlic, stir and cook for 2 minutes.
4. Add vinegar and half of the strawberries, stir and bring to a boil.
5. Reduce heat to medium and simmer for 10 minutes.
6. Add black pepper to the taste and the rest of the strawberries and stir.
7. Baste pork with some of the sauce and continue cooking over indirect heat until bacon is crispy enough.
8. Transfer pork to a cutting board, leave aside for a few minutes to cool down, slice and divide between plates. Serve with the strawberry sauce right away.

Nutrition: Calories: 279; Fat: 30g; Carbs: 8g; Fiber: 22g; Protein: 125

421. Beef And Veggies

Preparation Time: 3 hours 10 minutes
Servings: 4

Ingredients:
- 1 yellow onion; sliced
- 3 garlic cloves; minced
- 1 cup beef stock
- 2 tbsp. coconut oil
- 3 lbs. beef; cut into cubes
- A pinch of sea salt
- Black pepper to the taste
- 8 oz. carrots; sliced
- 8 oz. mushrooms; sliced
- 1 tsp. thyme; chopped

Instructions:
1. Heat up a Dutch oven with 1 tbsp. oil

over medium high heat, add beef cubes, season with a pinch of sea salt and black pepper, brown for 2 minutes on each side and transfer to a bowl.
2. Heat up the same Dutch oven over medium heat, add garlic, stir and cook for 2 minutes.
3. Add stock, stir well and heat it up.
4. Return meat to the pot, stir; place in the oven at 250 °F and roast for 3 hours.
5. In a bowl; mix carrots with mushrooms, 1 tbsp. oil, a pinch of sea salt, black pepper to the taste and thyme and stir well.
6. Spread these into a pan, place in the oven at 250 °F and roast them for 15 minutes. Divide beef and juices between plates and serve with roasted veggies on the side.

Nutrition: Calories: 200; Fat: 3g; Fiber: 4g; Carbs: 7g; Protein: 20g

422. Chicken Meatballs

Preparation Time: 30 minutes
Servings: 4

Ingredients:

- 1 tsp. sweet paprika
- 1 pineapple; diced
- 1 egg
- 2 lbs. chicken meat; ground
- A pinch of sea salt
- Black pepper to the taste
- 1 tsp. garlic powder
- 1 tsp. onion powder
- For the sauce:
- 1/4 cup coconut amino
- 4 tbsp. ketchup
- 1 tbsp. ginger; grated
- 1/2 cup pineapple juice
- 2 tsp. raw honey
- 1/2 tsp. red pepper flakes
- Salt and black pepper to the taste
- 1 tbsp. garlic; minced

Instructions:

1. In a pot, mix amino with ketchup, ginger, pineapple sauce, garlic, pepper flakes, honey, a pinch of sea salt and pepper to the taste, stir well, bring to a boil over medium heat, simmer for 8 minutes and take off heat.
2. In a bowl; mix chicken meat with paprika, egg, onion powder, garlic powder, salt and black pepper to the taste and stir well.
3. Shape meatballs, arrange them on a lined baking sheet, introduce them in the oven at 475 °F and bake for 15 minutes.
4. Heat up a pan over medium heat, add pineapple pieces, stir and cook for 2 minutes.
5. Add baked meatballs, pour sauce you've made at the beginnings, stir gently, cook for 5 minutes, divide between plates and serve.

Nutrition: Calories: 264; Fat: 20g; Carbs: 47g; Fiber: 2g; Protein: 47

423. Chicken And Veggies Stir Fry

Preparation Time: 35 minutes
Servings: 4

Ingredients:

- 1 red bell pepper; chopped
- 1 zucchini; chopped
- 1 yellow onion; finely chopped
- 1 broccoli head; florets separated
- 4 chicken breasts; skinless, boneless and chopped
- A pinch of sea salt
- Black pepper to the taste
- 1 tbsp. coconut oil

For the sauce:

- 1/4 cup chicken broth
- 2 garlic cloves; finely chopped
- 3 tbsp. coconut amino
- 1/2 cup orange juice
- 1 tbsp. orange zest
- 1 tsp. Sriracha sauce
- 1/4 tsp. ginger; grated
- A pinch of red pepper flakes

Instructions:

1. In a bowl; mix broth with orange juice, zest, amino, ginger, garlic, pepper flakes and Sriracha sauce and stir well.

2. Heat up a pan with the oil over medium heat, add chicken, cook for 8 minutes and transfer to a plate.
3. Heat up the same pan over medium heat, add bell pepper, broccoli florets, onion and zucchini, stir and cook for 4-5 minutes.
4. Add a pinch of sea salt, pepper, orange sauce you've made, stir; bring to a boil, add chicken, reduce heat and simmer for 8 minutes. Divide between plates and serve hot.

Nutrition: Calories: 320; Fat: 13g; Carbs: 17g; Protein: 45g; Fiber: 3.7; Sugar: 4

424. Beef And Brussels Sprouts

Preparation Time: 22 minutes
Servings: 4

Ingredients:

- 1 lb. beef; ground
- 1 apple; cored, peeled and chopped
- 1 yellow onion; chopped
- 3 cups Brussels sprouts; shredded
- A pinch of sea salt
- Black pepper to the taste
- 3 tbsp. ghee

Instructions:

1. Heat up a pan with the ghee over medium high heat, add beef, stir and brown for 2 minutes.
2. Add Brussels sprouts, stir and cook for 3 minutes more.
3. Add onion and apple, stir and cook for 5 minutes more.
4. Add a pinch of sea salt and black pepper to the taste, stir; cook for 1 minute more, divide among plates and serve.

Nutrition: Calories: 150; Fat: 1g; Fiber: 2g; Carbs: 3g; Protein: 9g

425. Steaks And Apricots

Preparation Time: 35 minutes
Servings: 2

Ingredients:

- 2 tbsp. Cajun spice
- 1/4 cup coconut oil
- 2 medium skirt steaks
- 1/3 cup lemon juice
- 1/4 cup apricot preserves
- 1/4 cup coconut aminos

Instructions:

1. In a bowl; mix half of the Cajun spice with lemon juice, aminos, oil and apricot preserves and stir well.
2. Pour this into a pan, bring to a boil over medium high heat and simmer for 8 minutes.
3. Blend this using an immersion blender and leave aside for now.
4. Season steaks with the rest of the Cajun spice, brush them with half of the apricots mix, place them on preheated grill over medium high heat and cook them for 6-minute son each side. Divide steaks on plates and top with the rest of the apricots mix.

Nutrition: Calories: 160; Fat: 6g; Fiber: 0.1g; Carbs: 1g; Protein: 22g

426. Beef And Wonderful Gravy

Preparation Time: 30 minutes
Servings: 4

Ingredients:

- 1 egg; whisked
- 1 tbsp. mustard
- 1 tbsp. tomato paste
- 1 tsp. garlic powder
- 1 tsp. onion powder
- Some coconut oil for cooking
- A pinch of sea salt and black pepper to the taste
- 1½ lb. beef; ground

For the gravy:

- 2 tsp. parsley; chopped
- 2 tbsp. ghee
- 1 tsp. tapioca
- 1 small yellow onion; chopped
- 1¼ cups beef stock
- Black pepper to the taste

Instructions:

1. In a bowl; mix beef with tomato paste, egg, mustard, onion powder, garlic powder, a pinch of salt and black pepper to the taste and stir well.
2. Heat up a pan with the ghee over medium heat, add onion, stir and cook for 2 minutes.
3. Add stock, some black pepper, tapioca mixed with water, stir; cook until it thickens and take off heat.
4. Shape 4 patties from the beef mix. Heat up a pan with the coconut oil over medium high heat, add beef patties and cook for 5 minutes on each side.
5. Pour the gravy over beef patties, sprinkle parsley on top, cook for a couple more minutes, divide between plates and serve.

Nutrition: Calories: 200; Fat: 4g; Fiber: 2g; Carbs: 4g; Protein: 20g

427. Sheppard's Pie

Preparation Time: 60 minutes
Servings: 6

Ingredients:

- 2 lbs. sweet potatoes; chopped
- 1½ lbs. beef; ground
- 2 cups beef stock
- 1 onion; chopped
- 2 carrots; chopped
- 2 thyme springs
- 2 bay leaves
- 2 garlic cloves; minced
- 2 celery stalks; chopped
- 1/4 cup ghee
- Bacon fat
- A handful parsley; chopped
- 2 tbsp. tomato paste
- A pinch of sea salt
- Black pepper to the taste

Instructions:

1. Put sweet potatoes in a pot, add water to cover, bring to a boil over medium high heat, cook for 20 minutes, drain, leave them to cool down and transfer to a bowl.
2. Add ghee, a pinch of salt and pepper and mash potatoes well.
3. Heat up a pan with the bacon fat over medium high heat, add beef, stir and cook for a couple of minutes.
4. Add carrots, garlic, onions, celery, stock, tomato paste, bay leaves, thyme springs, some black pepper and another pinch of salt, stir and cook for 10 minutes.
5. Discard bay leaves and thyme and spread beef mix on the bottom of a baking dish.
6. Top with mashed potatoes, spread well, place in the oven at 375 °F and bake for 25 minutes. Leave pie to cool down a bit before slicing and serving it.

Nutrition: Calories: 254; Fat: 7g; Fiber: 4g; Carbs: 7g; Protein: 14g

428. Barbeque Ribs

Preparation Time: 3 hour 2 minutes
Servings: 4

Ingredients:

- 1 tbsp. smoked paprika
- 1/2 tbsp. onion powder
- 1/2 tbsp. garlic powder
- 1/2 tsp. cayenne pepper
- 4 lbs. baby ribs
- 1 cup paleo BBQ sauce
- 2 tbsp. raw honey
- 4 tsp. Sriracha
- 1/4 cup cilantro; chopped
- 1/4 cup chives; chopped
- 1/4 cup parsley; chopped
- Black pepper to the taste

Instructions:

1. In a bowl; mix paprika with onion powder, garlic powder, pepper and cayenne and stir well.
2. Add ribs, toss to coat and arrange them on a lined baking sheet.
3. Introduce in the oven at 325 °F and bake them for 2 hours and 30 minutes.
4. In a bowl; mix BBQ sauce with honey and Sriracha and stir well.
5. Take ribs out of the oven, mix them with BBQ sauce, place them on preheated grill

over medium-high heat and cook for 7 minutes on each side. Divide ribs on plates, sprinkle chives, cilantro and parsley on top and serve.

Nutrition: Calories: 120; Fat: 6.4g; Carbs: 2g; Fiber: 03; Sugar: 0.3g; Protein: 6.2

429. Souvlaki

Preparation Time: 30 minutes
Servings: 4

Ingredients:

- 3 sweet potatoes; cubed
- 1 yellow onion; chopped
- 12 mini bell peppers; chopped
- 4 medium round steaks
- 1/2 cup sun dried tomatoes; chopped
- 1 tbsp. sweet paprika
- 2 tbsp. balsamic vinegar
- Juice of 1 lemon
- 1 tbsp. oregano; dried
- 1/4 cup olive oil
- 1 lemon; sliced
- 1/4 cup kalamata olives; pitted and chopped
- 4 dill springs
- 2 garlic cloves; minced
- Some bacon fat
- A pinch of sea salt and black pepper

Instructions:

1. Heat up a pan with some bacon fat over medium high heat, add steaks, season them with a pinch of sea salt and some black pepper, brown them for 2 minutes on each side and transfer to a baking dish.
2. Heat up the pan again over medium high heat, add sweet potatoes, cook them for 4 minutes and add them to the baking dish.
3. Also add bell peppers, tomatoes, onion, olives and lemon slices.
4. Meanwhile; in a bowl, mix lemon juice with olive oil, vinegar, garlic, paprika and oregano and whisk well.
5. Pour this over steak and veggies, add dill springs on top, toss to coat, place in the oven at 425 °F and bake for 12 minutes.

Divide steak and veggies between plates and serve.

Nutrition: Calories: 180; Fat: 11g; Fiber: 0g; Carbs: 0g; Protein: 21g

430. Turkey Casserole

Preparation Time: 1 hour 10 minutes
Servings: 6

Ingredients:

- 1/4 cup onion; chopped
- 1 lb. turkey meat; ground
- 1 sweet potato; cut with a spiralizer
- 1 eggplant; chopped
- 1 tbsp. garlic; minced
- 8 oz. tomato paste
- 15 oz. canned tomatoes; chopped
- A pinch of sea salt
- Black pepper to the taste
- A pinch of oregano; dried
- 1/4 tsp. chili powder
- 1/4 tsp. cumin; ground
- Cooking spray
- A pinch of cardamom; ground
- 1/2 tsp. tarragon flakes
- For the sauce:
- 1 tbsp. coconut flour
- 1 tbsp. almond flour
- 1 cup almond milk
- 1½ tbsp. olive oil

Instructions:

1. Heat up a pan over medium heat, add onion, turkey and garlic, stir and brown for a few minutes.
2. Add tomatoes, tomato paste and sweet potatoes, stir and cook for a few minutes more.
3. In a bowl; mix eggplant pieces with a pinch of sea salt, black pepper, chili powder, cumin, oregano, cardamom and tarragon flakes and stir well.
4. Spread eggplant into a baking dish after you sprayed it with some cooking spray and top with the turkey mix.
5. Place in the oven at 350 °F and bake for 15 minutes.

6. Meanwhile; heat up a pan with the oil over medium heat, add coconut and almond flour and stir for 1 minute.
7. Add almond milk and cook for 10 minutes stirring often.
8. Top turkey casserole with this sauce, place in the oven again and bake for 40 minutes more. Slice and serve hot.

Nutrition: Calories: 278; Fat: 3g; Fiber: 7g; Carbs: 9g; Protein: 18g

431. Moroccan Lamb

Preparation Time: 17 minutes
Servings: 4

Ingredients:
- 8 lamb chops
- 2 tbsp. ras el hanout
- 1 tsp. olive oil
- For the sauce:
- 1/4 cup parsley; chopped
- 2 tbsp. mint; chopped
- 3 garlic cloves; minced
- 2 tbsp. lemon zest
- 1/4 cup olive oil
- 1/2 tsp. smoked paprika
- 1 tsp. red pepper flakes
- 2 tbsp. lemon juice
- A pinch of sea salt
- Black pepper to the taste

Instructions:
1. Rub lamb chops with ras el hanout and 1 tsp. oil, place them on preheated grill over medium high heat, cook them for 2 minutes on each side and divide them between plates.
2. In your food processor, mix parsley with mint, garlic, lemon zest, 1/4 cup oil, paprika, pepper flakes, lemon juice, a pinch of salt and black pepper and pulse really well. Drizzle this over lamb chops and serve.

Nutrition: Calories: 400; Fat: 23g; Fiber: 1g; Carbs: 3g; Protein: 32

432. Carne Asada

Preparation Time: 55 minutes
Servings: 2

Ingredients:
- 1/4 cup olive oil
- 1/2 tsp. oregano; dried
- 2 garlic cloves; minced
- Juice from 1 lime
- 2 skirt steaks
- 1/4 tsp. cumin; ground
- 1 Serrano chili pepper; minced
- 1/4 cup cilantro; chopped
- A pinch of sea salt
- Black pepper to the taste

For the veggie mix:
- 2 red bell peppers; chopped
- 3 Portobello mushrooms; sliced
- 1 yellow onion; chopped
- 1 tbsp. olive oil
- 1 tbsp. lime juice
- 1 tbsp. taco seasoning

Instructions:
1. In a bowl; mix 1/4 cup oil with oregano, garlic, lime juice, cumin, cilantro, chili pepper, a pinch of salt and black pepper and whisk very well.
2. Add steaks, toss to coat and keep in the fridge for 30 minutes.
3. Place steaks on preheated grill over medium high heat, cook them for 4 minutes on each side and transfer to a plate.
4. Heat up a pan with 1 tbsp. oil over medium high heat, add bell pepper and onion, stir and cook for 3 minutes,
5. Add mushrooms, taco seasoning and lime juice, stir and cook for 6 minutes more. Divide steaks between plates and serve with mixed veggies on the side.

Nutrition: Calories: 190; Fat: 2g; Fiber: 1g; Carbs: 4g; Protein: 20g

433. Steak And Blueberry Sauce

Preparation Time: 30 minutes
Servings: 4

Ingredients:

- 1 cup beef stock
- 2 tbsp. shallots; chopped
- 2 garlic cloves; minced
- 1 cup blueberries
- 4 medium flank steaks
- 2 tbsp. ghee
- 1 tsp. thyme; chopped
- A pinch of sea salt
- Black pepper to the taste

Instructions:
1. Heat up a pan with the ghee over medium heat, add shallot and garlic, stir and cook for 4 minutes.
2. Add thyme, stock, a pinch of salt and black pepper, stir; bring to a simmer and cook for 10 minutes.
3. Add blueberries, stir and cook for 2 minutes more.
4. Place steaks on preheated grill over medium high heat, cook for 4 minutes son each side and transfer to plates. Drizzle the blueberry sauce on top and serve them.

Nutrition: Calories: 170; Fat: 4g; Fiber: 3g; Carbs: 7g; Protein: 15g

434. Filet Mignon And Special Sauce

Preparation Time: 35 minutes
Servings: 4

Ingredients:

- 12 mushrooms; sliced
- 1 shallot; chopped
- 4 fillet mignons
- 2 garlic cloves; minced
- 2 tbsp. olive oil
- 1/4 cup Dijon mustard
- 1/4 cup wine
- 1¼ cup coconut cream
- 2 tbsp. parsley; chopped
- Black pepper to the taste
- A pinch of sea salt

Instructions:
1. Heat up a pan with the oil over medium high heat, add garlic and shallots, stir and cook for 3 minutes.
2. Add mushrooms, stir and cook for 4 minutes more.
3. Add wine, stir and cook until it evaporates.
4. Add coconut cream, mustard, parsley, a pinch of salt and black pepper to the taste, stir and cook for 6 minutes more.
5. Heat up another pan over high heat, add fillets, season them with a pinch of salt and some black pepper and cook them for 4 minutes on each side. Divide fillets between plates and serve with the mushroom sauce on top.

Nutrition: Calories: 300; Fat: 12g; Fiber: 1g; Carbs: 4g; Protein: 23g

435. Veal Rolls

Preparation Time: 30 minutes
Servings: 4

Ingredients:

- 2 zucchinis; cut in quarters
- 8 veal scallops
- 2 tbsp. olive oil
- 2 tsp. garlic powder
- 1/4 cup balsamic vinegar
- A pinch of sea salt
- Black pepper to the taste

Instructions:
1. Flatten veal scallops with a meat tenderizer, season them with a pinch of sea salt and black pepper to the taste and leave aside.
2. Season zucchini with a pinch of sea salt, black pepper and garlic powder, place on preheated grill over medium high heat, cook for 2 minutes on each side and transfer to a working surface.
3. Roll veal around each zucchini piece.
4. In a bowl; mix oil with balsamic vinegar and whisk well.
5. Brush veal rolls with this mix, place them on your grill and cook for 3 minutes on each side. Serve right away.

Nutrition: Calories: 160; Fat: 3g; Fiber: 2g; Carbs: 5g; Protein: 14g

436. Roasted Lamb

Preparation Time: 2 hours 40 minutes
Servings: 4

Ingredients:

- 15 garlic cloves; peeled
- 2 tsp. onion powder
- 6 lamb shanks
- 2 tsp. cumin powder
- 1 cup water
- 3 tsp. oregano; dried
- 1/2 cup olive oil
- A pinch of sea salt
- Black pepper to the taste
- 1/2 cup lemon juice

Instructions:

1. Place garlic cloves in a roasting pan.
2. Add lamb on top, drizzle half of the oil and season with a pinch of salt and black pepper.
3. Also add onion powder and cumin and rub well.
4. Introduce this in the oven at 450 °F and roast for 35 minutes.
5. In a bowl mix the rest of the oil with the water, lemon juice and oregano and whisk very well.
6. Take lamb shanks out of the oven, drizzle this mix, toss to coat well and roast in the oven at 350 °F for 2 hours and 30 minutes. Divide lamb pieces between plates and serve.

Nutrition: Calories: 170; Fat: 2g; Fiber: 2g; Carbs: 4g; Protein: 12g

437. Beef Curry

Preparation Time: 45 minutes
Servings: 4

Ingredients:

- 1 tsp. mustard seeds
- 2 tbsp. coconut oil
- 2 curry leaves
- 1 Serrano pepper; chopped
- 1 onion; chopped
- 1 tbsp. garlic; minced
- 1/4 cup water
- 2 tsp. garam masala
- 1 small ginger piece; grated
- 1/4 tsp. chili powder
- 1/2 tsp. turmeric powder
- 1 tsp. coriander powder
- 1 lb. beef; ground
- A pinch of sea salt
- Black pepper to the taste
- 3 carrot; chopped
- 10 oz. canned coconut milk

Instructions:

1. Heat up a pan with the oil over medium high heat, add mustard seeds, stir and toast them for 1 minute.
2. Add Serrano pepper, onion and curry leaves, stir and cook for 5 minutes.
3. Add ginger and garlic, stir and cook for 1 minute.
4. Add beef, a pinch of salt, black pepper, coriander powder, turmeric, chili and garam masala, stir and cook for 10 minutes.
5. Add carrot and 1/4 cup water, stir and cook for 5 minutes more.
6. Add coconut milk, stir well and cook for 15 minutes. Divide curry into bowls and serve.

Nutrition: Calories: 260; Fat: 4g; Fiber: 5g; Carbs: 9g; Protein: 14g

438. Beef Teriyaki

Preparation Time: 30 minutes
Servings: 4

Ingredients:

- 2 green onions; chopped
- 1½ lbs. steaks; sliced
- 1/4 cup honey
- 1/2 cup coconut aminos
- 1 tbsp. ginger; minced
- 1 tbsp. tapioca flour
- 1 tbsp. water
- 2 garlic cloves; minced
- 1/4 cup pear juice
- Some bacon fat

- 4 tbsp. white wine

Instructions:
1. Heat up a pan with the bacon fat over medium heat, add ginger and garlic, stir and cook for 2 minutes.
2. Add wine, stir and cook until it evaporates.
3. Add honey, aminos, pear juice, stir; bring to a simmer and cook for 12 minutes.
4. Add tapioca mixed with the water, stir and cook until it thickens.
5. Heat up a pan with some bacon fat over medium high heat, add steak slices and brown them for 2 minutes on each side.
6. Add green onions and half of the sauce you've just made, stir gently and cook for 3 minutes more. Divide steaks between plates and serve with the rest of the sauce on top.

Nutrition: Calories: 170; Fat: 3g; Fiber: 2g; Carbs: 2g; Protein: 8g

439. Beef Skillet

Preparation Time: 50 minutes
Servings: 4

Ingredients:
- 1 lb. beef; ground
- 1 tbsp. parsley flakes
- 2 big tomatoes
- 2 yellow squash; chopped
- 2 green bell peppers; chopped
- 1 yellow onion; chopped
- A pinch of sea salt
- Black pepper to the taste

Instructions:
1. Place tomatoes on a lined baking sheet, place in preheated broiler for 5 minutes, leave them to cool down, peel and roughly chop them.
2. Heat up a pan over medium high heat, add onion and beef, stir and cook for 10 minutes.
3. Add tomatoes, stir and cook for a couple more minutes.
4. Add parsley flakes, black pepper and a pinch of sea salt, stir and cook for 10 minutes more.
5. Add bell pepper pieces and squash ones, stir and cook for 10 minutes. Divide between plates and serve.

Nutrition: Calories: 190; Fat: 3g; Fiber: 4g; Carbs: 6g; Protein: 20g

440. Thai Curry

Preparation Time: 40 minutes
Servings: 4

Ingredients:
- 1 yellow onion; chopped
- 3 Thai chilies; chopped
- 2 tbsp. avocado oil
- 1 lb. beef; ground
- 1 small ginger pieces; grated
- 3 garlic cloves; minced
- 1/2 tsp. cumin
- 1/2 tsp. turmeric
- A pinch of sea salt
- Black pepper to the taste
- A pinch of cayenne pepper
- 1 tbsp. red curry paste
- 1 cup tomato sauce
- 1 broccoli head; florets separated
- 1 handful basil; chopped
- 2 tsp. lime juice
- 2 tbsp. coconut aminos

Instructions:
1. Heat up a pan with the oil over medium heat, add chilies and onion, stir and cook for 5 minutes.
2. Add a pinch of salt, ginger, garlic, cumin, turmeric, black pepper, cayenneand beef, stir and cook for 10 minutes.
3. Add broccoli and curry paste, stir and cook for 1 minute more.
4. Add basil, tomato paste and coconut aminos, stir; bring to a simmer, cover, reduce heat to medium-low and cook for 15 minutes. Add lime juice, stir; divide into bowls and serve.

Nutrition: Calories: 200; Fat: 3g; Fiber: 5g; Carbs: 7g; Protein: 24g

441. Beef Casserole

Servings: 6
Preparation time: 10 minutes
Cooking time: 8 hours

Ingredients:

- 2 cups pearl onions
- 3 and ½ pounds grass fed beef meat, cubed
- 4 garlic cloves, minced
- 2 sweet potatoes, chopped
- 2 celery stalks, chopped
- A pinch of sea salt
- Black pepper to taste
- 2 tablespoons tomato paste
- 2 cups carrot, chopped
- 2 cups beef broth
- 1 teaspoon thyme, dried
- 1 tablespoon coconut oil

Directions:

1. Heat up a pan with the oil over medium-high heat, add beef, stir and brown for 2 minutes on each side and transfer to a slow cooker.
2. Add all the other ingredients, toss, cook on Low for 8 hours, divide between plates and serve.
3. Enjoy!

Nutritional value: calories 1689, fat 64,1, fiber 4,2, carbs 23,4, protein 239,1

442. Grilled Lamb Chops

Servings: 6
Preparation time: 10 minutes
Cooking time: 10 minutes

Ingredients:

- 3 tablespoons coconut aminos
- 4 tablespoons extra virgin olive oil
- 8 lamb chops
- A pinch of sea salt
- Black pepper to taste
- 2 garlic cloves, minced
- 2 tablespoons ginger, minced
- 1 tablespoon parsley leaves, chopped

Directions:

1. In a bowl, mix olive oil with coconut amino, garlic, ginger and parsley and stir well.
2. Season lamb chops with a pinch of sea salt and pepper to taste, place them on preheated grill over medium-high heat and cook for 4 minutes on each side, basting all the time with the marinade.
3. Divide lamb chops between plates and serve.
4. Enjoy!

Nutritional value: calories 601, fat 29,4, carbs 2,8, protein 76,8, fiber 0,3

443. Lamb Casserole

Servings: 4
Preparation time: 2 hours
Cooking time: 1 hour

Ingredients:

- 1 butternut squash, cubed
- 3 pounds lamb shoulder, chopped
- 4 shallots, chopped
- 4 carrots, chopped
- 4 tomatoes, chopped
- 2 Thai chilies, chopped
- 2 tablespoons tomato paste
- 1 cinnamon stick
- 2 and ½ cups warm beef broth
- 1 lemongrass stalk, finely chopped
- 1 teaspoon Chinese five spice powder
- 1 tablespoon ginger, minced
- 2 tablespoon coconut aminos
- 1 and ½ tablespoons coconut oil
- 3 garlic cloves, chopped
- Black pepper to taste

Directions:

1. In a bowl, mix lamb with coconut aminos, ginger, lemongrass, garlic and pepper, stir well, cover and keep in the fridge for 2 hours.
2. Heat up a pot with the oil over medium-high heat, add marinated lamb, stir and brown for 3 minutes.
3. Add tomato paste and tomatoes, stir and

cook for 2 more minutes.
4. Add squash, shallots, Thai chilies, carrots, cinnamon stick, beef stock and five spices, stir well, place in the oven at 325 degrees F and bake for 1 hour.
5. Divide between plates and serve hot.
6. Enjoy!

Nutritional value: calories 775, fat 29,6, fiber 33,9, carbs 22,1, protein 100,9

444. Lamb Chops with Mint Sauce

Servings: 4
Preparation time: 15 minutes
Cooking time: 20 minutes

Ingredients:

- 2 garlic cloves, minced
- 8 lamb chops
- 2/3 cup extra virgin olive oil
- 1 tablespoon oregano, finely chopped
- 3 tablespoons Dijon mustard
- 1 tablespoon lemon zest
- 2 tablespoons white wine vinegar
- 1/3 cup mint, chopped
- Black pepper to taste

Directions:

1. In a bowl, mix olive oil with oregano, garlic and lemon zest and stir well.
2. Season lamb with black pepper to taste and brush with the mix you've just made.
3. Heat up your grill over medium-high heat, add lamb chops, cook for 5 minutes on each side and transfer to plates.
4. In a bowl, mix mustard with vinegar, pepper and mint and whisk well.
5. Serve lamb chops with vinegar mix drizzled on top.
6. Enjoy!

Nutritional value/ serving: calories 765, fat 54,3, carbs 1,5, fiber 2,9, protein 63,5

445. Beef Tenderloin and Sauce

Servings: 4
Preparation time: 10 minutes
Cooking time: 40 minutes

Ingredients:

- 3 tablespoons Dijon mustard
- 3 pounds beef tenderloin
- A pinch of sea salt
- Black pepper to taste
- 1 tablespoon coconut oil
- 3 tablespoons balsamic vinegar

For the sauce:

- 3 tablespoons basil leaves, chopped
- ½ cup parsley leaves, chopped
- Zest of 1 lemon
- 2 garlic cloves, minced
- A pinch of sea salt
- Black pepper to taste
- ¼ cup extra virgin olive oil

Directions:

1. In a bowl, mix mustard with vinegar, stir well and leave to one side.
2. Season beef with a pinch of sea salt and pepper to the taste put in a pan heated with the coconut oil over medium-high heat and cook for 2 minutes on each side.
3. Transfer beef to a baking pan, cover with the mustard mix, place in the oven at 475 degrees F and bake for 25 minutes.
4. In a bowl, mix parsley with basil, lemon zest, garlic, olive oil, a pinch of sea salt, and pepper to taste and whisk very well.
5. Take beef tenderloin out of the oven, slice and divide between plates.
6. Serve with herbs sauce on the side.
7. Enjoy!

Nutritional value/ serving: calories 854, fat 47,6, fiber 0,8, carbs 1,8, protein 99,4

446. Beef Stir Fry

Servings: 4
Preparation time: 10 minutes
Cooking time: 20 minutes

Ingredients:

- 10 ounces mushrooms, sliced
- 10 ounces asparagus, sliced
- 1 and ½ pounds beef steak, thinly sliced
- 2 tablespoons coconut sugar
- 1/3 cup coconut amino
- 2 teaspoons apple cider vinegar

- ½ teaspoon ginger, minced
- 6 garlic cloves, minced
- 1 red chili, sliced
- 1 tablespoon coconut oil
- Black pepper to taste

Directions:
1. In a bowl, mix garlic with coconut amino, the sugar, ginger and vinegar and whisk well.
2. Put some water in a pan, heat up over medium-high heat, add asparagus and black pepper, cook for 3 minutes, transfer to a bowl filled with ice water, drain and leave aside.
3. Heat up a pan with the oil over medium-high heat, add mushrooms, cook for 2 minutes on each side, transfer to a bowl and leave aside.
4. Heat up the same pan over high heat, add meat, brown for a few minutes and mix with chili pepper.
5. Cook for 2 more minutes and mix with asparagus, mushrooms and vinegar sauce you've made at the beginning.
6. Stir well, cook for 3 minutes, take off heat, divide between plates and serve.
7. Enjoy!

Nutritional value: calories 284, fat 10,4, fiber 2,4, carbs 11,4, protein 36,4

447. Pork with Blueberry Sauce

Servings: 4
Preparation time: 10 minutes
Cooking time: 30 minutes

Ingredients:
- 1 cup blueberries
- ½ teaspoon thyme, dried
- 2 pounds pork loin
- 1 tablespoon balsamic vinegar
- ½ teaspoon red chili flakes
- 1 teaspoon ginger powder
- A pinch of sea salt
- Black pepper to taste
- 2 tablespoon water

Directions:
1. Put pork loin in a baking dish and season with a pinch of sea salt and pepper to taste.
2. Heat up a pan over medium heat, add blueberries and mix with vinegar, water, thyme, chili flakes and ginger.
3. Stir well, cook for 5 minutes and pour over pork loin.
4. Place in the oven at 375 degrees F and bake for 25 minutes.
5. Take pork out of the oven, leave aside for 5 minutes, slice, divide between plates and serve with blueberries sauce.
6. Enjoy!

Nutritional value/ serving: calories 572, fat 31,7, carbs 5,4, fiber 0,9, protein 62,3

448. Pulled Pork

Servings: 4
Preparation time: 12 hours and 10 minutes
Cooking time: 8 hours and 20 minutes

Ingredients:
- ½ cup paleo salsa
- ½ cup beef stock
- ½ cup enchilada sauce
- 3 pounds organic pork shoulder
- 2 green chilies, chopped
- 1 tablespoon garlic powder
- 1 tablespoon chili powder
- 1 teaspoon onion powder
- 1 teaspoon cumin, ground
- 1 teaspoon sweet paprika
- Black pepper to taste

Directions:
1. In a bowl, mix chili powder with onion and garlic one.
2. Add cumin, paprika and pepper to taste and stir everything.
3. Add pork, rub well and keep in the fridge for 12 hours.
4. Transfer pork to a slow cooker, add enchilada sauce, stock, salsa and green chilies, stir, cover and cook on Low for 8 hours.
5. Transfer pork to a plate, leave aside to cool down and shred.

6. Strain sauce from slow cooker into a pan, bring to a boil over medium heat and simmer for 8 minutes stirring all the time.
7. Add shredded pork to the sauce, stir, reduce heat to medium and cook for 20 more minutes.
8. Divide between plates and serve hot.
9. Enjoy!

Nutritional value: calories 1013, fat 73, carbs 4,3, fiber 1,6, protein 80,4

449. Barbeque Ribs

Servings: 4
Preparation time: 15 minutes
Cooking time: 2 hours and 47 minutes

Ingredients:

- 1 tablespoon smoked paprika
- ½ tablespoon onion powder
- ½ tablespoon garlic powder
- ½ teaspoon cayenne pepper
- 4 pounds baby ribs
- 1 cup paleo BBQ sauce
- 4 teaspoons Sriracha
- ¼ cup cilantro, chopped
- ¼ cup chives, chopped
- ¼ cup parsley, chopped
- Black pepper to taste

Directions:

1. In a bowl, mix paprika with onion powder, garlic powder, pepper and cayenne and stir well.
2. Add ribs, toss to coat and arrange them on a lined baking sheet.
3. Place in the oven at 325 degrees F and bake them for 2 hours and 30 minutes.
4. In a bowl, mix BBQ sauce with Sriracha and stir well.
5. Take ribs out of the oven, mix them with BBQ sauce, place them on preheated grill over medium-high heat and cook for 7 minutes on each side.
6. Divide ribs between plates, sprinkle chives, cilantro, and parsley on top and serve.
7. Enjoy!

Nutritional value/ serving: calories 1483, fat 122,3, fiber 1,1, carbs 9,5, protein 81,8

450. Flavored Pork Chops

Servings: 4
Preparation time: 10 minutes
Cooking time: 30 minutes

Ingredients:

- 8 sage springs
- 4 pork chops, bone-in
- 4 tablespoons ghee
- 4 garlic cloves, crushed
- 1 tablespoon coconut oil
- A pinch of sea salt
- Black pepper to taste

Directions:

1. Season pork chops with a pinch of sea salt and pepper to taste.
2. Heat up a pan with the oil over medium high heat, add pork chops and cook for 10 minutes turning them often.
3. Take pork chops off heat, add ghee, sage, and garlic and toss to coat.
4. Return to heat, cook for 4 minutes often stirring, divide between plates and serve.
5. Enjoy!

Nutritional value/ serving: calories 402, fat 36, fiber 0,1, carbs 1, protein 18,2

451. Pork with Pear Salsa

Servings: 4
Preparation time: 10 minutes
Cooking time: 45 minutes

Ingredients:

- 1 yellow onion, chopped
- 1 organic pork tenderloin
- 2 pears, chopped
- 2 garlic cloves, minced
- 1 tablespoon chives, chopped
- ¼ cup walnuts, chopped
- 3 tablespoons balsamic vinegar
- Black pepper to taste
- ½ cup chicken stock
- 1 tablespoon coconut oil

- 1 tablespoon lemon juice

Directions:
1. In a bowl, mix walnuts with pear, chives, pepper and lemon juice and stir well.
2. Heat up a pan with the oil over medium-high heat, add tenderloin and brown for 3 minutes on each side.
3. Reduce heat, add onion and garlic, stir and cook for 2 minutes.
4. Add balsamic vinegar, stock, pear mix, stir, place in the oven at 400 degrees F and bake for 20 minutes.
5. Take pork out of the oven, leave aside for 4 minutes, slice, divide between plates and serve with pear salsa on top.
6. Enjoy!

Nutritional value/ serving: calories 271, fat 11,2, fiber 4,4, carbs 20,1, protein 24,6

452. Pork Tenderloin with Carrot Puree

Servings: 4
Preparation time: 10 minutes
Cooking time: 45 minutes

Ingredients:
- 15 oz turkey mince
- A handful arugula
- Black pepper to taste
- 1 grass fed pork tenderloin
- 1 tablespoon coconut oil
- For the puree:
- 1 sweet potato, chopped
- 3 carrots, chopped
- A pinch of sea salt
- Black pepper to taste
- 1 tablespoon curry paste
- For the sauce:
- 2 tablespoons balsamic vinegar
- 1 teaspoon mustard
- 2 shallots, chopped
- Black pepper to taste
- 4 tablespoons extra virgin olive oil

Directions:
1. Slice pork tenderloin in half horizontally but not all the way and open it up.
2. Use a meat tenderizer to even it up.
3. Place turkey mince in the middle, roll pork around it, tie with twine, season pepper to taste and leave to one side.
4. Heat up an oven proof pan with the coconut oil over medium-high heat, add pork roll, cook for 3 minutes on each side, place in the oven at 350 degrees F and bake for 25 minutes.
5. Meanwhile, put potatoes and carrots in a large saucepan, add water to cover, bring to a boil over medium-high heat, cook for 20 minutes, drain and transfer to a food processor.
6. Pulse a few times until you obtain a puree, add a pinch of sea salt and pepper to taste, blend again, transfer to a bowl and leave aside.
7. Take pork roll out of the oven, slice and divide between plates.
8. Heat up a pan with the olive oil over medium-high heat, add shallots, stir and cook for 10 minutes.
9. Add balsamic vinegar, mustard, pepper, stir well and take off heat.
10. Divide carrots puree next to pork slices, drizzle vinegar sauce on to and serve with arugula on the side. Enjoy!

Nutritional value/ serving: calories 495, fat 29,5, carbs 2,2, fiber 17,5, protein 21,8

453. Pork with Strawberry Sauce

Servings: 4
Preparation time: 10 minutes
Cooking time: 35 minutes

Ingredients:
- 4 pounds pork tenderloin
- 1 cup strawberries, sliced
- 10 thin turkey fillet strips
- A pinch of sea salt
- Black pepper to taste
- 4 garlic cloves, minced
- ½ cup balsamic vinegar
- 2 tablespoons extra virgin olive oil

Directions:
1. Wrap turkey strips around tenderloin,

secure with toothpicks and season with salt and pepper.
2. Heat up your grill over indirect medium high heat, put tenderloin on it and cook for 30 minutes.
3. Heat up a pan with the oil over medium high heat, add garlic, stir and cook for 2 minutes.
4. Add vinegar and half of the strawberries, stir and bring to a boil.
5. Reduce heat to medium and simmer for 10 minutes.
6. Add black pepper to taste and the rest of the strawberries and stir.
7. Baste pork with some of the sauce and continue cooking over indirect heat until turkey is brown enough.
8. Transfer pork to a cutting board, leave aside for a few minutes to cool down, slice and divide between plates.
9. Serve with the strawberry sauce right away.
10. Enjoy!

Nutritional value/ serving: calories 981, fat 24,3, carbs 4, fiber 0,8, protein 174,1

454. Turkey Casserole

Servings: 6
Preparation time: 15 minutes
Cooking time: 45 minutes

Ingredients:

- 20 ounces ground turkey
- 2 green bell peppers, chopped
- 3 sweet potatoes, chopped
- 1-pint grape tomatoes, chopped
- A pinch of sea salt
- Black pepper to taste
- 2 garlic cloves, minced
- 1 red onion, chopped
- A few thyme springs

Directions:

1. In a baking dish, mix potatoes with tomatoes, onion, bell pepper, garlic, a pinch of sea salt and pepper and stir gently.
2. Heat up a pan over high heat, add turkey mince, brown it for 15 minutes side and transfer on top of veggies in the baking dish.
3. Add thyme, introduce in the oven at 400 degrees F and bake for 45 minutes.
4. Divide between plates and serve hot.
5. Enjoy!

Nutritional value/ serving: calories 306, fat 10,8, carbs 28,4, fiber 4,8, protein 28,2

455. Greek Souvlaki

Preparation time: 10 minutes
Cooking time: 20 minutes
Servings: 4

Ingredients:

- 3 sweet potatoes, cubed
- 1 yellow onion, chopped
- 12 mini bell peppers, chopped
- 4 medium round steaks
- ½ cup sun dried tomatoes, chopped
- 1 tablespoon sweet paprika
- 2 tablespoons balsamic vinegar
- Juice of 1 lemon
- 1 tablespoons oregano, dried
- ¼ cup olive oil+ a drizzle
- 1 lemon, sliced
- ¼ cup kalamata olives, pitted and chopped
- 4 dill springs
- 2 garlic cloves, minced
- A pinch of sea salt and black pepper

Directions:

1. Heat up a pan with a drizzle of oil over medium-high heat, add steaks, season them with salt and some black pepper, brown them for 2 minutes on each side and transfer to a baking dish.
2. Heat up the pan again over medium-high heat, add sweet potatoes, cook them for 4 minutes and add them to the baking dish.
3. Also add bell peppers, tomatoes, onion, olives and lemon slices.
4. Meanwhile, in a bowl, mix lemon juice with rest of the olive oil, vinegar, garlic, paprika and oregano and whisk well.

5. Pour this over steak and veggies, add dill springs on top, toss to coat, place in the oven at 425 degrees F and bake for 12 minutes.
6. Divide steak and veggies between plates and serve.
7. Enjoy!

Nutrition: calories 869, fat 30,8, fiber 10,9, carbs 56,5, protein 89,1

456. Mexican Steaks

Preparation time: 10 minutes
Cooking time: 15 minutes
Servings: 4

Ingredients:
- 2 tablespoons chili powder
- 4 medium sirloin steaks
- 1 teaspoon cumin, ground
- ½ tablespoon sweet paprika
- 1 teaspoon onion powder
- 1 teaspoon garlic powder
- A pinch of sea salt and black pepper

For the Pico de gallo:
- 1 small red onion, chopped
- 2 tomatoes, chopped
- 2 garlic cloves, minced
- 2 tablespoons lime juice
- 1 small green bell pepper, chopped
- 1 jalapeno, chopped
- ¼ cup cilantro, chopped
- ¼ teaspoon cumin, ground
- Black pepper to taste

Directions:
1. In a bowl, mix chili powder with a pinch of salt, black pepper, onion powder, garlic powder, paprika and 1 teaspoon cumin and stir well.
2. Season steaks with this mix, rub well and place them on preheated grill over medium high heat.
3. Cook steaks for 5 minutes on each side and divide them between plates.
4. In a bowl, mix red onion with tomatoes, garlic, lime juice, bell pepper, jalapeno, cilantro, black pepper to taste and ¼ teaspoon cumin and stir well.
5. Top steaks with this mix and serve.
6. Enjoy!

Nutrition: calories 285, fat 9, fiber 3,1 carbs 10,2, protein 40,5

457. ` `Grilled Steaks

Preparation time: 10 minutes
Cooking time: 10 minutes
Servings: 4

Ingredients:
- 1 and ½ tablespoons coffee, ground
- 4 rib eye steaks
- ½ tablespoon sweet paprika
- 2 tablespoons chili powder
- 2 teaspoons garlic powder
- 2 teaspoons onion powder
- ¼ teaspoon ginger, ground
- ¼ teaspoon, coriander, ground
- A pinch of cayenne pepper
- Black pepper to the taste

Directions:
1. In a bowl, mix coffee with paprika, chili powder, garlic powder, onion powder, ginger, coriander, cayenne and black pepper and stir well.
2. Rub steaks with the coffee mix, place them on your preheated grill over medium high heat, cook them for 5 minutes on each side and divide between plates.
3. Leave steaks to cool down for 5 minutes before serving them with a side salad!
4. Enjoy!

Nutrition: calories 621, fat 50, fiber 0, carbs 0, protein 40

458. Beef Lasagna

Preparation time: 10 minutes
Cooking time: 6 hours
Servings: 6

Ingredients:
- 1 red bell pepper, chopped
- 1 eggplant, sliced lengthwise

- 2 zucchinis, sliced lengthwise
- 1 pound beef, ground
- 2 cups tomatoes, chopped
- 2 teaspoons oregano, dried
- 4 cups tomato sauce
- ¼ cup basil, chopped
- 2 garlic cloves, minced
- 1 yellow onion, chopped
- 2 tablespoons tomato paste
- 1 tablespoon parsley, chopped
- 2 tablespoons olive oil
- A pinch of sea salt
- Black pepper to taste

Directions:
1. Heat up a pan with the oil over medium-high heat, add onion and garlic, stir and cook for 2 minutes.
2. Add beef, stir and brown for 5 minutes more.
3. Add bell pepper, tomatoes, oregano, basil, tomato paste and parsley, stir and cook for 4 minutes more.
4. Add tomato sauce, black pepper to taste and a pinch of salt and stir well again.
5. Arrange layers of eggplant and zucchini slices with the sauce you've made in your slow cooker.
6. Cover and cook on Low for 4 hours and 45 minutes.
7. Divide your lasagna between plates and serve.
8. Enjoy!

Nutrition: calories 281, fat 10,2, fiber 7,7, carbs 22,7, protein 28

459. Steak and Apricots

Preparation time: 10 minutes
Cooking time: 25 minutes
Servings: 2

Ingredients:
- 2 tablespoons Cajun spice
- ¼ cup coconut oil
- 2 medium skirt steaks
- 1/3 cup lemon juice
- ¼ cup apricot preserves
- ¼ cup coconut aminos

Directions:
1. In a bowl, mix half of the Cajun spice with lemon juice, aminos, oil and apricot preserves and stir well.
2. Pour this into a pan, bring to a boil over medium high heat and simmer for 8 minutes.
3. Blend this using an immersion blender and leave aside for now.
4. Season steaks with the rest of the Cajun spice, brush them with half of the apricots mix, place them on preheated grill over medium- high heat and cook them for 6-minute son each side.
5. Divide steaks on plates and top with the rest of the apricots mix.
6. Enjoy!

Nutrition: calories 887, fat 53,3, fiber 0,3, carbs 31,1, protein 68,7

460. Filet Mignon and Sauce

Preparation time: 10 minutes
Cooking time: 25 minutes
Servings: 4

Ingredients:
- 12 mushrooms, sliced
- 1 shallot, chopped
- 4 fillet mignons
- 2 garlic cloves, minced
- 2 tablespoons olive oil
- ¼ cup Dijon mustard
- ¼ cup veggie stock
- 1 and ¼ cup coconut cream
- 2 tablespoons parsley, chopped
- Black pepper to taste
- A pinch of sea salt

Directions:
1. Heat up a pan with the oil over medium-high heat, add garlic and shallots, stir and cook for 3 minutes.
2. Add mushrooms, stir and cook for 4 minutes more.
3. Add the stock, coconut cream, mustard, parsley, a pinch of salt and black pepper

to taste, stir and cook for 6 minutes more.
4. Heat up another pan over high heat, add fillets, season them with a pinch of salt and some black pepper and cook them for 4 minutes on each side.
5. Divide fillets between plates and serve with the mushroom sauce on top.
6. Enjoy!

Nutrition: calories 873, fat 53, fiber 1,3, carbs 44, protein 54,6

461. Beef Kabobs

Preparation time: 10 minutes
Cooking time: 12 minutes
Servings: 4

Ingredients:

- 2 red bell peppers, chopped
- 2 pounds sirloin steak, cut into medium pieces
- 1 red onion, chopped
- 1 zucchini, sliced
- Juice of 1 lime
- 2 tablespoons chili powder
- 2 tablespoon hot sauce
- ½ tablespoons cumin powder
- ¼ cup olive oil
- ¼ cup Paleo Salsa
- A pinch of sea salt and black pepper

Directions:

1. In a bowl, mix the salsa with lime juice, oil, hot sauce, chili powder, cumin, salt and black pepper and whisk well.
2. Layer steaks pieces, bell peppers, zucchini and onion on skewers.
3. Brush kabobs with the salsa mix you made earlier, place them on preheated grill over medium-high heat and cook them for 5 minutes on each side.
4. Divide kabobs between plates and serve.
5. Enjoy!

Nutrition: calories 590, fat 27,9, fiber 3,6, carbs 12,2, protein 71,2

462. Steak and Veggies

Preparation time: 10 minutes
Cooking time: 30 minutes
Servings: 4

Ingredients:

- 2 sweet potatoes, chopped
- 4 sirloin steaks
- 1 red onion, chopped
- 1 broccoli head, florets separated
- 8 cherry tomatoes, halved
- 4 thyme springs
- 4 garlic cloves, minced
- A pinch of sea salt
- Black pepper to taste
- 4 tablespoons olive oil
- ½ tablespoon sweet paprika

Directions:

1. In a bowl, mix oil with a pinch of salt, black pepper, garlic and paprika and stir well.
2. Spread broccoli and sweet potatoes on a lined baking sheet, place in the oven at 425 degrees f and bake for 10 minutes.
3. Heat up a pan over medium-high heat, add steaks, season them with a pinch of sea salt and black pepper, cook for 2 minutes on each side and add to the baking sheet.
4. Also add onions and tomatoes, drizzle the oil and garlic mix, toss to coat, top with thyme and bake in the oven for 15 minutes more.
5. Divide everything between plates and serve.
6. Enjoy!

Nutrition: calories 614, fat 25,7, fiber 9,3, carbs 40, protein 57,7

463. Beef Teriyaki

Preparation time: 10 minutes
Cooking time: 20 minutes
Servings: 4

Ingredients:

- 2 green onions, chopped
- 1 and ½ pounds steaks, sliced
- ¼ cup coconut sugar
- ½ cup coconut aminos

- 1 tablespoon ginger, minced
- 2 garlic cloves, minced
- ¼ cup pear juice
- 2 tablespoons olive oil

Directions:
1. Heat up a pan with half of the oil over medium heat, add ginger and garlic, stir and cook for 2 minutes.
2. Add the sugar, aminos, pear juice, stir, bring to a simmer and cook for 12 minutes.
3. Add tapioca mixed with the water, stir and cook until it thickens.
4. Heat up a pan with the rest of the oil over medium-high heat, add steak slices and brown them for 2 minutes on each side.
5. Add green onions and half of the sauce you've just made, stir gently and cook for 3 minutes more.
6. Divide steaks between plates and serve with the rest of the sauce on top.
7. Enjoy!

Nutrition: calories 487, fat 19,1, fiber 0,4, carbs 17,6, protein 58,5

464. Beef and Gravy

Preparation time: 10 minutes
Cooking time: 20 minutes
Servings: 4

Ingredients:
- 1 egg, whisked
- 1 tablespoon mustard
- 1 tablespoon tomato paste
- 1 teaspoon garlic powder
- 1 teaspoon onion powder
- Some coconut oil for cooking
- A pinch of sea salt and black pepper to taste
- 1 and ½ pound beef, ground
- For the gravy:
- 2 teaspoons parsley, chopped
- 2 tablespoons ghee
- 1 small yellow onion, chopped
- 1 and ¼ cups beef stock
- Black pepper to taste

Directions:
1. In a bowl, mix beef with tomato paste, egg, mustard, onion powder, garlic powder, a pinch of salt and black pepper to taste and stir well.
2. Heat up a pan with the ghee over medium heat, add onion, stir and cook for 2 minutes.
3. Add stock and the black pepper, stir and take off the heat.
4. Shape 4 patties from the beef mix.
5. Heat up a pan with the coconut oil over medium high heat, add beef patties and cook for 5 minutes on each side.
6. Pour the gravy over beef patties, sprinkle parsley on top, cook for a couple more minutes, divide between plates and serve.
7. Enjoy!

Nutrition: calories 502, fat 31,8, fiber 1,3, carbs 4,9, protein 42,2

465. Steak and Scallops

Preparation time: 10 minutes
Cooking time: 20 minutes
Servings: 2

Ingredients:
- 10 sea scallops
- 4 garlic cloves, minced
- 2 beef steaks
- 1 shallot, chopped
- 2 tablespoons lemon juice
- 2 tablespoons parsley, chopped
- 2 tablespoons basil, chopped
- 1 teaspoon lemon zest
- ¼ cup ghee
- ¼ cup veggie stock
- 1 tablespoon olive oil
- A pinch of sea salt
- Black pepper to taste

Directions:
1. Heat up a pan with the oil over medium-high heat, add steaks, season them with a pinch of salt and black pepper and cook for 4 minutes on each side.
2. Add shallot and garlic, stir and cook for 2

minutes more.
3. Add the ghee and stir everything.
4. Add stock, basil, lemon juice, parsley and lemon zest and stir.
5. Add scallops, season them with some black pepper and cook for a couple more minutes.
6. Divide steaks and scallops between plates and serve with pan juices.
7. Enjoy!

Nutrition: calories 835, fat 47,4, fiber 0,4, carbs 8,3, protein 90,7

466. Sheppard's Pie

Preparation time: 15 minutes
Cooking time: 45 minutes
Servings: 6

Ingredients:
- 2 pounds sweet potatoes, chopped
- 1 and ½ pounds beef, ground
- 2 cups beef stock
- 1 onion, chopped
- 2 carrots, chopped
- 2 garlic cloves, minced
- 2 celery stalks, chopped
- ¼ cup ghee
- 1 tablespoon olive oil
- A handful parsley, chopped
- 2 tablespoons tomato paste
- A pinch of sea salt
- Black pepper to taste

Directions:
1. Put sweet potatoes in a large saucepan, add water to cover, bring to a boil over medium high heat, cook for 20 minutes, drain, leave them to cool down and transfer to a bowl.
2. Add ghee, a pinch of salt and pepper and mash potatoes well.
3. Heat up a pan with the oil over medium high heat, add beef, stir and cook for a couple of minutes.
4. Add carrots, garlic, onions, celery, stock, tomato paste, salt and pepper, stir and cook for 10 minutes.
5. Spread the beef mix on the bottom of a baking dish, top with mashed potatoes, spread well, place in the oven at 375 degrees F and bake for 25 minutes.
6. Slice and serve.
7. Enjoy!

Nutrition: calories 535, fat 25,4, fiber 7,8, carbs 48, protein 28,7

467. Ginger Lamb Chops

Preparation time: 10 minutes
Cooking time: 10 minutes
Servings: 6

Ingredients:
- 3 tablespoons coconut aminos
- 4 tablespoons olive oil
- 2 tablespoons ginger, grated
- 8 lamb chops
- 1 tablespoon parsley, chopped
- 2 garlic cloves, minced
- A pinch of sea salt
- Black pepper to taste

Directions:
1. In a bowl, mix oil with aminos, parsley, ginger and garlic and stir well.
2. Place lamb chops on a preheated grill over medium high heat, season them with a pinch of salt and black pepper to taste and grill them for 4 minutes on each side basting them with the oil and ginger mix you've made.
3. Leave lamb chops to cool down for a couple of minutes and then serve.
4. Enjoy!

Nutrition: calories 904, fat 41,4, fiber 0,3, carbs 2,6, protein 122,7

468. Hungarian Sausages

Preparation Time: 15 minutes
Cooking time: 45 minutes
Servings: 4

Ingredients:
- 1 sausage casing
- 1 teaspoon minced garlic
- 1-pound pork shoulder, finely chopped

- 1 teaspoon dried dill
- 1 teaspoon ground black pepper
- 1 teaspoon salt
- ½ teaspoon ground nutmeg
- 1 teaspoon olive oil
- ¼ cup of water

Directions:
1. Preheat the oven to 365F.
2. In the mixing bowl, mix up together minced garlic, finely chopped pork shoulder, dried dill, ground black pepper, salt, and ground nutmeg.
3. Mix up the mixture well.
4. Fill the sausage casing with the meat mixture and secure the edges.
5. Then place the sausage in the tray and brush it with the olive oil.
6. Make the small pins in the sausage.
7. Add water and transfer it in the preheated oven.
8. Cook the sausage for 45 minutes.
9. When the time is over, remove the sausage from the oven and let it chill in the tray for 10-15 minutes.

Nutrition value/serving: calories 346, fat 25.6, fiber 0.2, carbs 0.9, protein 26.6

469. Sesame Pork Tenderloin

Preparation Time: 20 minutes
Cooking time: 30 minutes
Servings:4
Ingredients:
- 1-pound pork tenderloin
- ½ teaspoon cumin seeds
- 1 teaspoon sesame seeds
- 1 tablespoon sesame oil
- 1 teaspoon chili flakes
- 1 teaspoon chili powder
- 1 teaspoon dried marjoram
- 1 teaspoon dried oregano
- 1 teaspoon rosemary
- 4 tablespoons butter, softened

Directions:
1. Churn the butter with the chili flakes, chili powder, dried marjoram, oregano, and rosemary.
2. Then rub the pork tenderloin with the mixture and place it in the freezer for 10 minutes.
3. After this, remove the meat from the freezer and brush it with the sesame oil.
4. Sprinkle the surface of the meat with cumin seeds and sesame seeds.
5. Wrap the meat in the foil and bake in the preheated to the 375F oven for 30 minutes.
6. When the meat is cooked, remove it from the oven and discard the foil.
7. Transfer the meat into the big serving plate and slice it into the servings.

Nutrition value/serving: calories 304, fat 19.5, fiber 0.7, carbs 1.2, protein 30.1

470. Kalua Pork

Preparation Time: 10 minutes
Cooking time: 2 hours
Servings:6

Ingredients:
- 2-pound pork butt shoulder
- 2 tablespoons liquid smoke flavoring
- 1 tablespoon salt
- 1 teaspoon ground black pepper

Directions:
1. Pin the pork shoulder with the help of the knife. Make a lot of small holes.
2. Then rub the meat with salt and ground black pepper.
3. Place the meat in the pan and sprinkle with the liquid smoke flavoring.
4. Massage the meat gently and cover the pan with foil. Secure the edges.
5. Place the pan with meat in the oven and cook it for 2 hours at 360F.
6. When the meat is cooked, it will be tender. If the time is over and the meat is not cooked yet, continue to cook it for 30-40 minutes more.

Nutrition value/serving: calories 368, fat 23.4, fiber 0.1, carbs 0.2, protein 36.7

471. Pork Belly with Crunchy Crust

Preparation Time: 10 minutes
Cooking time: 40 minutes
Servings: 4

Ingredients:

- 10 oz pork belly
- ½ tablespoon salt
- 1 teaspoon minced garlic
- 1 teaspoon butter
- 1 teaspoon dried cilantro

Directions:

1. Rub the pork belly with salt, minced garlic, and dried cilantro.
2. Then rub the meat with butter and wrap in the foil.
3. Bake the pork belly for 30 minutes at 365F.
4. After this, discard the foil and set the grill mode of the oven.
5. Grill the pork belly for 10 minutes from each side.
6. Slice the pork belly.

Nutrition value/serving: calories 337, fat 20, fiber 0, carbs 0.2, protein 32.8

472. Sauteed Pork with Garlic Cloves

Preparation Time: 7 minutes
Cooking time: 60 minutes
Servings: 4

Ingredients:

- 9 oz pork loin, chopped
- ¼ cup garlic cloves, halved
- 1 teaspoon salt
- 3 tablespoons butter
- ¼ cup of coconut milk

Directions:

1. Toss the butter in the saucepan and melt it.
2. When the butter starts to boil, add chopped pork loin and roast it for 5 minutes over the medium heat.
3. Then add coconut milk, salt, and halved garlic cloves.
4. Mix up the meat and close the lid.
5. Saute the meat over the low heat for 55 minutes.

Nutrition value/serving: calories 278, fat 21.1, fiber 0.5, carbs 3.7, protein 18.4

473. Eastern Aromatic Stew

Preparation Time: 10 minutes
Cooking time: 35 minutes
Servings: 3

Ingredients:

- 8 oz beef fillet, chopped
- ½ teaspoon ground cardamom
- ½ teaspoon ground cinnamon
- 1 teaspoon salt
- 1 teaspoon harissa
- ½ teaspoon chili flakes
- ½ cup organic almond milk
- 1 teaspoon olive oil
- 1 bell pepper, chopped
- ¾ cup of water
- 1 teaspoon coconut flakes
- 1 teaspoon ground turmeric

Directions:

1. Put olive oil in the pan. Add chopped beef fillet and roast it for 2 minutes.
2. Stir the meat and add chopped bell pepper.
3. Cook the ingredients for 3 minutes more.
4. After this, sprinkle the meat with ground cardamom, cinnamon, salt, harissa, chili flakes, and ground turmeric. Mix up well.
5. Then add water and almond milk.
6. Add coconut flakes and mix up.
7. Close the lid and saute the stew for 30 minutes with the closed lid over the medium-low heat.
8. Let the cooked stew rest with the closed lid for at least 15 minutes before serving.

Nutrition value/serving: calories 134, fat 5.6, fiber 1.2, carbs 7.8, protein 12.8

474. Pork Rollatini

Preparation Time: 15 minutes
Cooking time: 25 minutes
Servings: 6

Ingredients:

- 1-pound pork cutlet, sliced
- 2 oz prosciutto, sliced
- 2 teaspoons ricotta cheese
- 1 tablespoon cream cheese
- 1 tablespoon dried dill
- 3 oz Mozzarella, sliced
- ¼ cup tomatoes, crushed
- 1 teaspoon minced garlic
- 1 teaspoon Italian seasoning
- ½ cup of water
- 1 teaspoon butter

Directions:

1. Spread the sliced pork cutlets with ricotta and cream cheese from one side.
2. Then place on them sliced Mozzarella, dried dill, prosciutto, and roll the cutlets.
3. Secure them with toothpicks and place in the skillet.
4. Add butter and roast the meal for 2 minutes from each side.
5. Then add water, Italian seasoning, and minced garlic.
6. After this, add crushed tomatoes.
7. Close the lid and cook the meal for 20 minutes over the medium heat.

Nutrition value/serving: calories 76, fat 4.3, fiber 0.8, carbs 2.4, protein 7.2

475. Chipotle Lamb Ribs

Preparation Time: 15 minutes
Cooking time: 16 minutes
Servings: 6

Ingredients:

- 2-pound lamb ribs
- 1 tablespoon chipotle pepper, minced
- 1 teaspoon salt
- 2 tablespoons olive oil
- 1 teaspoon ground paprika
- 1 teaspoon garlic powder
- ¼ cup of water

Directions:

1. Preheat the grill to 375F.
2. Meanwhile, rub the lamb ribs with the salt, minced chipotle pepper, olive oil, ground paprika, and garlic powder.
3. Place the ribs in the water and mix up well. Pierce the meat with the help of the knife.
4. Marinate the meat for 10 minutes.
5. After this, transfer the meat in the grill and roast it for 8 minutes from each side.
6. The cooked lamb ribs will have a light crunchy surface.

Nutrition value/serving: calories 397, fat 24.9, fiber 0.5, carbs 1.4, protein 39.8

476. Sweet Spare Ribs

Preparation Time: 10 minutes
Cooking time: 1.5 hours
Servings: 6

Ingredients:

- 2 racks of pork ribs (6 servings
- 1 tablespoon chili flakes
- 1 teaspoon salt
- 1 teaspoon cayenne pepper
- 2 tablespoon olive oil
- 1 teaspoon dried thyme
- 1 teaspoon garlic powder
- 3 tablespoons lemon juice
- 1 teaspoon Erythritol

Directions:

1. Preheat the oven to 345F.
2. Meanwhile, rub the pork ribs with the chili flakes, salt, cayenne pepper, olive oil, dried thyme, garlic powder, lemon juice, and Erythritol.
3. Massage the pork ribs well and place in the tray.
4. Transfer the tray in the preheated oven and cook for 1.5 hours.
5. When the ribs are cooked, sprinkle them with the meat juice from the tray and remove from the oven.

Nutrition value/serving: calories 365, fat 31.8, fiber 0.2, carbs 0.8, protein 18.2

477. Grilled Beef Steaks

Preparation Time: 15 minutes

Cooking time: 16 minutes
Servings: 2

Ingredients:
- 2 beef steaks (7 oz each)
- 1 teaspoon peppercorns, grinded
- 1 teaspoon of sea salt
- 1 tablespoon olive oil
- 1 teaspoon fresh rosemary, chopped

Directions:
1. Rub the beef with peppercorns, sea salt, and chopped rosemary. Let the meat for 15 minutes to marinate.
2. Meanwhile, preheat the grill to 375F.
3. Sprinkle the beefsteaks with the olive oil and place in the grill.
4. Cook the steaks for 8 minutes from each side.
5. Slice the meat before serving.

Nutrition value/serving: calories 527, fat 23.7, fiber 0.5, carbs 1.1, protein 73.6

478. Indian Style Pork Saute

Preparation Time: 10 minutes
Cooking time: 25 minutes
Servings: 4

Ingredients:
- 2 cups ground pork
- 1 teaspoon curry powder
- 1 teaspoon curry paste
- ½ teaspoon salt
- 1 teaspoon ground paprika
- 3 garlic cloves, diced
- 1 tablespoon almond butter
- 1 tablespoon dried cilantro

Directions:
1. Place almond butter in the saucepan and melt it.
2. Add diced garlic, ground paprika, salt, curry paste, and curry powder.
3. Mix up the mixture and bring it to boil.
4. Add ground pork and stir well.
5. Close the lid and simmer the saute for 20 minutes over the low heat.
6. If the saute doesn't form enough liquid, add a ¼ cup of water and simmer it for an extra 10 minutes over the medium heat.

Nutrition value/serving: calories 272, fat 19.4, fiber 0.8, carbs 2.4, protein 21.3

479. Lamb Fillet with Cream Sauce

Preparation Time: 10 minutes
Cooking time: 18 minutes
Servings: 4

Ingredients:
- 1 tablespoon fresh parsley, chopped
- 1 tablespoon fresh dill, chopped
- 4 tablespoon cream cheese
- 1 tablespoon Psyllium Husk
- 1 teaspoon ground turmeric
- 1 teaspoon salt
- 1 tablespoon olive oil
- 4 lamb fillets (3 oz each)
- ½ teaspoon chili powder
- 1 tablespoon apple cider vinegar

Directions:
1. Sprinkle the lamb fillets with chili powder, salt, and apple cider vinegar from each side.
2. After this, pour olive oil in the skillet and preheat it.
3. Roast the lamb fillets for 4 minutes from each side over the medium heat.
4. After this, transfer the meat in the bowl.
5. Put cream cheese in the skillet.
6. Add parsley and dill.
7. Then add ground turmeric and Psyllium Husk.
8. Whisk the mixture and simmer for 1 minute.
9. Then add cooked lamb fillets and coat them in the mixture well.
10. Close the lid and cook lamb in the cream sauce for 10 minutes over the low heat.
11. Serve the lamb fillets with the cream sauce.

Nutrition value/serving: calories 250, fat 13.4, fiber 7.4, carbs 9.8, protein 24.9

480. Rosemary Lamb Roast

Preparation Time: 10 minutes

Cooking time: 47 minutes
Servings: 4

Ingredients:
- 1-pound lamb loin
- 1 tablespoon fresh rosemary
- ½ cup of coconut milk
- ¼ cup of water
- 1 teaspoon peppercorns
- 1 teaspoon salt
- 1 teaspoon butter

Directions:
1. Rub the lamb loin with salt well and pierce it with the help of the knife.
2. Place butter in the saucepan and melt it.
3. Place the lamb loin in the saucepan and roast it for 3 minutes from each side over the high heat.
4. Then add fresh rosemary and coconut milk.
5. Add water and peppercorns.
6. Close the lid and cook meat on medium heat for 40 minutes.
7. When the time is over, you will get only ½ part of all added liquid.
8. Slice the cooked lamb roast and sprinkle it with the remaining coconut milk juice.
9. It is recommended to serve the meat only hot.

Nutrition value/serving: calories 471, fat 27.1, fiber 1.2, carbs 2.5, protein 52.1

481. Lamb Ragu

Preparation Time: 10 minutes
Cooking time: 35 minutes
Servings: 6

Ingredients:
- 14 oz lamb fillet, cubed
- 4 oz celery stalk, chopped
- 1 cup white mushrooms, chopped
- 1 teaspoon paprika
- ½ teaspoon salt
- ¾ teaspoon rosemary
- 1 teaspoon ground black pepper
- 1 teaspoon dried dill
- 1 tablespoon tomato sauce
- 1 cup of water
- 1 cup of coconut milk
- 1 teaspoon butter

Directions:
1. Place the butter in the pan and preheat it for 1 minute over the medium heat.
2. Then add cubed lamb fillet, and cook it for 3 minutes.
3. Stir the meat and add chopped celery stalk and mushrooms. Mix up well.
4. Sprinkle the ragu mixture with paprika, salt, rosemary, ground black pepper, and dill.
5. Mix up well and add tomato sauce and water.
6. Stir the ingredients very carefully.
7. Then add coconut milk and close the lid.
8. Simmer ragu for 30 minutes over the medium-low heat.

Nutrition value/serving: calories 230, fat 15.2, fiber 1.6, carbs 3.9, protein 20.2

482. Spiced Lamb Shoulder

Preparation Time: 10 minutes
Cooking time: 45 minutes
Servings: 5

Ingredients:
- 1 ½ pound lamb shoulder
- 1 tablespoon fresh rosemary
- 1 tablespoon mustard
- 1 teaspoon salt
- 1 teaspoon garlic powder
- 1 teaspoon chili flakes
- 1 teaspoon chili powder
- 3 tablespoons apple cider vinegar
- 1 white onion, peeled
- 2 cups of water
- ¼ cup heavy cream
- 1/3 teaspoon cumin

Directions:
1. In the shallow bowl mix up together fresh rosemary, mustard, salt, garlic powder, chili flakes, chili powder, apple cider

vinegar, and cumin.
2. Then rub the lamb shoulder with the spice mixture and let the meat marinate for 25 minutes.
3. After this, pour water and heavy cream in the pan and bring the liquid to boil.
4. Place the meat and all the remaining marinade in the boiling water-cream liquid.
5. Chop the onion roughly and add it in the pan too.
6. Close the lid and cook it for 40 minutes over the medium heat or bake in the preheated to the 365F oven for 30 minutes.

Nutrition value/serving: calories 301, fat 13.1, fiber 1.3, carbs 4.3, protein 39.3

483. Butter Lamb Shank

Preparation Time: 10 minutes
Cooking time: 55 minutes
Servings:3

Ingredients:
- 3 lamb shanks (10 oz each)
- 1 tablespoon fresh cilantro, chopped
- 1 tablespoon minced garlic
- ¾ teaspoon minced ginger
- 1 teaspoon salt
- 4 tablespoons butter, softened
- ½ cup organic almond milk
- 1 teaspoon dried dill

Directions:
1. Churn together chopped cilantro, minced garlic, minced ginger, salt, and dried dill.
2. Then rub the lamb shanks with the butter mixture generously and place in the tray.
3. Add almond milk and cover the tray with foil.
4. Bake the lamb shanks for 40 minutes at 365F.
5. Then discard the foil and coat the meat in the butter juice (from the tray carefully.
6. Cook the lamb shanks for 15 minutes more.

Nutrition value/serving: calories 235, fat 25, fiber 1.1, carbs 3.7, protein 1.4

484. Lamb Vindaloo

Preparation Time: 15 minutes
Cooking time: 50 minutes
Servings:4

Ingredients:
- 1 teaspoon ground cumin
- 1 tablespoon mustard
- ½ teaspoon paprika
- 1 teaspoon turmeric
- 1 teaspoon chili flakes
- 1 tablespoon apple cider vinegar
- 15 oz lamb fillet, chopped
- ½ cup of coconut milk
- 1 tablespoon butter
- 2 garlic cloves, peeled
- ½ teaspoon Pink salt

Directions:
1. Place lamb fillet in the skillet and roast it over the high heat for 3 minutes. Stir it from time to time.
2. Then sprinkle the meat with ground cumin, mustard, paprika, turmeric, chili flakes, apple cider vinegar, and add butter.
3. Mix up the meat well and roast it for 2 minutes more.
4. After this, transfer the meat in the tray.
5. Add peeled garlic cloves, salt, and coconut milk. Mix up the meat mixture and cover with foil.
6. Secure the edges of the tray well and transfer the tray in the oven.
7. Cook the meal for 45 minutes at 360F.

Nutrition value/serving: calories 313, fat 18.8, fiber 1.4, carbs 3.9, protein 31.6

485. Meat Bread

Preparation Time: 15 minutes
Cooking time: 50 minutes
Servings:8

Ingredients:
- 3 cups ground beef
- 1 teaspoon garlic, diced
- 1 teaspoon ground nutmeg
- 1 tablespoon flaxseeds meal

- 3 eggs, beaten
- 1 tablespoon almond flour
- 1 oz pecans, chopped
- 1 teaspoon salt
- 1 teaspoon ground black pepper

Directions:
1. In the mixing bowl, mix up together ground beef, diced garlic, ground nutmeg, flaxseeds meal, eggs, almond flour, chopped pecans, salt, and ground black pepper.
2. When you get homogenous meat mixture, transfer it in the bread mold and flatten well.
3. Preheat the oven to 370F.
4. Place the meat bread inside the oven and cook it for 50 minutes.
5. Chill the cooked meat bread well and slice it into the servings.

Nutrition value/serving: calories 301, fat 20.6, fiber 1.2, carbs 2.1, protein 26.3

486. Saddle of Lamb

Preparation Time: 10 minutes
Cooking time: 60 minutes
Servings:5

Ingredients:
- 1-pound saddle of lamb
- 2 oz pancetta, chopped
- 1 tablespoon butter
- ½ white onion, diced
- 1 teaspoon salt
- 1 teaspoon ground black pepper
- 1 teaspoon rosemary
- 1 tablespoon sesame oil

Directions:
1. Beat the saddle of lamb gently with the help of the kitchen hammer.
2. Then rub the meat with salt, ground black pepper, and rosemary.
3. Place pancetta on the meat. Add diced onion and butter.
4. Roll the saddle of lamb and secure with the toothpicks if needed.
5. Then brush the meat with the sesame oil.
6. Cover the meat in the foil and transfer in the preheated to the 365F oven.
7. Cook the meal for 60 minutes.
8. Discard the foil from the cooked meat and slice it into the servings.

Nutrition value/serving: calories 281, fat 16.5, fiber 0.5, carbs 1.6, protein 29.9

487. Herbed Beef Pie

Preparation Time: 10 minutes
Cooking time: 45 minutes
Servings:8

Ingredients:
- 15 oz pork steak, cubed
- 1 onion, diced
- 1 tablespoon butter
- 1 teaspoon tomato paste
- 1 teaspoon salt
- 1 teaspoon chili powder
- ½ teaspoon ground paprika
- ¾ cup heavy cream
- 1 cup almond flour
- 1 egg, beaten
- 1 teaspoon baking powder
- ¼ cup of coconut milk
- 1 teaspoon olive oil
- 1 teaspoon ground cumin

Directions:
1. Make the dough: in the mixing bowl, mix up together coconut milk, baking powder, egg, and almond flour. Knead the dough. Leave the dough to rest.
2. Meanwhile, toss the butter in the pan and melt it.
3. Add cubed pork steak and diced onion. Add heavy cream.
4. Sprinkle the ingredients with salt, chili powder, ground paprika, and mix up well.
5. Then add tomato paste and mix up the meat again. Cook it for 10 minutes with the closed lid.
6. Meanwhile, cut the dough into 2 halves.
7. Roll up the dough in the shape of the pie crust.
8. Place the first pie crust in the springform mold.

9. Then sprinkle it with ground cumin. Add pork mixture and flatten it.
10. Cover the meat with the second part of the dough and secure the edges.
11. Brush the pie with the olive oil and pierce it with the help of kife.
12. Bake the pie for 30 minutes in the preheated to the 360F oven.
13. Chill the cooked pie to the room temperature and cut into the servings.

Nutrition value/serving: calories 191, fat 14.2, fiber 1.1, carbs 3.6, protein 12.5

488. Turmeric Rack of Lamb

Preparation Time: 15 minutes
Cooking time: 16 minutes
Servings: 4

Ingredients:
- 13 oz rack of lamb
- 1 tablespoon ground turmeric
- ½ teaspoon chili flakes
- 3 tablespoons olive oil
- 1 tablespoon balsamic vinegar
- 1 teaspoon salt
- ½ teaspoon peppercorns
- ¾ cup of water

Directions:
1. In the shallow bowl, mix up together ground turmeric, chili flakes, olive oil, balsamic vinegar, salt, and peppercorns.
2. Brush the rack of lamb with the oily mixture generously.
3. After this, preheat grill to 380F.
4. Place the rack of lamb in the grill and cook it for 8 minutes from each side.
5. The cooked rack of lamb should have a light crunchy crust.

Nutrition value/serving: calories 252 fat 18.8, fiber 0.4, carbs 1.3, protein 18.9

489. Sausage Casserole

Preparation Time: 10 minutes
Cooking time: 35 minutes
Servings: 6

Ingredients:
- 2 jalapeno peppers, sliced
- 5 oz Cheddar cheese, shredded
- 9 oz sausages, chopped
- 1 tablespoon olive oil
- ½ cup spinach, chopped
- ½ cup heavy cream
- ½ teaspoon salt

Directions:
1. Brush the casserole mold with the olive oil from inside.
2. Then put the chopped sausages in the casserole mold in one layer.
3. Add chopped spinach and sprinkle it with salt.
4. After this, add sliced jalapeno pepper.
5. Then make the layer of shredded Cheddar cheese.
6. Pour the heavy cream over the cheese.
7. Preheat the oven to 355F.
8. Transfer the casserole in the oven and cook it for 35 minutes.
9. Use the kitchen torch to make the crunchy cheese crust of the casserole.

Nutrition value/serving: calories 296, fat 26, fiber 0.3, carbs 1, protein 14.5

490. Cajun Pork Sliders

Preparation Time: 10 minutes
Cooking time: 45 minutes
Servings: 4

Ingredients:
- 4 low carb bread slices
- 14 oz pork loin
- 2 tablespoons Cajun spices
- 1 tablespoon olive oil
- 1/3 cup water
- 1 teaspoon tomato sauce

Directions:
1. Rub the pork loin with Cajun spices and place in the skillet.
2. Add olive oil and roast it over the high heat for 5 minutes from each side.
3. After this, transfer the meat in the saucepan, add tomato sauce and water.
4. Stir gently and close the lid.

5. Simmer the meat for 35 minutes.
6. Slice the cooked pork loin.
7. Place the pork sliders over the bread slices and transfer in the serving plates.

Nutrition value/serving: calories 382, fat 22.4, fiber 4.5, carbs 2.4, protein 38.9

491. Stuffed Beef Loin in Sticky Sauce

Preparation Time: 15 minutes
Cooking time: 6 minutes
Servings: 4

Ingredients:
- 1 tablespoon Erythritol
- 1 tablespoon lemon juice
- 4 tablespoons water
- 1 tablespoon butter
- ½ teaspoon tomato sauce
- ¼ teaspoon dried rosemary
- 9 oz beef loin
- 3 oz celery root, grated
- 3 oz bacon, sliced
- 1 tablespoon walnuts, chopped
- ¾ teaspoon garlic, diced
- 2 teaspoons butter
- 1 tablespoon olive oil
- 1 teaspoon salt
- ½ cup of water

Directions:
1. Cut the beef loin into the layer and spread it with the dried rosemary, butter, and salt.
2. Then place over the beef loin: grated celery root, sliced bacon, walnuts, and diced garlic.
3. Roll the beef loin and brush it with olive oil.
4. Secure the meat with the help of the toothpicks.
5. Place it in the tray and add a ½ cup of water.
6. Cook the meat in the preheated to 365F oven for 40 minutes.
7. Meanwhile, make the sticky sauce: mix up together Erythritol, lemon juice, 4 tablespoons of water, and butter.
8. Preheat the mixture until it starts to boil.
9. Then add tomato sauce and whisk it well.
10. Bring the sauce to boil and remove from the heat.
11. When the beef loin is cooked, remove it from the oven and brush with the cooked sticky sauce very generously.
12. Slice the beef roll and sprinkle with the remaining sauce.

Nutrition value/serving: calories 248, fat 17.5, fiber 0.5, carbs 2.2, protein 20.7

492. BBQ Pork Tenders

Preparation Time: 15 minutes
Cooking time: 7 minutes
Servings: 4

Ingredients:
- 1 teaspoon Erythritol
- 3 tablespoons ground paprika
- 1 teaspoon ground black pepper
- 1 teaspoon salt
- ½ teaspoon chili powder
- ¼ teaspoon cayenne pepper
- 1 teaspoon garlic powder
- 14 oz pork loins
- 1 tablespoon olive oil
- 1 tablespoon almond butter

Directions:
1. Make the BBQ mix: in the shallow bowl, mix up together ground paprika, Erythritol, ground black pepper, salt, chili powder, cayenne pepper, garlic powder.
2. Cut the pork loin into the tenders.
3. Rub every pork loin with BBQ mix and sprinkle with olive oil.
4. Leave the meat to marinate for at least 15 minutes.
5. After this, place almond butter in the skillet and melt it.
6. Place the pork tenders in the almond butter and cook them for 5 minutes.
7. Then flip the meat onto another side and cook for 2 minutes more. The time of cooking depends on meat thickness.

Nutrition value/serving: calories 315, fat 20.3,

fiber 2.7, carbs 4.7, protein 29

Vegetables

493. Spinach Dip

Serving: 2
Preparation Time: 4 minutes
Cook Time: 0 minutes

Ingredients:

- 5 ounces Spinach, raw
- 1 cup Greek yogurt
- 1/2 tablespoon onion powder
- 1/4 teaspoon garlic sunflower seeds
- Black pepper to taste
- 1/4 teaspoon Greek Seasoning

Directions:

1. Add the listed ingredients in a blender.
2. Emulsify.
3. Season and serve.

Nutrition:

Calories: 101
Fat: 4g
Carbohydrates: 4g
Protein: 10g

494. Cauliflower Rice

Serving: 2
Preparation Time: 5 minutes
Cook Time: 6 minutes

Ingredients:

- 1 head grated cauliflower head
- 1 tablespoon coconut aminos
- 1 pinch of sunflower seeds
- 1 pinch of black pepper
- 1 tablespoon Garlic Powder
- 1 tablespoon Sesame Oil

Directions:

1. Add cauliflower to a food processor and grate it.
2. Take a pan and add sesame oil, let it heat up over medium heat.
3. Add grated cauliflower and pour coconut aminos.
4. Cook for 4-6 minutes.
5. Season and enjoy!

Nutrition:

Calories: 329
Fat: 28g
Carbohydrates: 13g
Protein: 10g

495. Grilled Sprouts and Balsamic Glaze

Serving: 2
Preparation Time: 10 minutes
Cook Time: 30 minutes
Smart Points: 4

Ingredients:

- ½ pound Brussels sprouts, trimmed and halved
- Fresh cracked black pepper
- 1 tablespoon olive oil
- Sunflower seeds to taste
- 2 teaspoons balsamic glaze
- 2 wooden skewers

Directions:

1. Take wooden skewers and place them on a largely sized foil.
2. Place sprouts on the skewers and drizzle oil, sprinkle sunflower seeds and pepper.
3. Cover skewers with foil.
4. Pre-heat your grill to low and place skewers (with foil in the grill.
5. Grill for 30 minutes, making sure to turn after every 5-6 minutes.
6. Once done, uncovered and drizzle balsamic glaze on top.
7. Enjoy!

Nutrition:

Calories: 440
Fat: 27g
Carbohydrates: 33g
Protein: 26g

496. Amazing Green Creamy Cabbage

Serving: 4
Preparation Time: 10 minutes

Cook Time: 10 minutes

Ingredients:

- 2 ounces almond butter
- 1 ½ pounds green cabbage, shredded
- 1 ¼ cups coconut cream
- Sunflower seeds and pepper to taste
- 8 tablespoons fresh parsley, chopped

Directions:

1. Take a skillet and place it over medium heat, add almond butter and let it melt.
2. Add cabbage and sauté until brown.
3. Stir in cream and lower the heat to low.
4. Let it simmer.
5. Season with sunflower seeds and pepper.
6. Garnish with parsley and serve.
7. Enjoy!

Nutrition:

Calories: 432
Fat: 42g
Carbohydrates: 8g
Protein: 4g

497. Simple Rice Mushroom Risotto

Serving: 4
Preparation Time: 5 minutes
Cook Time: 15 minutes

Ingredients:

- 4 ½ cups cauliflower, riced
- 3 tablespoons coconut oil
- 1 pound Portobello mushrooms, thinly sliced
- 1 pound white mushrooms, thinly sliced
- 2 shallots, diced
- ¼ cup organic vegetable broth
- Sunflower seeds and pepper to taste
- 3 tablespoons chives, chopped
- 4 tablespoons almond butter
- ½ cup kite ricotta/cashew cheese, grated

Directions:

1. Use a food processor and pulse cauliflower florets until riced.
2. Take a large saucepan and heat up 2 tablespoons oil over medium-high flame.
3. Add mushrooms and sauté for 3 minutes until mushrooms are tender.
4. Clear saucepan of mushrooms and liquid and keep them on the side.
5. Add the rest of the 1 tablespoon oil to skillet.
6. Toss shallots and cook for 60 seconds.
7. Add cauliflower rice, stir for 2 minutes until coated with oil.
8. Add broth to riced cauliflower and stir for 5 minutes.
9. Remove pot from heat and mix in mushrooms and liquid.
10. Add chives, almond butter, parmesan cheese.
11. Season with sunflower seeds and pepper.
12. Serve and enjoy!

Nutrition:

Calories: 438
Fat: 17g
Carbohydrates: 15g
Protein: 12g

498. Hearty Green Bean Roast

Serving: 4
Preparation Time: 10 minutes
Cook Time: 20 minutes

Ingredients:

- 1 whole egg
- 2 tablespoons olive oil
- Sunflower seeds and pepper to taste
- 1 pound fresh green beans
- 5 ½ tablespoons grated parmesan cheese

Directions:

1. Pre-heat your oven to 400 degrees F.
2. Take a bowl and whisk in eggs with oil and spices.
3. Add beans and mix well.
4. Stir in parmesan cheese and pour the mix into baking pan (lined with parchment paper.
5. Bake for 15-20 minutes.
6. Serve warm and enjoy!

Nutrition:

Calories: 216
Fat: 21g
Carbohydrates: 7g

Protein: 9g

499. Almond and Blistered Beans

Serving: 4
Preparation Time: 10 minutes
Cook Time: 20 minutes

Ingredients:

- 1 pound fresh green beans, ends trimmed
- 1 ½ tablespoon olive oil
- ¼ teaspoon sunflower seeds
- 1 ½ tablespoons fresh dill, minced
- Juice of 1 lemon
- ¼ cup crushed almonds
- Sunflower seeds as needed

Directions:

1. Pre-heat your oven to 400 degrees F.
2. Add the green beans with your olive oil and also the sunflower seeds.
3. Then spread them in one single layer on a large sized sheet pan.
4. Roast it for 10 minutes and stir, then roast for another 8-10 minutes.
5. Remove from the oven and keep stirring in the lemon juice alongside the dill.
6. Top it with crushed almonds and some flaked sunflower seeds and serve.

Nutrition:

Calories: 347
Fat: 16g
Carbohydrates: 6g
Protein: 45g

500. Tomato Platter

Serving: 8
Preparation Time: 10 minutes + Chill time
Cook Time: Nil

Ingredients:

- 1/3 cup olive oil
- 1 teaspoon sunflower seeds
- 2 tablespoons onion, chopped
- ¼ teaspoon pepper
- ½ a garlic, minced
- 1 tablespoon fresh parsley, minced
- 3 large fresh tomatoes, sliced
- 1 teaspoon dried basil
- ¼ cup red wine vinegar

Directions:

1. Take a shallow dish and arrange tomatoes in the dish.
2. Add the rest of the ingredients in a mason jar, cover the jar and shake it well.
3. Pour the mix over tomato slices.
4. Let it chill for 2-3 hours.
5. Serve!

Nutrition:

Calories: 350
Fat: 28g
Carbohydrates: 10g
Protein: 14g

501. Lemony Sprouts

Serving: 4
Preparation Time: 10 minutes
Cook Time: Nil

Ingredients:

- 1 pound Brussels sprouts, trimmed and shredded
- 8 tablespoons olive oil
- 1 lemon, juice and zested
- Sunflower seeds and pepper to taste
- ¾ cup spicy almond and seed mix

Directions:

1. Take a bowl and mix in lemon juice, sunflower seeds, pepper and olive oil.
2. Mix well.
3. Stir in shredded Brussels sprouts and toss.
4. Let it sit for 10 minutes.
5. Add nuts and toss.
6. Serve and enjoy!

Nutrition:

Calories: 382
Fat: 36g
Carbohydrates: 9g
Protein: 7g

502. Cool Garbanzo and Spinach Beans

Serving: 4
Preparation Time: 5-10 minutes

Cook Time: Nil

Ingredients:

- 1 tablespoon olive oil
- ½ onion, diced
- 10 ounces spinach, chopped
- 12 ounces garbanzo beans
- ½ teaspoon cumin

Directions:

1. Take a skillet and add olive oil, let it warm over medium-low heat.
2. Add onions, garbanzo and cook for 5 minutes.
3. Stir in spinach, cumin, garbanzo beans and season with sunflower seeds.
4. Use a spoon to smash gently.
5. Cook thoroughly until heated, enjoy!

Nutrition:

Calories: 90
Fat: 4g
Carbohydrates:11g
Protein:4g

503. Delicious Garlic Tomatoes

Serving: 4
Preparation Time: 10 minutes
Cook Time: 50 minutes

Ingredients:

- 4 garlic cloves, crushed
- 1 pound mixed cherry tomatoes
- 3 thyme sprigs, chopped
- Pinch of sunflower seeds
- Black pepper as needed
- ¼ cup olive oil

Directions:

1. Preheat your oven to 325 degrees F.
2. Take a baking dish and add tomatoes, olive oil and thyme.
3. Season with sunflower seeds and pepper and mix.
4. Bake for 50 minutes.
5. Divide tomatoes and pan juices and serve.
6. Enjoy!

Nutrition:

Calories: 100
Fat: 0g
Carbohydrates: 1g
Protein: 6g

504. Mashed Celeriac

Serving: 4
Preparation Time: 10 minutes
Cook Time: 20 minutes

Ingredients:

- 2 celeriac, washed, peeled and diced
- 2 teaspoons extra-virgin olive oil
- 1 tablespoon honey
- ½ teaspoon ground nutmeg
- Sunflower seeds and pepper as needed

Directions:

1. Pre-heat your oven to 400 degrees F.
2. Line a baking sheet with aluminum foil and keep it on the side.
3. Take a large bowl and toss celeriac and olive oil.
4. Spread celeriac evenly on a baking sheet.
5. Roast for 20 minutes until tender.
6. Transfer to a large bowl.
7. Add honey and nutmeg.
8. Use a potato masher to mash the mixture until fluffy.
9. Season with sunflower seeds and pepper.
10. Serve and enjoy!

Nutrition:

Calories: 136
Fat: 3g
Carbohydrates: 26g
Protein: 4g

505. Spicy Wasabi Mayonnaise

Serving: 4
Preparation Time: 15 minutes
Cook Time: Nil

Ingredients:

- 1 cup mayonnaise
- ½ tablespoon wasabi paste

Directions:

1. Take a bowl and mix wasabi paste and

mayonnaise.
2. Mix well.
3. Let it chill and use as needed.

Nutrition:

Calories: 388
Fat: 42g
Carbohydrates: 1g
Protein: 1g

506. Mediterranean Kale Dish

Serving: 6
Preparation Time: 15 minutes
Cook Time: 10 minutes

Ingredients:

- 12 cups kale, chopped
- 2 tablespoons lemon juice
- 1 tablespoon olive oil
- 1 teaspoon coconut aminos
- Sunflower seeds and pepper as needed

Directions:

1. Add a steamer insert to your saucepan.
2. Fill the saucepan with water up to the bottom of the steamer.
3. Cover and bring water to boil (medium-high heat.
4. Add kale to the insert and steam for 7-8 minutes.
5. Take a large bowl and add lemon juice, olive oil, sunflower seeds, coconut aminos, and pepper.
6. Mix well and add the steamed kale to the bowl.
7. Toss and serve.
8. Enjoy!

Nutrition:

Calories: 350
Fat: 17g
Carbohydrates: 41g
Protein: 11g

507. Spicy Kale Chips

Serving: 4
Preparation Time: 10 minutes
Cook Time: 25 minutes

Ingredients:

- 3 cups kale, stemmed and thoroughly washed, torn in 2-inch pieces
- 1 tablespoon extra-virgin olive oil
- ½ teaspoon chili powder
- ¼ teaspoon sea sunflower seeds

Directions:

1. Pre-heat your oven to 300 degrees F.
2. Line 2 baking sheets with parchment paper and keep it on the side.
3. Dry kale entirely and transfer to a large bowl.
4. Add olive oil and toss.
5. Make sure each leaf is covered.
6. Season kale with chili powder and sunflower seeds, toss again.
7. Divide kale between baking sheets and spread into a single layer.
8. Bake for 25 minutes until crispy.
9. Cool the chips for 5 minutes and serve.
10. Enjoy!

Nutrition:

Calories: 56
Fat: 4g
Carbohydrates: 5g
Protein: 2g

508. Seemingly Easy Portobello Mushrooms

Serving: 4
Preparation Time: 10 minutes
Cook Time: 10 minutes

Ingredients:

- 12 cherry tomatoes
- 2 ounces scallions
- 4 portabella mushrooms
- 4 ¼ ounces almond butter
- Sunflower seeds and pepper to taste

Directions:

1. Take a large skillet and melt almond butter over medium heat.
2. Add mushrooms and sauté for 3 minutes.
3. Stir in cherry tomatoes and scallions.
4. Sauté for 5 minutes.
5. Season accordingly.
6. Sauté until veggies are tender.

7. Enjoy!

Nutrition:

Calories: 154
Fat: 10g
Carbohydrates: 2g
Protein: 7g

509. The Garbanzo Bean Extravaganza

Serving: 5
Preparation Time: 10 minutes
Cook Time: Nil
Smart Points: 5

Ingredients:

- 1 can garbanzo beans, chickpeas
- 1 tablespoon olive oil
- 1 teaspoon sunflower seeds
- 1 teaspoon garlic powder
- ½ teaspoon paprika

Directions:

1. Pre-heat your oven to 375 degrees F.
2. Line a baking sheet with a silicone baking mat.
3. Drain and rinse garbanzo beans, pat garbanzo beans dry and put into a large bowl.
4. Toss with olive oil, sunflower seeds, garlic powder, paprika and mix well.
5. Spread over a baking sheet.
6. Bake for 20 minutes.
7. Turn chickpeas so they are roasted well.
8. Place back in oven and bake for another 25 minutes at 375 degrees F.
9. Let them cool and enjoy!

Nutrition:

Calories: 395
Fat: 7g
Carbohydrates: 52g
Protein: 35g

510. Classic Guacamole

Serving: 6
Preparation Time: 15 minutes
Cook Time: Nil

Ingredients:

- 3 large ripe avocados
- 1 large red onion, peeled and diced
- 4 tablespoons freshly squeezed lime juice
- Sunflower seeds as needed
- Freshly ground black pepper as needed
- Cayenne pepper as needed

Directions:

1. Halve the avocados and discard stone.
2. Scoop flesh from 3 avocado halves and transfer to a large bowl.
3. Mash using a fork.
4. Add 2 tablespoons of lime juice and mix.
5. Dice the remaining avocado flesh (remaining half and transfer to another bowl.
6. Add remaining juice and toss.
7. Add diced flesh with the mashed flesh and mix.
8. Add chopped onions and toss.
9. Season with sunflower seeds, pepper and cayenne pepper.
10. Serve and enjoy!

Nutrition:

Calories: 172
Fat: 15g
Carbohydrates: 11g
Protein: 2g

511. Apple Slices

Serving: 4
Preparation Time: 10 minutes
Cook Time: 10 minutes
Smart Points: 1

Ingredients:

- 1 cup of coconut oil
- ¼ cup date paste
- 2 tablespoons ground cinnamon
- 4 granny smith apples, peeled and sliced, cored

Directions:

1. Take a large sized skillet and place it over medium heat.
2. Add oil and allow the oil to heat up.
3. Stir in cinnamon and date paste into the oil.

4. Add cut up apples and cook for 5-8 minutes until crispy.
5. Serve and enjoy!

Nutrition:

Calories: 368
Fat: 23g
Carbohydrates: 44g
Protein: 1g

512. Elegant Cashew Sauce

Serving: 4
Preparation Time: 5 minutes
Cook Time: Nil

Ingredients:

- 3 ounces cashew nuts
- ¼ cup water
- ½ cup olive oil
- 1 tablespoons lemon juice
- ½ teaspoon onion powder
- ½ teaspoon sunflower seeds
- 1 pinch cayenne pepper

Directions:

1. Add nuts to your blender and process.
2. Add other ingredients (except oil and process until smooth .
3. Add a little bit of oil and puree .
4. Serve as needed!

Nutrition:

Calories: 361
Fat: 37g
Carbohydrates: 6g
Protein: 3g

513. Lovely Japanese Cabbage Dish

Serving: 6
Preparation Time: 25 minute
Cook Time: Nil

Ingredients:

- 3 tablespoons sesame oil
- 3 tablespoons rice vinegar
- 1 garlic clove, minced
- 1 teaspoon fresh ginger root, grated
- 1 teaspoon sunflower seeds
- 1 teaspoon pepper
- ½ large head cabbage, cored and shredded
- 1 bunch green onions, thinly sliced
- 1 cup almond slivers
- ¼ cup toasted sesame seeds

Directions:

1. Add all listed ingredients to a large bowl, making sure to add the wet ingredients first, followed by the dried ingredients.
2. Toss well to ensure that the cabbages are coated well.
3. Let it chill and enjoy!

Nutrition:

Calories: 126
Fat: 10g
Carbohydrates: 9g
Protein: 4g

514. Almond Buttery Green Cabbage

Serving: 4
Preparation Time: 10 minutes
Cook Time: 15 minutes

Ingredients:

- 1 ½ pounds shredded green cabbage
- 3 ounces almond butter
- Sunflower seeds and pepper to taste
- 1 dollop, whipped cream

Directions:

1. Take a large skillet and place it over medium heat.
2. Add almond butter and melt.
3. Stir in cabbage and sauté for 15 minutes.
4. Season accordingly.
5. Serve with a dollop of cream.
6. Enjoy!

Nutrition:

Calories: 199
Fat: 17g
Carbohydrates: 10g
Protein: 3g

515. Mesmerizing Brussels and Pistachios

Serving: 4
Preparation Time: 15 minutes
Cook Time: 15 minutes

Ingredients:

- 1 pound Brussels sprouts, tough bottom trimmed and halved lengthwise
- 1 tablespoon extra-virgin olive oil
- Sunflower seeds and pepper as needed
- ½ cup roasted pistachios, chopped
- Juice of ½ lemon

Directions:

1. Pre-heat your oven to 400 degrees F.
2. Line a baking sheet with aluminum foil and keep it on the side.
3. Take a large bowl and add Brussels sprouts with olive oil and coat well.
4. Season sea sunflower seeds, pepper, spread veggies evenly on sheet.
5. Bake for 15 minutes until lightly caramelized.
6. Remove from oven and transfer to a serving bowl.
7. Toss with pistachios and lemon juice.
8. Serve warm and enjoy!

Nutrition:

Calories: 126
Fat: 7g
Carbohydrates: 14g
Protein: 6g

516. Brussels's Fever

Serving: 4
Preparation Time: 10 minutes
Cook Time: 20 minutes

Ingredients:

- 2 tablespoons olive oil
- 1 yellow onion, chopped
- 2 pounds Brussels sprouts, trimmed and halved
- 4 cups vegetable stock
- ¼ cup coconut cream

Directions:

1. Take a pot and place it over medium heat.
2. Add oil and let it heat up.
3. Add onion and stir-cook for 3 minutes.
4. Add Brussels sprouts and stir, cook for 2 minutes.
5. Add stock and black pepper, stir and bring to a simmer.
6. Cook for 20 minutes more.
7. Use an immersion blender to make the soup creamy.
8. Add coconut cream and stir well.
9. Ladle into soup bowls and serve.
10. Enjoy!

Nutrition:

Calories: 200
Fat: 11g
Carbohydrates: 6g
Protein: 11g

517. Hearty Garlic and Kale Platter

Serving: 4
Preparation Time: 5 minutes
Cook Time: 10 minutes

Ingredients:

- 1 bunch kale
- 2 tablespoons olive oil
- 4 garlic cloves, minced

Directions:

1. Carefully tear the kale into bite sized portions, making sure to remove the stem.
2. Discard the stems.
3. Take a large sized pot and place it over medium heat.
4. Add olive oil and let the oil heat up.
5. Add garlic and stir for 2 minutes.
6. Add kale and cook for 5-10 minutes.
7. Serve!

Nutrition:

Calories: 121
Fat: 8g
Carbohydrates: 5g
Protein: 4g

518. Acorn Squash with Mango Chutney

Serving: 4
Preparation Time: 10 minutes

Cook Time: 3 hours 10 minutes

Ingredients:
- 1 large acorn squash
- ¼ cup mango chutney
- ¼ cup flaked coconut
- Salt and pepper as needed

Directions:
1. Cut the squash into quarters and remove the seeds, discard the pulp.
2. Spray your cooker with olive oil.
3. Transfer the squash to the Slow Cooker and place lid.
4. Take a bowl and add coconut and chutney, mix well and divide the mixture into the center of the Squash.
5. Season well.
6. Place lid on top and cook on LOW for 2-3 hours.
7. Enjoy !

Nutrition:
Calories: 226
Fat: 6g
Carbohydrates: 24g
Protein: 17g

519. Satisfying Honey and Coconut Porridge

Serving: 8
Preparation Time: 10 minutes
Cook Time: 8 hours

Ingredients:
- 4 cups light coconut milk
- 3 cups apple juice
- 2 ¼ cups coconut flour
- 1 teaspoon ground cinnamon
- ¼ cup honey

Directions:
1. In a Slow Cooker, add the coconut milk, apple juice, flour, cinnamon and honey.
2. Stir well.
3. Close lid and cook on LOW for 8 hours.
4. Open lid and stir.
5. Serve with an additional seasoning of fresh fruits.

6. Enjoy!

Nutrition:
Calories: 372
Fat: 14g
Carbohydrates: 56g
Protein: 8g

520. Pure Maple Glazed Carrots

Serving: 6
Preparation Time: 10 minutes
Cook Time: 8 hours

Ingredients:
- ¼ cup pure maple syrup
- ½ teaspoon ground ginger
- ¼ teaspoon ground nutmeg
- ½ teaspoon salt
- Juice of 1 orange
- 1 pound baby carrots

Directions:
1. Take a small bowl and whisk in syrup, nutmeg, ginger, salt, orange juice.
2. Add carrots to your Slow Cooker and pour the maple syrup.
3. Toss to coat.
4. Close lid and cook on LOW for 8 hours.
5. Serve and enjoy!

Nutrition:
Calories: 76
Fat: 1g
Carbohydrates: 19g
Protein: 76g

521. Ginger and Orange "Beets"

Serving: 6
Preparation Time: 20 minutes
Cook Time: 8 hours

Ingredients:
- 2 pounds beets, peeled and cut into wedges
- Juice of 2 oranges
- Zest of 1 orange
- 1 teaspoon fresh ginger, grated
- 1 tablespoon honey
- 1 tablespoon apple cider vinegar

- 1/8 teaspoon fresh ground black pepper
- Sea salt

Directions:
1. Add beets, zest, orange juice, ginger, honey, pepper, salt and vinegar to your Slow Cooker.
2. Stir well.
3. Close lid and cook on LOW for 8 hours.
4. Serve and enjoy!

Nutrition:
Calories: 108
Fat: 1g
Carbohydrates: 25g
Protein: 3g

522. Pineapple Rice

Serving: 2
Preparation Time: 10 minutes
Cook Time: 2 hours

Ingredients:
- 1 cup rice
- 2 cups water
- 1 small cauliflower, florets separated and chopped
- ½ small pineapple, peeled and chopped
- Salt and pepper as needed
- 1 teaspoon olive oil

Directions:
1. Add rice, cauliflower, pineapple, water, oil, salt and pepper to your Slow Cooker.
2. Gently stir.
3. Place lid and cook on HIGH for 2 hours.
4. Fluff the rice with fork and season with more salt and pepper if needed.
5. Divide between serving platters and enjoy!

Nutrition:
Calories: 152
Fat: 4g
Carbohydrates: 18g
Protein: 4g

523. Creative Lemon and Broccoli Dish

Serving: 6
Preparation Time: 10 minutes
Cook Time: 15 minutes

Ingredients:
- 2 heads broccocli, separated into florets
- 2 teaspoons extra virgin olive oil
- 1 teaspoon sunflower seeds
- ½ teaspoon black pepper
- 1 garlic clove, minced
- ½ teaspoon lemon juice

Directions:
1. Pre-heat your oven to 400 degrees F.
2. Take a large sized bowl and add broccoli florets.
3. Drizzle olive oil and season with pepper, sunflower seeds and garlic.
4. Spread broccoli out in a single even layer on a baking sheet.
5. Bake for 15-20 minutes until fork tender.
6. Squeeze lemon juice on top.
7. Serve and enjoy!

Nutrition:
Calories: 49
Fat: 1.9g
Carbohydrates: 7g
Protein: 3g

524. Baby Potatoes

Serving: 4
Preparation Time: 10 minutes
Cook Time: 35 minutes

Ingredients:
- 2 pounds new yellow potatoes, scrubbed and cut into wedges
- 2 tablespoons extra virgin olive oil
- 2 teaspoons fresh rosemary, chopped
- 1 teaspoon garlic powder
- ½ teaspoon freshly ground black pepper and sunflower seeds

Directions:
1. Pre-heat your oven to 400 degrees F.
2. Line a baking sheet with aluminum foil and set it aside.
3. Take a large bowl and add potatoes, olive oil, garlic, rosemary, sea sunflower seeds

and pepper.
4. Spread potatoes in a single layer on a baking sheet and bake for 35 minutes.
5. Serve and enjoy!

Nutrition:
Calories: 225
Fat: 7g
Carbohydrates: 37g
Protein: 5g

525. Cauliflower Cakes

Serving: 4
Preparation Time: 10 minutes
Cook Time: 10 minutes

Ingredients:
- 4 cups cauliflowers, cut into florets
- 1 cup kite ricotta/cashew cheese, grated
- 2 eggs, lightly beaten
- 1 teaspoon paprika
- 1 teaspoon chili powder
- Sunflower seeds and pepper to taste
- ½ cup fresh parsley, chopped
- 1 tablespoon olive oil

Directions:
1. Add cauliflower, cheese, paprika, eggs, chili, sunflower seeds, pepper and parsley into a large sized bowl.
2. Mix well.
3. Drizzle olive oil into frying pan and place over medium-high heat.
4. Shape cauliflower mixture into 12 even patties.
5. Once oil is hot, fry cakes until both sides are golden brown.
6. Serve hot and enjoy!

Nutrition:
Calories: 180
Fat: 8g
Carbohydrates: 6g
Protein: 8g

526. Tender Coconut and Cauliflower Rice with Chili

Serving: 4
Preparation Time: 20 minutes
Cook Time: 20 minutes

Ingredients:
- 3 cups cauliflower, riced
- 2/3 cups full-fat coconut almond milk
- 1-2 teaspoons sriracha paste
- ¼- ½ teaspoon onion powder
- Sunflower seeds as needed
- Fresh basil for garnish

Directions:
1. Take a pan and place it over medium low heat.
2. Add all of the ingredients and stir them until fully combined.
3. Cook for about 5-10 minutes, making sure that the lid is on.
4. Remove the lid and keep cooking until any excess liquid is absorbed.
5. Once the rice is soft and creamy, enjoy!

Nutrition:
Calories: 95
Fat: 7g
Carbohydrates: 4g
Protein: 1g

527. Apple Slices

Serving: 4
Preparation Time: 10 minutes
Cook Time: 10 minutes
Smart Points: 1

Ingredients:
- 1 cup of coconut oil
- ¼ cup date paste
- 2 tablespoons ground cinnamon
- 4 Granny Smith apples, peeled and sliced, cored

Directions:
1. Take a large sized skillet and place it over medium heat.
2. Add oil and allow the oil to heat up.
3. Stir cinnamon and date paste into the oil.
4. Add sliced apples and cook for 5-8 minutes until crispy.
5. Serve and enjoy!

Nutrition:

Calories: 368
Fat: 23g
Carbohydrates: 44g
Protein: 1g

528. The Exquisite Spaghetti Squash

Serving: 6
Preparation Time: 5 minutes
Cooking Time: 7-8 hours

Ingredients:

- 1 spaghetti squash
- 2 cups water

Directions:

1. Wash squash carefully with water and rinse it well.
2. Puncture 5-6 holes in the squash using a fork.
3. Place squash in Slow Cooker.
4. Place lid and cook on LOW for 7-8 hours.
5. Remove squash to cutting board and let it cool.
6. Cut squash in half and discard seeds.
7. Use two forks and scrape out squash strands and transfer to bowl.
8. Serve and enjoy!

Nutrition:

Calories: 52
Fat: 0g
Carbohydrates: 12g
Protein: 1g

529. The Hearty Garlic and Mushroom Crunch

Serving: 6
Preparation Time: 10 minutes
Cooking Time: 8 hours

Ingredients:

- ¼ cup vegetable stock
- 2 tablespoons extra virgin olive oil
- 1 tablespoon Dijon mustard
- 1 teaspoon dried thyme
- 1 teaspoon sea salt
- ½ teaspoon dried rosemary
- ¼ teaspoon fresh ground black pepper
- 2 pounds cremini mushrooms, cleaned
- 6 garlic cloves, minced
- ¼ cup fresh parsley, chopped

Directions:

1. Take a small bowl and whisk in vegetable stock, mustard, olive oil, salt, thyme, pepper and rosemary.
2. Add mushrooms, garlic and stock mix to your Slow Cooker.
3. Close lid and cook on LOW for 8 hours.
4. Open lid and stir in parsley.
5. Serve and enjoy!

Nutrition:

Calories: 92
Fat: 5g
Carbohydrates: 8g
Protein: 4g

530. Easy Pepper Jack Cauliflower

Serving: 6
Preparation Time: 10 minutes
Cooking Time: 3 hours 35 minutes

Ingredients:

- 1 head cauliflower
- ¼ cup whipping cream
- 4 ounces cream cheese
- ½ teaspoon pepper
- 1 teaspoon salt
- 2 tablespoons butter
- 4 ounces pepper jack cheese

Directions:

1. Grease slow cooker and add listed ingredients.
2. Stir and place lid, cook on LOW for 3 hours.
3. Remove lid and add cheese, stir.
4. Place lid and cook for 1 hour more.
5. Enjoy!

Nutrition:

Calories: 272
Fat: 21g
Carbohydrates: 5g
Protein: 10g

531. The Brussels Platter

Serving: 4
Preparation Time: 15 minutes
Cooking Time: 4 hours

Ingredients:

- 1 pound Brussels sprouts, bottoms trimmed and cut
- 1 tablespoon olive oil
- 1 ½ tablespoons Dijon mustard
- Salt and pepper to taste
- ½ teaspoon dried tarragon

Directions:

1. Add Brussels sprouts, mustard, water, salt and pepper to your Slow Cooker
2. Add dried tarragon.
3. Stir well and cover.
4. Cook on LOW for 5 hours, making sure to keep cooking until the Brussels sprouts are tender.
5. Stir well and arrange.
6. Add Dijon over the Brussels sprouts.
7. Enjoy!

Nutrition:

Calories: 83
Fat: 4g
Carbohydrates: 11g
Protein: 4g

532. The Crazy Southern Salad

Serving: 2
Preparation Time: 10 minutes
Cook Time: nil

Ingredients:

- 5 cups Romaine lettuce
- ½ cup sprouted black beans
- 1 cup cherry tomatoes, halved
- 1 avocado, diced
- ¼ cup almonds, chopped
- ½ cup of fresh cilantro
- ½ cup of Salsa Fresca

Directions:

1. Take a large sized bowl and add lettuce, tomatoes, beans, almonds, cilantro, avocado, Salsa Fresco
2. Toss everything well and mix them
3. Divide the salad into serving bowls and serve!
4. Enjoy!

Nutrition:

Calories: 211
Fat: 16g
Carbohydrates: 6g
Protein: 10g

533. Kale and Carrot with Tahini Dressing

Serving: 1
Preparation Time: 15 minutes
Cook Time: nil

Ingredients:

- Handful of kale
- 1 tablespoon tahnini
- ½ head lettuce
- Pinch of garlic powder
- 1 tablespoon olive oil
- Juice of ½ lime
- 1 carrot, grated

Directions:

1. Add kale and roughly chopped lettuce to a bowl.
2. Add grated carrots to the greens and mix.
3. Take a small bowl and add the remaining ingredients, mix well.
4. Pour dressing on top of greens and toss.
5. Enjoy!

Nutrition:

Calories: 249
Fat: 11g
Carbohydrates: 35g
Protein: 10g

534. Crispy Kale

Serving: 4
Preparation Time: 10 minutes
Cook Time: 25 minutes

Ingredients:

- 3 cups kale, stemmed and thoroughly washed, torn in 2-inch pieces

- 1 tablespoon extra-virgin olive oil
- ½ teaspoon chili powder
- ¼ teaspoon sea salt

Directions:
1. Prepare your oven by pre-heating to 300 degrees F.
2. Line 2 baking sheets with parchment paper and keep them on the side.
3. Dry kale and transfer to a large bowl.
4. Add olive oil and toss, making sure to cover the leaves well.
5. Season kale with salt, chili powder and toss.
6. Divide kale between baking sheets and spread into single layer.
7. Bake for 25 minutes until crispy.
8. Let them cool for 5 minutes, serve.
9. Enjoy!

Nutrition:
Calories: 56
Fat: 4g
Carbohydrates: 5g
Protein: 2g

535. Juicy Summertime Veggies

Serving: 6
Preparation Time: 10 minutes
Cooking Time: 3 hours 5 minutes

Ingredients:
- 1 cup grape tomatoes
- 2 cups okra
- 1 cup mushrooms
- 2 cups yellow bell peppers
- 1 ½ cup red onions
- 2 ½ cups zucchini
- ½ cup olive oil
- ½ cup balsamic vinegar
- 1 tablespoon fresh thyme, chopped
- 2 tablespoons fresh basil, chopped

Directions:
1. Slice and chop okra, onions, tomatoes, zucchini, mushrooms.
2. Add veggies to a large container and mix.
3. Take another dish and add oil and vinegar, mix in thyme and basil.
4. Toss the veggies into the Slow Cooker and pour marinade.
5. Stir well.
6. Close lid and cook on 3 hours on HIGH, making sure to stir after every hour.

Nutrition:
Calories: 233
Fat: 18g
Carbohydrates: 14g
Protein: 3g

536. Crazy Caramelized Onion

Serving: 4
Preparation Time: 10 minutes
Cooking Time: 9-10 hours

Ingredients:
- 6 onions, sliced
- 2 tablespoons oil
- ½ teaspoon salt

Directions:
1. Add onions, oil and salt to your Slow Cooker.
2. Close lid and cook on LOW for 8 hours.
3. Open lid and keep simmering for 1-2 hours until any excess water has evaporated.
4. Serve and enjoy!

Nutrition:
Calories: 126
Fat: 15g
Carbohydrates: 15g
Protein: 2g

537. Kidney Beans and Cilantro

Serving: 6
Preparation Time: 5 minutes
Cook Time: nil

Ingredients:
- 1 can (15 ounces kidney beans, drained and rinsed
- ½ English cucumber, chopped
- 1 medium heirloom tomato, chopped
- 1 bunch fresh cilantro, stems removed and chopped

- 1 red onion, chopped
- Juice of 1 large lime
- 3 tablespoons Dijon mustard
- ½ teaspoon fresh garlic paste
- 1 teaspoon Sumac
- Salt and pepper as needed

Directions:
1. Take a medium-sized bowl and add kidney beans, chopped up veggies and cilantro.
2. Take a small bowl and make the vinaigrette by adding lime juice, oil, fresh garlic, pepper, mustard and Sumac.
3. Pour the vinaigrette over the salad and give it a gentle stir.
4. Add some salt and pepper.
5. Cover and allow to chill for half an hour.
6. Serve!

Nutrition:
Calories: 74
Fat: 0.7g
Carbohydrates: 16g
Protein: 21g

538. Broccoli Crunchies

Serving: 4
Preparation Time: 10 minutes
Cooking Time: 3 hours

Ingredients:
- 2 cups broccoli florets
- 2 ounces cream of celery soup
- 2 tablespoons cheddar cheese, shredded
- 1 small yellow onion, chopped
- ¼ teaspoon Worcestershire sauce
- Salt and pepper as needed
- ½ tablespoon butter

Directions:
1. Add broccoli, cream, cheese, onion, cheddar to Slow Cooker.
2. Stir and season with salt and pepper.
3. Place lid and cook on LOW for 3 hours.
4. Serve and enjoy!

Nutrition:
Calories: 162
Fat: 11g
Carbohydrates: 11g
Protein: 5g

539. Ultimate Buffalo Cashews

Serving: 4
Preparation Time: 10 minutes
Cook Time: 55 minutes

Ingredients:
- 2 cups raw cashews
- ¾ cup red hot sauce
- 1/3 cup avocado oil
- ½ teaspoon garlic powder
- ¼ teaspoon turmeric

Directions:
1. Take a bowl, mix the wet ingredients in a bowl and stir in seasoning.
2. Add cashews to the bowl and mix.
3. Soak cashews in hot sauce mix for 2-4 hours.
4. Pre-heat your oven to 325 degrees F.
5. Spread cashews onto baking sheet.
6. Bake for 35-55 minutes, turning after every 10-15 minutes.
7. Let them cool and serve!

Nutrition:
Calories: 268
Fat: 16g
Carbohydrates: 20g
Protein: 14g

540. A Green Bean Mixture

Serving: 2
Preparation Time: 10 minutes
Cooking Time: 2 hours

Ingredients:
- 4 cups green beans, trimmed
- 2 tablespoons butter, melted
- 1 tablespoon date paste
- Salt and pepper as needed
- ¼ teaspoon coconut aminos

Directions:
1. Add green beans, date paste, pepper, salt, coconut aminos to the Slow Cooker,

gently stir.
2. Toss and place lid.
3. Cook on LOW for 2 hours.
4. Serve and enjoy!

Nutrition:

Calories: 236
Fat: 6g
Carbohydrates: 10g
Protein: 6g

541. Decisive Cauliflower and Mushroom Risotto

Serving: 4
Preparation Time: 10 minutes
Cook Time: 20 minutes

Ingredients:

- 1 cup vegetable stock
- head cauliflower, grated
- 9 ounces mushroom, chopped
- tablespoons almond butter
- Sunflower seeds and black pepper, to taste
- 1 cup coconut cream

Directions:

1. Take a saucepan and pour stock into it.
2. Bring it to boil and set it aside.
3. Then take a skillet and melt almond butter over medium heat.
4. Add mushroom to sauté until it turns golden brown.
5. Stir in stock and grated cauliflower.
6. Bring the mixture to a simmer and add cream.
7. Cook until liquid is reduced and cauliflower is al dente.
8. Serve warm and enjoy!

Nutrition:

Calories: 186
Fat: 16.5g
Carbohydrates: 6.7g
Protein: 2.8g

542. Authentic Zucchini Boats

Serving: 4
Preparation Time: 10 minutes
Cook Time: 25 minutes
Smart Points: 3

Ingredients:

- medium zucchini
- ½ cup marinara sauce
- ¼ red onion, sliced
- ¼ cup kalamata olives, chopped
- ½ cup cherry tomatoes, sliced
- 2 tablespoons fresh basil

Directions:

1. Pre-heat your oven to 400 degrees F.
2. Cut the zucchini half-lengthwise and shape them in boats.
3. Take a bowl and add tomato sauce, spread 1 layer of sauce on top of each of the boat.
4. Top with onion, olives, and tomatoes.
5. Bake for 20-25 minutes.
6. Top with basil and enjoy!

Nutrition:

Calories: 278
Fat: 20g
Carbohydrates: 10g
Protein: 15g

543. Roasted Onions and Green Beans

Serving: 6
Preparation Time: 10 minutes
Cook Time: 15 minutes

Ingredients:

- 1 yellow onion, sliced into rings
- ½ teaspoon onion powder
- 2 tablespoons coconut flour
- 1 1/3 pounds fresh green beans, trimmed and chopped

Directions:

1. Take a large bowl and mix sunflower seeds with onion powder and coconut flour.
2. Add onion rings.
3. Mix well to coat.
4. Spread the rings in the baking sheet, lined with parchment paper.
5. Drizzle with some oil.

6. Bake for 10 minutes at 400 degrees F.
7. Parboil the green beans for 3 to 5 minutes in the boiling water.
8. Drain and serve the beans with baked onion rings.
9. Serve warm and enjoy!

Nutrition:
Calories: 214
Fat: 19.4g
Carbohydrates: 3.7g
Protein: 8.3g

Soups and stews

544. Turkey Soup

Servings: 6
Preparation time: 15 minutes
Cooking time: 40 minutes

Ingredients:

- 1 yellow onion, chopped
- 1 tablespoon avocado oil
- 3 thyme springs, chopped
- 3 garlic cloves, finely minced
- 25 oz fresh tomatoes, peeled, chopped
- 6 ounces tomato paste
- ¼ cup water
- 1 pound turkey meat, ground, fried
- 14 ounces beef stock
- 6 mushrooms, chopped
- 1 small red bell pepper, chopped
- ½ cup black olives, chopped

Directions:

1. Heat a saucepan with the oil over medium-high heat, add half of the onion, garlic and thyme. Stir and cook for 5 minutes.
2. Add tomatoes, tomato paste and the water, stir, bring to a boil, reduce heat to medium-low and simmer for 20 minutes.
3. Pour this mixture into a blender and pulse well.
4. Heat up a saucepan over medium-high heat, add the turkey, stir and cook for 4 minutes, breaking it into small pieces with a fork.
5. Add the rest of the onion, mushrooms and the bell pepper, stir and cook for 5 minutes.
6. Add blended soup and beef stock, stir and cook for 5 more minutes.
7. Ladle the soup into bowls, top with the olives and serve.
8. Enjoy!

Nutritional value: calories 218, fat 6, fiber 4,6, carbs 16,3, protein 18,3

545. Tomato and Basil Soup

Servings: 4
Preparation time: 10 minutes
Cooking time: 35 minutes

Ingredients:

- 56 oz fresh tomatoes, peeled, crushed
- 2 cups tomato juice
- 2 cups chicken stock
- ¼ pound coconut butter, melted
- 14 basil leaves, torn
- 1 cup coconut milk
- Salt and black pepper to the taste

Directions:

1. Put tomatoes, tomato juice and stock in a saucepan, heat up over medium-high heat, bring to a boil, reduce heat, stir and simmer for 30 minutes.
2. Pour this into a blender, add basil, pulse very well and return to saucepan.
3. Heat up the soup again, add the butter, salt, pepper and coconut milk, stir, cook over low heat for 4 minutes more, divide into bowls and serve.
4. Enjoy!

Nutritional value: calories 421, fat 33,5, fiber 11,6, carbs 31,3, protein 8,2

546. Chicken and Mushroom Soup

Servings: 4
Preparation time: 15 minutes
Cooking time: 60 minutes

Ingredients:

- 2 teaspoons coconut oil, melted
- 3 carrots, chopped
- 1 yellow onion, chopped
- 1 zucchini, chopped
- 15 ounces mushrooms, chopped
- 4 cups chicken meat, already cooked and shredded
- 2 teaspoons rosemary, dried

- 1 teaspoon thyme, dried
- 1 tablespoon apple cider vinegar
- 1 teaspoon cumin, ground
- 2 and ½ cups chicken stock
- A pinch of sea salt and black pepper

Directions:
1. Heat up a saucepan with the oil over medium heat, add carrots and onion, stir and cook for 5 minutes.
2. Add zucchini, and mushrooms, stir and cook for 10 more minutes.
3. Add the chicken meat, rosemary, thyme, vinegar, cumin and the stock, stir, bring to a boil, reduce heat to medium-low and simmer for 40 minutes.
4. Add salt and pepper to the taste, stir again, ladle into bowls and serve.
5. Enjoy!

Nutritional value/ serving: calories 459, fat 16,9, carbs 23,6, protein 52,8, fiber 3,7

547. Cauliflower Soup

Servings: 6
Preparation time: 10 minutes
Cooking time: 60 minutes

Ingredients:
- 1 yellow onion, chopped
- 2 tablespoons extra virgin olive oil
- 2 pounds cauliflower florets
- A pinch of sea salt and black pepper
- ½ teaspoon turmeric powder
- 2 garlic cloves, minced
- 5 cups veggie stock

Directions:
1. Heat up a saucepan with the oil over medium heat, add the onion and garlic, stir and sauté for 10 minutes.
2. Add cauliflower, salt and pepper, stir and cook for 12 more minutes.
3. Add the stock, stir, bring to a boil, reduce heat to medium and simmer for 25 minutes.
4. Transfer to a blender, add the turmeric powder, pulse well, ladle into bowls and serve.
5. Enjoy!

Nutritional value/ serving: calories 100, fat 6,8, carbs 12,4, fiber 4,3, protein 3,3

548. Beef Soup

Servings: 6
Preparation time: 10 minutes
Cooking time: 1 hour

Ingredients:
- 2 pounds organic beef, ground
- 4 cups beef stock
- 25 oz fresh tomatoes, peeled, chopped
- 1 green bell pepper, chopped
- 3 zucchinis, chopped
- 1 cup celery, chopped
- 1 teaspoon Italian seasoning
- ½ yellow onion, chopped
- ½ teaspoon oregano, dried
- ½ teaspoon basil, dried
- ¼ teaspoon garlic powder
- A pinch of sea salt and black pepper

Directions:
1. Heat up a saucepan over medium heat, add the beef, stir, cook for 5 minutes and drain excess grease
2. Add all the other ingredients, reduce heat to medium-low and simmer for 1 hour.
3. Ladle the soup into bowls and serve right away.
4. Enjoy!

Nutritional value/ serving: calories 345, fat 10,5, fiber 3,3, carbs 11,1, protein 50,4

549. Root Vegetable Soup

Servings: 8
Preparation time: 10 minutes
Cooking time: 1 hour and 30 minutes

Ingredients:
1. 1 sweet onion, chopped
2. 2 tablespoons ghee, melted
3. 5 carrots, chopped
4. 3 parsnips, chopped
5. 3 beets, chopped
6. 3 small shallots, chopped, cooked and

crumbled
7. 1-quart chicken stock
8. A pinch of sea salt and black pepper
9. 2 quarts water
10. ½ teaspoon chili flakes
11. 1 tablespoons rosemary, chopped

Directions:
1. Heat up a Dutch oven with the ghee over medium-high heat, add the onion, stir and cook for 5 minutes.
2. Add all the other ingredients, stir, bring to a boil, reduce heat to medium-low and simmer for 1 hour and 30 minutes.
3. Ladle the soup into bowls and serve hot.
4. Enjoy!

Nutritional value/ serving: calories 139, fat 3,9, fiber 6,2, carbs 25,4, protein 2,6

550. Coconut Chicken Soup

Servings: 6
Preparation time: 15 minutes
Cooking time: 30 minutes

Ingredients:
- 2 celery stalks, chopped
- ½ cup coconut oil, melted
- 2 carrots, chopped
- ½ cup arrowroot powder
- 6 cups chicken stock
- 1 teaspoon parsley, dried
- ½ cup water
- 1 bay leaf
- A pinch of sea salt and black pepper
- ½ teaspoon thyme, dried
- 1 and ½ cups coconut milk
- 3 cups organic chicken meat, already cooked and cubed

Directions:
1. Heat up a large saucepan with the oil over medium-high heat, add carrots and celery, stir and cook for 10 minutes.
2. Add stock, stir and bring to a boil.
3. In a bowl, mix arrowroot with ½ cup water, whisk well and add to the pot.
4. Also add parsley, sea salt, pepper, bay leaf and thyme, stir and simmer over medium heat for 15 minutes.
5. Add the meat and coconut milk, stir, cook 1 more minute, ladle into bowls and serve.
6. Enjoy!

Nutritional value: calories 793, fat 71,7, fiber 5,1, carbs 19,6, protein 25,8

551. Lemon Soup

Servings: 4
Preparation time: 10 minutes
Cooking time: 10 minutes

Ingredients:
- 6 cups shellfish stock
- 1 tablespoons garlic, minced
- 1 tablespoon coconut oil, melted
- 2 eggs
- ½ cup lemon juice
- A pinch of sea salt and black pepper
- 1 tablespoon arrowroot powder
- 1 tablespoon cilantro, chopped

Directions:
1. Heat up a saucepan with the oil over medium-high heat, add the garlic, stir and cook for 2 minutes.
2. Add the stock, stir and bring to a simmer.
3. In a bowl, mix eggs with salt, pepper, lemon juice and arrowroot, whisk very well, pour into the pot, stir, cook for 4 minutes more, ladle into bowls and serve with chopped cilantro on top.
4. Enjoy!

Nutritional value/ serving: calories 64, fat 4,7, carbs 5, fiber 0,2, protein 1,8

552. Spinach and Watermelon Soup

Servings: 3
Preparation time: 10 minutes
Cooking time: 0

Ingredients:
- 1 avocado, pitted and chopped
- 1 cucumber, chopped
- 2 bunches spinach
- 1 and ½ cups watermelon, chopped

- 1 bunch cilantro, roughly chopped
- Juice of 2 lemons
- ½ cup coconut aminos
- ½ cup lime juice

Directions:
1. In your blender, combine all the ingredients, pulse them well, divide into bowls and serve.

Nutritional value/ serving: calories 288, fat 14,2, carbs 42,9, fiber 11,8, protein 9,5

553. Cream of Carrot Soup

Servings: 4
Preparation time: 10 minutes
Cooking time: 45 minutes

Ingredients:
- 2 sweet potatoes, peeled and chopped
- 2 yellow onions, cut into wedges
- 2 pounds carrots, diced
- 4 tablespoons coconut oil, melted
- 1 head garlic, cloves peeled
- A pinch of sea salt and black pepper
- 2 cups chicken stock
- 3 tablespoons maple syrup

Directions:
1. Put onions, carrots, sweet potatoes and garlic in a baking dish, add the oil, salt and pepper, toss to coat, place in the oven at 425 degrees F and bake for 35 minutes.
2. Transfer the veggies to a large saucepan, add chicken stock, heat everything over medium-high heat, reduce to medium-low and cook for 10 minutes.
3. Transfer soup to a blender, add the maple syrup, pulse well, divide into soup bowls and serve.
4. Enjoy!

Nutritional value/ serving: calories 371, fat 14,1, carbs 60,3, fiber 9,9, protein 4,3

554. Beef Stew

Servings: 4
Preparation time: 10 minutes
Cooking time: 2 hours

Ingredients:
- 2 pounds beef stew meat, cubed
- 1 red chili, seeded and chopped
- 1 brown onion, chopped
- 1 teaspoon ghee, melted
- 2 tablespoons extra virgin olive oil
- A pinch of sea salt and black pepper
- 2/3 teaspoon nutmeg, ground
- 1 garlic clove, minced
- ½ cup white mushrooms, sliced
- 1 teaspoon rosemary, dried
- ¼ teaspoon fennel seeds
- 2 celery stick, chopped
- 2 carrots, thinly sliced
- 1-quart beef stock
- 2 tablespoons almond flour
- 1 sweet potato, chopped

Directions:
1. Heat up a large saucepan with the ghee and the olive oil over medium-high heat, add onion, chili, salt and pepper, stir and cook for 2-3 minutes.
2. Add the meat, stir and brown it for 5 minutes.
3. Add the mushrooms, garlic, stock, fennel, rosemary and the nutmeg, stir, bring to a boil, cover, reduce heat to low and cook for 1 hour and 10 minutes.
4. Add celery, carrots, and the potato, stir, cover and cook for 30 minutes.
5. In a bowl, mix the flour with a cup of liquid from the stew, stir well, pour over the stew, cook for 15 more minutes, divide into bowls and serve.
6. Enjoy!

Nutritional value/ serving: calories 574, fat 23,6, carbs 13,8, fiber 3,3, protein 73,5

555. Slow Cooked Beef Stew

Servings: 6
Preparation time: 10 minutes
Cooking time: 8 hours

Ingredients:
- 2 pounds beef stew meat, cubed
- 3 cups beef stock

- 7 garlic cloves, minced
- A pinch of sea salt and black pepper
- 4 carrots, chopped
- 1 cup coconut flour
- 2 yellow onions, chopped
- ½ green cabbage head, chopped
- 25 ounces tomatoes, peeled, chopped

Directions:
1. In a slow cooker, combine all the ingredients, toss, cover and cook on Low for 8 hours.
2. Divide into bowls and serve.
3. Enjoy!

Nutritional value/ serving: calories 412, fat 11,3, carbs 25, fiber 9,8, protein 21,7

556. Veggie and Turkey Stew

Servings: 3
Preparation time: 10 minutes
Cooking time: 30 minutes

Ingredients:
- 1 yellow onion, chopped
- 1 tablespoon coconut oil, melted
- 15 ounces turkey meat, cooked, thinly sliced
- 1 red bell pepper, chopped
- 1 carrot, thinly sliced
- 1 celery stick, chopped
- 1 tomato, chopped
- 2 garlic cloves, minced
- 2 cups chicken stock
- 1 tablespoon lemon juice
- Black pepper to the taste
- 1 zucchini, chopped
- A handful parsley leaves, chopped

Directions:
1. Heat up a pan with the oil over medium-high heat, add turkey, onion, celery and carrot, stir and cook for 3 minutes.
2. Add red bell pepper, tomatoes and garlic, stir and cook 1 minute.
3. Add lemon juice, stock and pepper, stir, bring to a boil, cover pan, reduce heat to medium and cook for 10 minutes.
4. Add zucchini, stir, cook for 12 more minutes, divide into bowls, sprinkle the parsley on top and serve.
5. Enjoy!

Nutritional value/ serving: calories 345, fat 12,4, fiber 3,3, carbs 13,5, protein 44,3

557. Beef and Plantain Stew

Servings: 4
Preparation time: 10 minutes
Cooking time: 5 hours

Ingredients:
- 6 plantains, skinless and cubed
- 2 pounds beef meat, cubed
- 3 cups collard greens, chopped
- A pinch of sea salt and black pepper
- 3 cups water
- ½ cup sweet paprika
- 3 tablespoons allspice
- ¼ cup garlic powder
- 1 teaspoon chili powder
- 1 teaspoon cayenne pepper

Directions:
1. In a slow cooker, mix all the ingredients, toss, cover and cook on High for 5 hours.
2. Divide into bowls and serve.
3. Enjoy!

Nutritional value/ serving: calories 827, fat 19,6, fiber 14,2, carbs 104,5, protein 19,9

558. Chicken Stew

Servings: 6
Preparation time: 15 minutes
Cooking time: 8 hours

Ingredients:
- 5 garlic cloves, minced
- 2 celery stalks, chopped
- 2 yellow onions, chopped
- 2 carrots, chopped
- 30 ounces homemade pumpkin puree
- 2 quarts chicken stock
- 2 cups chicken breast, skinless, boneless and cubed

- ¼ cup coconut flour
- Black pepper to taste
- ½ pound baby spinach
- ¼ teaspoon cayenne pepper

Directions:
1. In a slow cooker, combine all the ingredients except the spinach, cover and cook on Low for 7 hours and 50 minutes.
2. Add the spinach, cook on Low for 10 more minutes, divide into bowls and serve.
3. Enjoy!

Nutritional value/ serving: calories 222, fat 3,6, fiber 10,8, carbs 30, protein 18,6

559. Lamb and Coconut Stew

Servings: 4
Preparation time: 15 minutes
Cooking time: 1 hour and 50 minutes

Ingredients:
- 1 and ½ pounds lamb meat, cubed
- 1 tablespoon coconut oil, melted
- ½ red chili, seedless and chopped
- 1 brown onion, chopped
- 3 garlic cloves, minced
- 2 celery sticks, chopped
- 2 and ½ teaspoons garam masala powder
- 1 teaspoon fennel seeds
- A pinch of sea salt and black pepper
- 1 and ¼ teaspoons turmeric powder
- 1 and ½ teaspoons ghee, melted
- 14 ounces coconut milk
- 1 cup water
- 1 tablespoon lemon juice
- 2 carrots, chopped
- A handful parsley leaves, finely chopped

Directions:
1. Heat up a pan with the oil over medium-high heat, add the lamb, stir and brown for 4 minutes.
2. Add celery, chili and onion, stir and cook 1 minute more.
3. Reduce heat to medium, add garam masala, garlic, ghee, fennel, and turmeric, stir and cook 1 minute.
4. Add salt, pepper, tomato paste, coconut milk and water, stir, bring to a boil, reduce heat to low, cover and cook for 1 hour.
5. Add carrots and cook for 40 minutes more, stirring occasionally.
6. Add lemon juice and parsley, stir, transfer to bowls and serve.
7. Enjoy!

Nutritional value/ serving: calories 829, fat 54, fiber 9,5, carbs 38,7, protein 45,1

560. Veggie and Kale Stew

Servings: 6
Preparation time: 10 minutes
Cooking time: 1 hour and 10 minutes

Ingredients:
- 4 pounds mixed root vegetables (parsnips, carrots, rutabagas, beets, celery root, turnips, chopped
- 6 tablespoons extra virgin olive oil
- 1 garlic head, cloves separated and peeled
- ½ cup yellow onion, chopped
- Black pepper to taste
- 25 ounces fresh tomatoes, peeled, chopped
- 1 tablespoon tomato paste
- 2 cups kale leaves, torn
- 1 teaspoon oregano, dried

Directions:
1. In a baking dish, mix all root vegetables with black pepper, half of the oil and garlic, toss to coat, and bake at 450 degrees F for 45 minutes.
2. Heat up a pot with the rest of the oil over medium-high heat, add onions and sauté for 2-3 minutes
3. Add tomato paste, tomatoes, salt, pepper and the oregano, stir, bring to a simmer, reduce heat to low and cook for 10 minutes.
4. Add baked veggies and kale, toss, cook for 5 more minutes, divide into bowls and serve.
5. Enjoy!

Nutritional value/ serving: calories 293, fat

19,2, fiber 9,8, carbs 32,7, protein 2,2

561. French Chicken Stew

Servings: 4
Preparation time: 15 minutes
Cooking time: 2 hours

Ingredients:

- 10 garlic cloves, peeled
- 30 black olives, pitted
- 2 pounds chicken breasts, skinless, boneless and cubed
- 2 cups chicken stock
- 25 ounces tomatoes, peeled, chopped
- 2 tablespoon rosemary, chopped
- 2 tablespoons parsley, chopped
- 2 tablespoons basil, chopped
- A pinch of sea salt and black pepper
- A drizzle of extra virgin olive oil

Directions:

1. Heat up a large saucepan with a drizzle of olive oil over medium-high heat, add the chicken, salt and pepper, and cook for 4 minutes.
2. Add garlic, stir and brown for 2 minutes more.
3. Add chicken stock, tomatoes, olives, thyme, and rosemary, stir, cover saucepan and bake in the oven at 325 degrees F for 1 hour.
4. Add parsley and basil, stir, bake for 45 more minutes, divide into bowls and serve.
5. Enjoy!

Nutritional value/ serving: calories 553, fat 24,8, fiber 4,1, carbs 13, protein 68,5

562. Oxtail Stew

Servings: 8
Preparation time: 15 minutes
Cooking time: 6 hours

Ingredients:

- 4 and ½ pounds oxtail, cut into medium chunks
- 2 tablespoons extra virgin olive oil
- 2 leeks, chopped
- 4 carrots, chopped
- 2 celery sticks, chopped
- 4 thyme springs, chopped
- 4 rosemary springs, chopped
- 4 cloves
- 4 bay leaves
- Black pepper to taste
- 2 tablespoons coconut flour
- 25 ounces plum tomatoes, peeled, chopped
- 1-quart beef stock

Directions:

1. In a roasting pan, mix oxtail with black pepper and half of the oil, toss and bake at 425 degrees F for 20 minutes.
2. Heat up a large saucepan with the rest of the oil over medium heat, add leeks, celery, and carrots, stir and cook for 4 minutes.
3. Add thyme, rosemary and bay leaves, stir and cook everything for 20 minutes.
4. Add flour and cloves to veggies and stir.
5. Also add tomatoes, the oxtail, its cooking juices and stock, stir, increase heat to high, bring to a boil, place the pot in the oven and bake at 325 degrees F for 5 hours.
6. Take the oxtail out of the pot, discard bones, return it to the pot, toss, divide the stew into bowls and serve.
7. Enjoy!

Nutritional value/ serving: calories 580, fat 32,6, fiber 3,1, carbs 12,8, protein 59,7

563. Eggplant Stew

Servings: 3
Preparation time: 10 minutes
Cooking time: 30 minutes

Ingredients:

- 1 eggplant, chopped
- 1 yellow onion, chopped
- 2 tomatoes, chopped
- 1 teaspoon cumin powder
- A pinch of sea salt and black pepper

- 1 cup tomato puree
- A pinch of cayenne pepper
- ½ cup water

Directions:
1. Heat up a saucepan over medium-high heat, add the water, tomato paste, salt, pepper, cayenne and cumin and stir well.
2. Add the eggplant, tomato, and onion, stir, bring to a boil, reduce heat to medium, cook for 30 minutes, divide into bowls and serve.
3. Enjoy!

Nutritional value/ serving: calories 102, fat 0,8, fiber 8,8, carbs 23,4, protein 4,1

564. Squash Soup

Preparation time: 10 minutes
Cooking time: 50 minutes
Servings: 4

Ingredients:
- 1 butternut squash, halved lengthwise and deseeded
- 14 ounces coconut milk
- A pinch of sea salt and black pepper
- A handful parsley, chopped
- A pinch of nutmeg, ground

Directions:
1. Arrange the butternut squash halves on a lined baking sheet, place in the oven at 350 degrees F, bake for 45 minutes, cool down, scoop the flesh and transfer it to a large saucepan.
2. Add half of the coconut milk, blend using an immersion blender and then heat everything up over medium-low heat.
3. Add the rest of the coconut milk, salt, black pepper, nutmeg and parsley, blend using your immersion blender for a few seconds, cook for about 4 minutes, ladle into bowls and serve.
4. Enjoy!

Nutrition: calories 245, fat 23,7, fiber 3, carbs 9,8, protein 2,7

565. Broccoli Soup

Preparation time: 10 minutes
Cooking time: 20 minutes
Servings: 4

Ingredients:
- 1 yellow onion, chopped
- 2 tablespoons olive oil
- 1 celery stick, chopped
- Zest of ½ lemon, grated
- 1-quart veggie stock
- 17 ounces water
- 1 teaspoon cumin, ground
- 1 broccoli head, florets separated
- 3 garlic cloves, minced
- 2 bay leaves
- Juice of ½ lemon
- A pinch of sea salt and black pepper
- For the pesto:
- ½ cup almonds, chopped
- 1 garlic clove
- 2 tablespoons lemon juice
- 2 tablespoons olive oil
- 4 tablespoons green olives, pitted and chopped

Directions:
1. Heat up a large saucepan with 2 tablespoons olive oil over medium-high heat, add onion, lemon zest and a pinch of salt, stir and cook for 3 minutes.
2. Add celery and 3 garlic cloves, stir and cook for 1 minute more.
3. Add stock, cumin, water, and black pepper, stir, cover, bring to a boil and simmer for 10 minutes.
4. Add bay leaves and broccoli, stir, cover again and cook for 6 minutes more.
5. Take soup off the heat, discard bay leaves, transfer to a blender and pulse well.
6. Add juice from ½ lemon, pulse again, return to the pot and heat up again over medium-low heat.
7. Meanwhile, in a food processor, blend the almonds with 1 garlic clove, 2 tablespoon lemon juice, 2 tablespoons olive oil and the green olives.
8. Ladle the soup into bowls, top with the pesto you've just made and serve hot.

9. Enjoy!

Nutrition: calories 201, fat 16,8, fiber 4,8, carbs 14,6, protein 5,4

566. Tomato Gazpacho

Preparation time: 10 minutes
Cooking time: 0 minutes
Servings: 4

Ingredients:

- 8 tomatoes
- 1 red onion, chopped
- 1 cucumber, peeled and chopped
- 1 red bell pepper, chopped
- 1 green bell pepper, chopped
- 1 red chili pepper, chopped
- 3 garlic cloves
- 1 cup tomato juice
- 1 cup water
- 2 tablespoon apple cider vinegar
- Zest of ½ orange, grated
- ¾ cup olive oil
- A pinch of sea salt and black pepper

Directions:

1. In a blender, combine all the ingredients and pulse them well.
2. Divide the gazpacho into bowls and serve it cold.
3. Enjoy!

Nutrition: calories 417, fat 38,5, fiber 5,2, carbs 21, protein 3,9

567. Veggie Soup

Preparation time: 10 minutes
Cooking time: 15 minutes
Servings: 4

Ingredients:

- 1 yellow onion, chopped
- 2 carrots, chopped
- 6 mushrooms, chopped
- 1 red chili pepper, chopped
- 2 celery sticks, chopped
- 1 tablespoon coconut oil
- A pinch of sea salt and black pepper
- 4 garlic cloves, minced
- 4 ounces kale, chopped
- 15 oz fresh tomatoes, peeled, chopped
- 1 zucchini, chopped
- 1-quart veggie stock
- 1 bay leaf
- A handful parsley, chopped for serving

Directions:

1. Set your instant pot on Sauté mode, add oil and heat it up.
2. Add celery, carrots, onion, a pinch of salt and black pepper, stir and cook for 2 minutes.
3. Add chili pepper, garlic and the mushrooms, stir and cook for 2 minutes.
4. Add tomatoes, stock, bay leaf, kale and zucchinis, stir, cover pot and cook on High for 10 minutes.
5. Release pressure, stir soup again, discard the bay leaf, ladle into bowls, sprinkle the parsley on top and serve.
6. Enjoy!

Nutrition: calories 109, fat 3,9, fiber 4,3, carbs 16,9, protein 4,1

568. Jalapeno Chicken Soup

Preparation time: 10 minutes
Cooking time: 15 minutes
Servings: 2

Ingredients:

- 1 red bell pepper, chopped
- 1 teaspoon coconut oil
- 1 yellow onion, chopped
- ¼ cup pickled jalapeno peppers, chopped
- 2 garlic cloves, minced
- 1 tablespoon ghee, melted
- 1 teaspoon cumin, ground
- 1 teaspoon coriander, ground
- 1 teaspoon oregano, dried
- 1 and ½ cups chicken breast, skinless, boneless, cooked and shredded
- 2 and ½ cups chicken stock
- 2 cups kale, torn
- Zest of 1 lime, grated
- Juice of 1 lime

- A pinch of sea salt and black pepper
- 15 ounces fresh tomatoes, peeled, chopped
- 2 tablespoons spring onions, chopped
- 3 tablespoons pumpkin seeds, toasted
- 1 avocado, peeled, pitted and sliced
- 1 teaspoon sweet paprika
- 3 tablespoons coriander, chopped

Directions:
1. Heat up a large saucepan with the oil over medium heat, add the onion, stir and sauté for 2 minutes.
2. Add red bell peppers, the garlic, jalapenos, oregano, cumin, coriander, and ghee, stir and cook for 1 minute more.
3. Add tomatoes, kale, chicken, lime zest, stock, lime juice, salt and pepper, stir, bring to a boil, cook for 5 minutes and take off the heat.
4. Ladle the soup into bowls, top with pumpkin seeds, green onion, paprika, chopped coriander and avocado and serve.
5. Enjoy!

Nutrition: calories 1227, fat 53,2, fiber 14,2, carbs 60,7, protein 127,6

Meatless

569. Avocado Zucchini Noodles

Preparation Time: 10 minutes
Cooking Time: 5 minutes
Servings: 1

Ingredients:

- 1 zucchini, spiralized using slicer
- 1/2 avocado
- 3 tbsp parmesan cheese, shredded
- 2 tbsp mascarpone
- Pepper
- Salt

Directions:

1. In a bowl, add avocado and mascarpone and mash until smooth.
2. Add avocado mixture to the small saucepan and heat until warm.
3. Add zucchini noodles into the saucepan and cook until heated through.
4. Season with pepper and salt. Stir in parmesan cheese and serve.

Nutritional Value (Amount per Serving:

Calories 325
Fat 29 g
Carbohydrates 12 g
Sugar 2 g
Protein 7 g
Cholesterol 25 mg

570. Sweet & Tangy Green Beans

Preparation Time: 10 minutes
Cooking Time: 10 minutes
Servings: 4

Ingredients:

- 1 lb green beans, washed and trimmed
- 1/2 tsp whole grain mustard
- 1 tbsp erythritol
- 2 tbsp apple cider vinegar
- 1 small onion, chopped
- 1 tbsp olive oil
- 1/4 tsp pepper
- 1/4 tsp salt

Directions:

1. Steam green beans in microwave until tender.
2. Meanwhile, in a pan heat olive oil over medium heat.
3. Add onion in a pan sauté until softened.
4. Add water, sweetener, apple cider vinegar, and mustard in the pan and stir well.
5. Add green beans and stir to coat well. Season with pepper and salt.
6. Serve and enjoy.

Nutritional Value (Amount per Serving:

Calories 70
Fat 4 g
Carbohydrates 9 g
Sugar 2 g
Protein 2 g
Cholesterol 0 mg

571. Tomato Cauliflower Rice

Preparation Time: 10 minutes
Cooking Time: 15 minutes
Servings: 3

Ingredients:

- 1 medium cauliflower head, cut into florets
- 2 tbsp olive oil
- 1 tomato, chopped
- 1 small onion, chopped
- 2 tbsp tomato paste
- 1 tsp white pepper
- 1 tsp black pepper
- 1/2 tbsp dried thyme
- 2 green chilies, chopped
- 3 garlic cloves, chopped
- 1/2 tsp salt

Directions:

1. Preheat the oven to 400 F.
2. Add cauliflower florets into the food processor and process until it looks like rice.

3. Stir in tomato paste, tomatoes, and spices and mix well.
4. Spread cauliflower mixture on a baking tray and drizzle with olive oil.
5. Bake for 15 minutes.
6. Serve and enjoy.

Nutritional Value (Amount per Serving:

Calories 135
Fat 10 g
Carbohydrates 13 g
Sugar 6 g
Protein 3 g
Cholesterol 0 mg

572. Spinach Pie

Preparation Time: 10 minutes
Cooking Time: 30 minutes
Servings: 8

Ingredients:

- 6 eggs, beaten
- 2 cup cheddar cheese, shredded
- 20 oz frozen spinach, chopped
- 15 oz cottage cheese
- 1 tsp black pepper
- 1 tsp salt

Directions:

1. Preheat the oven to 375 F.
2. Spray 8*8-inch baking dish with cooking spray and set aside.
3. In a large bowl, mix together spinach, eggs, cheddar cheese, cottage cheese, pepper, and salt.
4. Pour spinach mixture into the baking dish and bake for 10 minutes.
5. Serve and enjoy.

Nutritional Value (Amount per Serving:

Calories 225
Fat 14 g
Carbohydrates 5 g
Sugar 1 g
Protein 20 g
Cholesterol 155 mg

573. Zucchini Eggplant with Cheese

Preparation Time: 10 minutes
Cooking Time: 40 minutes
Servings: 6

Ingredients:

- 1 medium eggplant, sliced
- 4 tbsp parsley, chopped
- ½ cup fresh basil, chopped
- 3 zucchini, sliced
- 3 oz Parmesan cheese, grated
- 1 tbsp olive oil
- 1 cup cherry tomatoes, cut in half
- 2 garlic cloves, minced
- 1/4 tsp pepper
- 1/4 tsp salt

Directions:

1. Preheat the oven to 350 F.
2. In a bowl, add cherry tomatoes, eggplant, zucchini, olive oil, garlic, cheese, basil, pepper and salt toss well.
3. Transfer the eggplant mixture into the baking dish and bake for 35 minutes.
4. Garnish with chopped parsley and serve.

Nutritional Value (Amount per Serving:

Calories 111
Fat 6 g
Carbohydrates 11 g
Sugar 5 g
Protein 7 g
Cholesterol 10 mg

574. Turnips Mashed

Preparation Time: 10 minutes
Cooking Time: 10 minutes
Servings: 4

Ingredients:

- 3 cups turnip, diced
- 3 tbsp butter, melted
- 1/4 cup heavy cream
- 2 garlic cloves, minced
- ¼ tsp garlic powder
- ¼ tsp onion powder
- Pepper
- Salt

Directions:

1. Boil turnips in a saucepan until tender. Drain well and mashed turnips until smooth.
2. Add remaining ingredients and mix well.
3. Serve and enjoy.

Nutritional Value (Amount per Serving:

Calories 130
Fat 12 g
Carbohydrates 7 g
Sugar 9 g
Protein 2 g
Cholesterol 30 mg

575. Tasty Coconut Cauliflower Rice

Preparation Time: 10 minutes
Cooking Time: 7 minutes
Servings: 2

Ingredients:

- 2 cups cauliflower, chopped
- 2 tbsp water
- 2 tbsp unsweetened shredded coconut
- 2 tbsp coconut oil
- 1 tsp lime zest
- 1 tbsp fresh cilantro, chopped
- 3 tbsp coconut milk powder

Directions:

1. Add cauliflower, water, shredded coconut, coconut oil, and coconut milk powder in a microwave-safe dish and microwave on high for 7 minutes.
2. Add lime zest and cilantro and stir well.
3. Serve and enjoy.

Nutritional Value (Amount per Serving:

Calories 195
Fat 19 g
Carbohydrates 6 g
Sugar 3 g
Protein 2 g
Cholesterol 0 mg

576. Parmesan Zucchini Chips

Preparation Time: 10 minutes
Cooking Time: 15 minutes
Servings: 3

Ingredients:

- 2 medium zucchinis, sliced
- ½ tsp garlic powder
- ¼ tsp onion powder
- 1/2 cup parmesan cheese, grated
- Pepper
- Salt

Directions:

1. Arrange sliced zucchinis on a baking tray. Season with garlic powder, onion powder, pepper, and salt.
2. Sprinkle parmesan cheese on top of zucchini slices.
3. Bake at 425 F for 15 minutes.
4. Serve and enjoy.

Nutritional Value (Amount per Serving:

Calories 45
Fat 2 g
Carbohydrates 6 g
Sugar 2 g
Protein 4 g
Cholesterol 5 mg

577. Zucchini Carrot Patties

Preparation Time: 10 minutes
Cooking Time: 5 minutes
Servings: 4

Ingredients:

- 1 large egg, lightly beaten
- 1/2 cup mozzarella cheese, shredded
- 1 carrot, grated
- 1 cup zucchini, grated
- 1/3 cup parmesan cheese, grated
- 2 tsp olive oil
- 1/4 tsp pepper
- 1 tsp salt

Directions:

1. Add all ingredients except oil into the bowl and mix until well combined.
2. Heat oil in a pan over medium-high heat.
3. Drop tablespoon of zucchini mixture on a hot pan and cook for 2 minutes on each side.
4. Serve and enjoy.

Nutritional Value (Amount per Serving:

Calories 102
Fat 7 g
Carbohydrates 2 g
Sugar 2 g
Protein 7 g
Cholesterol 55 mg

578. Cauliflower Mac n Cheese

Preparation Time: 10 minutes
Cooking Time: 20 minutes
Servings: 4

Ingredients:

- 1 medium cauliflower head, cut into florets
- 3/4 cup cheddar cheese, shredded
- 3 tbsp butter, melted
- 1/4 cup unsweetened coconut milk
- 1/4 cup heavy cream
- ¼ tsp garlic powder
- Pepper
- Salt

Directions:

1. Preheat the oven to 450 F.
2. Add cauliflower florets and 2 tbsp butter in a large bowl and toss well. Season with pepper and salt.
3. Spread cauliflower florets on a baking tray and roast in oven for 15 minutes.
4. Add roasted cauliflower into the large bowl and set aside.
5. In a saucepan, add remaining ingredients and heat over medium heat until cheese is melted.
6. Pour saucepan mixture over cauliflower and mix well.
7. Serve and enjoy.

Nutritional Value (Amount per Serving:

Calories 265
Fat 25 g
Carbohydrates 5 g
Sugar 2 g
Protein 9 g
Cholesterol 60 mg

579. Stir Fried Zucchini

Preparation Time: 10 minutes
Cooking Time: 5 minutes
Servings: 4

Ingredients:

- 2 zucchini, cut into slices
- ¼ tsp garlic powder
- 1 tsp butter
- 1 tsp dried basil
- 2 medium tomatoes, chopped
- 1 medium onion, chopped
- 1/4 tsp pepper
- 1/2 tsp salt

Directions:

1. Melt butter in a pan over medium heat.
2. Add onion and cook until softened.
3. Add zucchini and cook for 3 minutes.
4. Add tomatoes, garlic powder, and basil and cook until zucchini is tender.
5. Season with pepper and salt.
6. Serve and enjoy.

Nutritional Value (Amount per Serving:

Calories 40
Fat 1 g
Carbohydrates 8 g
Sugar 4 g
Protein 2 g
Cholesterol 3 mg

580. Stir Fry Cauliflower & Cabbage

Preparation Time: 10 minutes
Cooking Time: 15 minutes
Servings: 6

Ingredients:

- 2 cups cauliflower florets, chopped
- 3 cups cabbage, chopped
- 2/3 cup unsweetened coconut milk
- 1 tbsp olive oil
- ½ tsp garlic powder
- ¼ tsp onion powder
- 2 tbsp parsley, chopped
- Pepper
- Salt

Directions:

- Heat olive oil in a pan over medium heat.
- Add cauliflower, cabbage, onion powder, and garlic powder in a pan and sauté until softened.
- Add coconut milk and stir well. Bring to boil.
- Turn heat to low and simmer for 15 minutes or until sauce thickened.
- Season with pepper and salt.
- Garnish with parsley and serve.

Nutritional Value (Amount per Serving:

Calories 95
Fat 9 g
Carbohydrates 5 g
Sugar 3 g
Protein 2 g
Cholesterol 0 mg

581. Avocado Salsa

Preparation Time: 10 minutes
Cooking Time: 10 minutes
Servings: 8

Ingredients:

- 4 avocados, peeled and diced
- 1 onion, diced
- 1 chili, chopped
- 1 fresh lemon juice
- 2 tbsp fresh parsley, chopped
- 1 tbsp lemon juice
- 2 tomatoes, diced
- Pepper
- Salt

Directions:

1. Add all ingredients into the mixing bowl and mix well.
2. Serve and enjoy.

Nutritional Value (Amount per Serving:

Calories 215
Fat 20 g
Carbohydrates 10 g
Sugar 2 g
Protein 2 g
Cholesterol 0 mg

582. Cabbage Stir Fry

Preparation Time: 10 minutes
Cooking Time: 10 minutes
Servings: 4

Ingredients:

- 1 head cabbage, chopped
- 1 small onion, chopped
- 2 tbsp olive oil
- 1/8 tsp turmeric
- 2 tbsp shredded coconut
- 2 tbsp fresh parsley, chopped
- ¼ tsp cumin powder
- Pepper
- Salt

Directions:

1. Heat olive oil in a pan over medium heat.
2. Add onion to the pan and sauté until softened.
3. Add cabbage, shredded coconut, turmeric, and cumin powder and stir until cooked. Season with pepper and salt.
4. Serve and enjoy.

Nutritional Value (Amount per Serving:

Calories 110
Fat 7.2 g
Carbohydrates 12 g
Sugar 7 g
Protein 2.5 g
Cholesterol 0 mg

588. Cauliflower Fried Rice

Preparation Time: 10 minutes
Cooking Time: 5 minutes
Servings: 6

Ingredients:

- 3 cups cauliflower rice
- 3 eggs, lightly beaten
- 2 garlic cloves, minced
- 3 tbsp olive oil
- ¼ cup carrots, peeled and chopped
- 1 small onion, chopped
- 1/2 tbsp coconut aminos
- 2 tbsp unsweetened coconut milk

- Pepper
- Salt

Directions:
1. Heat olive oil in a pan over medium-high heat.
2. Add onion and garlic and sauté until softened.
3. Add cauliflower rice and carrots and stir well and set cauliflower rice to one side of pan.
4. Whisk together coconut milk and eggs and pour into the pan and stir until eggs are scrambled.
5. Stir scrambled eggs into the cauliflower rice.
6. Add coconut aminos and stir well and cook for 2 minutes more.
7. Serve and enjoy.

Nutritional Value (Amount per Serving:

Calories 115
Fat 9 g
Carbohydrates 5 g
Sugar 2 g
Protein 5 g
Cholesterol 80 mg

584. Basil Eggplant Casserole

Preparation Time: 10 minutes
Cooking Time: 40 minutes
Servings: 6

Ingredients:

- 3 zucchini, sliced
- ¼ cup fresh basil, chopped
- 1 cup cherry tomatoes, halved
- 1 medium eggplant, sliced
- 1 tbsp olive oil
- 2 garlic cloves, minced
- 3 oz parmesan cheese, grated
- 1/4 cup parsley, chopped
- 1/4 tsp pepper
- 1/4 tsp salt

Directions:
1. Preheat the oven to 350 F.
2. Add all ingredients into the large bowl and toss well to combine.
3. Pour eggplant mixture into baking dish and bake for 35 minutes.
4. Serve and enjoy.

Nutritional Value (Amount per Serving:

Calories 105
Fat 6 g
Carbohydrates 10 g
Sugar 4 g
Protein 7 g
Cholesterol 10 mg

585. Broccoli Fritters

Preparation Time: 10 minutes
Cooking Time: 10 minutes
Servings: 4

Ingredients:

- 8 oz broccoli, chopped
- 1 cup cheddar cheese, shredded
- ¼ tsp garlic powder
- ¼ tsp onion powder
- ¼ tsp dried thyme
- 1 tbsp olive oil
- 2 tbsp almond flour
- 2 eggs, beaten
- ¼ tsp paprika
- Pepper
- Salt

Directions:
1. Steam chopped broccoli in the microwave and drain excess water.
2. Add broccoli, almond flour, spices, cheese, eggs, and salt in a bowl and stir until combined.
3. Heat olive oil in a pan over medium heat.
4. Pour tablespoon of batter onto hot pan and cook until lightly brown and crusty about 2-3 minutes.
5. Turn to another side and cook until lightly brown.
6. Serve and enjoy.

Nutritional Value (Amount per Serving:

Calories 212
Fat 16 g
Carbohydrates 5.5 g
Sugar 1 g
Protein 13 g

Cholesterol 110 mg

586. Simple Stir Fry Brussels sprouts

Preparation Time: 10 minutes
Cooking Time: 15 minutes
Servings: 4

Ingredients:

- 1 lb Brussels sprouts, trimmed and halved
- 1 onion, chopped
- 1 tbsp olive oil
- 2 jalapeno pepper, seeded and chopped
- 2 tbsp parsley, chopped
- Pepper
- Salt

Directions:

1. Heat olive oil in a pan over medium heat.
2. Add onion and jalapeno and sauté until softened.
3. Add Brussels sprouts and stir fry for 10 minutes.
4. Season with pepper and salt.
5. Garnish with parsley and serve.

Nutritional Value (Amount per Serving:

Calories 90
Fat 4 g
Carbohydrates 13 g
Sugar 4 g
Protein 4 g
Cholesterol 0 mg

587. Sautéed Mushrooms & Zucchini

Preparation Time: 10 minutes
Cooking Time: 7 minutes
Servings: 4

Ingredients:

- 1/2 cup mushrooms, sliced
- 1 squash, diced
- 1 zucchini, diced
- 3 tbsp olive oil
- ¼ tsp coriander powder
- ¼ tsp garlic powder
- ¼ tsp cumin powder
- ¼ tsp paprika
- ¼ tsp chili powder
- 2 tsp pepper
- Salt

Directions:

1. In a medium bowl, whisk together spices, pepper, olive oil, and salt.
2. Add vegetables to a bowl and toss well to coat.
3. Heat pan over medium-high heat.
4. Add vegetables in pan and sauté for 5-7 minutes or until vegetables are tender.
5. Serve and enjoy.

Nutritional Value (Amount per Serving:

Calories 105
Fat 10 g
Carbohydrates 3.6 g
Sugar 1.5 g
Protein 1 g
Cholesterol 0 mg

588. Healthy Spinach Stir Fry

Preparation Time: 10 minutes
Cooking Time: 15 minutes
Servings: 2

Ingredients:

- 4 cups spinach
- 1/2 onion, sliced
- 2 tsp olive oil
- 5 mushrooms, sliced
- 1 garlic clove, diced
- 1/2 tsp lemon zest
- 1/2 cup cherry tomatoes, halved
- 1 tsp butter
- Pepper
- Salt

Directions:

1. Heat butter in a pan over medium heat.
2. Add mushrooms and sauté for 3-4 minutes or until lightly browned.
3. Remove mushrooms to a dish and set aside.
4. Heat oil in same pan over medium heat.
5. Add onion and sauté for 2-3 minutes.
6. Add tomatoes, garlic, lemon zest, pepper, and salt and cook for 2-3 minutes.
7. Add mushrooms and spinach and cook

until spinach is wilted.
8. Drizzle with lemon juice and serve.

Nutritional Value (Amount per Serving:

Calories 102
Fat 7 g
Carbohydrates 9 g
Sugar 3 g
Protein 4 g
Cholesterol 5 mg

589. Roasted Carrots

Preparation Time: 10 minutes
Cooking Time: 35 minutes
Servings: 6

Ingredients:

- 15 baby carrots
- 2 tbsp fresh parsley, chopped
- 5 garlic cloves, minced
- 1/2 tbsp dried basil
- 4 tbsp olive oil
- 1 1/2 tsp salt

Directions:

1. Preheat the oven to 375 F.
2. In a bowl, combine together oil, carrots, basil, garlic, and salt.
3. Spread the carrots onto a baking tray and bake for 35 minutes.
4. Garnish with parsley and serve.

Nutritional Value (Amount per Serving:

Calories 140
Fat 9 g
Carbohydrates 13 g
Sugar 6 g
Protein 2 g
Cholesterol 0 mg

590. Creamy Garlic Basil Mushrooms

Preparation Time: 10 minutes
Cooking Time: 35 minutes
Servings: 4

Ingredients:

- 1 1/2 lbs mushrooms, rinsed and quartered
- 3 garlic cloves, minced
- 1 onion, sliced
- 2 tbsp butter
- 1/2 cup heavy cream
- 1/2 cup dry red wine
- 1 tbsp dried basil
- 1/2 tsp pepper
- 1 1/2 tsp salt

Directions:

1. Melt butter in a large pan over medium-high heat.
2. Add onion and sauté for 15 minutes.
3. Add mushrooms and season with pepper and salt and cook for 15 minutes.
4. Add basil and garlic and stir well.
5. Add wine and stir well.
6. Turn heat to low and cook until wine reduced.
7. Add cream and stir for a minute.
8. Serve and enjoy.

Nutritional Value (Amount per Serving:

Calories 175
Fat 12 g
Carbohydrates 10.1 g
Sugar 5 g
Protein 6.2 g
Cholesterol 35 mg

591. Zucchini Noodles with Spinach

Preparation Time: 10 minutes
Cooking Time: 15 minutes
Servings: 4

Ingredients:

- 2 medium zucchini, spiralized using slicer
- 1 cup baby spinach
- 1/4 cup basil leaves
- 2 garlic cloves, chopped
- 1 tbsp olive oil
- 1/3 cup parmesan cheese, grated
- 4 oz cream cheese
- 1/2 tsp pepper
- 1/2 tsp salt

Directions:

1. Heat oil in a saucepan over medium heat.
2. Add garlic and sauté for 3-5 minutes.
3. Add zucchini noodles and cook for 10

minutes.
   4. Add cream cheese, basil, and spinach and stir until cream cheese is melted.
   5. Add parmesan cheese and season with pepper and salt.
   6. Serve and enjoy.

Nutritional Value (Amount per Serving:

Calories 175
Fat 15 g
Carbohydrates 6 g
Sugar 2 g
Protein 6 g
Cholesterol 35 mg

592. Parmesan Pepper Eggs

Preparation Time: 5 minutes
Cooking Time: 5 minutes
Servings: 4

Ingredients:

- 4 eggs
- 1/4 cup parmesan cheese, grated
- 1 bell pepper, cut into rings
- ¼ tsp garlic powder
- 1 tbsp olive oil
- Pepper
- Salt

Directions:

1. Heat olive oil in a pan over medium heat.
2. Add bell pepper rings to the pan and sauté for minute.
3. Add 1 egg into the center of each pepper slice.
4. Season with garlic powder, pepper and salt and cook for 3 minutes, then turn it carefully.
5. Sprinkle with parmesan cheese and cook for a minute.
6. Serve and enjoy.

Nutritional Value (Amount per Serving:

Calories 141
Fat 11 g
Carbohydrates 3 g
Sugar 2 g
Protein 9 g
Cholesterol 170 mg

593. Vegetable Egg Scramble

Preparation Time: 10 minutes
Cooking Time: 10 minutes
Servings: 1

Ingredients:

- 3 eggs, beaten
- 1/2 cup baby spinach, chopped
- 1 bell pepper, chopped
- 5 mushrooms, sliced
- 1 tbsp olive oil
- Pepper
- Salt

Directions:

1. Heat half tbsp oil in a pan over medium heat.
2. Add vegetables and sauté for 5 minutes.
3. Heat remaining oil in another pan and add beaten eggs into the pan and cook over medium heat, stirring constantly.
4. Season with pepper and salt.
5. Add sautéed vegetables to egg mixture and mix well.
6. Serve and enjoy.

Nutritional Value (Amount per Serving:

Calories 320
Fat 27 g
Carbohydrates 4.5 g
Sugar 3 g
Protein 18 g
Cholesterol 490 mg

Salads

594. Shrimp and Asparagus Salad

Preparation Time: 10 mins
Servings: 4

Ingredients:

- 2 c. halved cherry tomatoes
- Cracked black pepper
- 12 oz. trimmed fresh asparagus spears
- 16 oz. frozen peeled and cooked shrimp
- Cracker bread
- 4 c. watercress
- ½ c. bottled light raspberry

Directions:

1. In a large skillet, cook asparagus, covered, in a small amount of boiling lightly salted water for 3 minutes or until crisp-tender; drain in a colander. Run under cold water until cool.
2. Divide asparagus among 4 dinner plates; top with watercress, shrimp, and cherry tomatoes. Drizzle with dressing.
3. Sprinkle with cracked black pepper and serve with cracker bread.

Nutrition:
Calories: 155.5, Fat:1.4 g, Carbs:15 g, Protein:22 g, Sugars:1 g, Sodium:324 mg

595. Carrot and walnut salad

Preparation Time: 10 mins
Servings: 2

Ingredients:

- ¼ c. chopped walnuts
- 1 peeled, cored and sliced apple
- Parsley leaves
- 1 peeled and grated carrot
- 1 tbsp. honey

Directions:

1. Coat the grated carrots with honey.
2. Arrange the carrots, apples and walnuts in a salad bowl.
3. Decorate with parsley leaves.

Nutrition:
Calories: 193, Fat:8.7 g, Carbs:27.2 g, Protein:1.4 g, Sugars:238 g, Sodium:632 mg

596. Pickled onion salad

Preparation Time: 1 hour
Servings: 4

Ingredients:

- 4 chopped spring onions
- ½ c. chopped fresh cilantro
- 2 tbsps. brown sugar
- 1 tbsp. lime juice
- ½ c. cider vinegar
- 2 thinly sliced red onions
- 4 lettuce leaves
- 2 tsps. olive oil

Directions:

1. In a salad bowl combine the onions, vinegar, oil and sugar.
2. Cover and refrigerate for 1 hr.
3. Add cilantro and lime juice.
4. Serve on lettuce leaves.

Nutrition:
Calories: 223, Fat:14.1 g, Carbs:20 g, Protein:1.8 g, Sugars:0 g, Sodium:0.5 mg

597. Chicken Raisin Salad

Preparation Time: 15-20 mins
Servings: 2

Ingredients:

- 2 tbsps. lemon juice
- 2 tbsps. raisins
- 1 peeled, cored and cubed apple
- ¼ c. chopped celery
- 2 tbsps. olive oil
- 3 ¼ c. skinless and sliced chicken meat

Directions:

1. In a saucepan or skillet, cook the cubed chicken meat in olive oil until golden.
2. Transfer the cooked meat to a mixing

bowl of medium-large size and add all other ingredients. Stir to combine
3. Serve while the chicken is warm.

Nutrition:
Calories: 382, Fat:16 g, Carbs:41 g, Protein:25.7 g, Sugars:21 g, Sodium:125 mg

598. Pickled Grape Salad with Pear, Taleggio and Walnuts

Preparation Time: 15 mins
Servings: 3

Ingredients:
- 200g sliced taleggio cheese
- 4 tbsps. red wine vinegar
- 2 tbsps. light brown sugar
- 2 handfuls fresh watercress
- 100g halved red grapes
- 1 wedged pear
- 50g halved walnut

Directions:
1. Heat a cast-iron skillet or frying pan and toast the walnut halves, until they are slightly brown and give off a lovely nutty aroma. Set aside to cool.
2. Stir together the red wine vinegar and light brown sugar in a bowl, and leave for 5 minutes to allow the sugar to dissolve.
3. Add the grapes to this sweet and tangy mixture, and toss. Marinate for 10 minutes while you work on the rest of the recipe.
4. Scatter the watercress onto 3 plates or onto one large sharing platter, and then top evenly with the taleggio cheese and pear wedges.
5. Drain the grapes from their marinade, but do not discard the marinade.
6. Whisk 2 tablespoons of olive oil into the pickling marinade.
7. Scatter the pickled grapes all over the salad, and then drizzle over 3-4 tablespoons of the dressing.
8. Finish with the toasted walnut halves, and enjoy immediately.

Nutrition:
Calories: 421, Fat:28.4 g, Carbs:24.1 g, Protein:15.9 g, Sugars:23.9 g, Sodium:1 mg

599. Mango salad

Preparation Time: 5 mins
Servings: 2

Ingredients:
- ½ seeded and minced jalapeño pepper
- 2 tbsps. chopped fresh cilantro
- Juice of 1 lime
- 3 pitted and cubed ripe mangos
- 1 tsp. minced red onion

Directions:
1. Combine all ingredients in a salad bowl.
2. Toss well.

Nutrition:
Calories: 331, Fat:5 g, Carbs:28.1 g, Protein:1 g, Sugars:27 g, Sodium:3.4 mg

600. Fresh Fruit Salad

Preparation Time: 15 mins
Servings: 3

Ingredients:
- 1 halved and sliced ripe banana
- 170 g sliced and halved strawberries,
- 170 g julienned granny smith apples
- 1 g salt
- 340 g chopped ripe pineapple
- 170 g sliced and quartered kiwi
- 340 g chopped ripe mango

Directions:
1. Cut the mangoes and kiwis into small cubes to get that full burst of flavor.
2. Slice the bananas about a centimeter thick and then halve them.
3. Once you have all the fruits cut up, put them in a bowl, and top with salt.
4. Stir it all together and you are ready to serve!

Nutrition:
Calories: 203, Fat:0.9 g, Carbs:51 g, Protein:2 g, Sugars:16 g, Sodium:26 mg

601. Dried apricot sauce

Preparation Time: 2 hours
Servings: 4

Ingredients:

- ½ c. sugar
- 4 oz. dried apricots
- 3½ tbsps. cornstarch

Directions:

1. Place the dried apricots into enough hot water to cover them and let soak for 1-2 hours.
2. Bring the water with dried apricots to a boil and cook on low heat for 30 minutes.
3. Add sugar and bring back to a boil, constantly stirring.
4. Prepare the cornstarch solution: add the cornstarch to water in a 1:4 ratio, mix well.
5. Add the cornstarch solution to the boiling dried apricot sauce. Stir and remove from heat after 5 minutes.
6. Serve as topping for your favorite desserts.

Nutrition:

Calories: 153, Fat:0.2 g, Carbs:3.8 g, Protein:0.5 g, Sugars:7 g, Sodium:0.7 mg

602. Tomato, Cucumber, and Basil Salad

Preparation Time: 10 mins | Serves 4

Ingredients:

- 1 minced garlic clove
- ¼ tsp. freshly ground black pepper
- 1 tbsp. olive oil
- 1 thinly sliced small onion
- 2 medium cucumbers
- 4 quartered ripe medium tomatoes
- ¼ c. chopped fresh basil
- 3 tbsps. red wine vinegar

Directions:

1. Peel the cucumbers, slice in half lengthwise, and then use a spoon to gently scrape out the seeds.
2. Slice the cucumber halves and place in a bowl. Add the tomatoes, onion, and basil.
3. Place the remaining ingredients into a small bowl and whisk well to combine.
4. Pour the dressing over the salad and toss to coat. Serve immediately or cover and refrigerate until ready to serve.

Nutrition:

Calories: 66, Fat:4 g, Carbs:7 g, Protein:1 g, Sugars:8 g, Sodium:15 mg

603. Strawberries and Avocado Salad

Preparation Time: 5 mins
Servings: 2

Ingredients:

- 2 c. halved strawberries
- 2 pitted and peeled avocados
- 3 tbsps. chopped mint
- 1 peeled and sliced banana

Directions:

1. In a bowl, combine the banana while using the strawberries, mint and avocados, toss and serve cold.
2. Enjoy!

Nutrition:

Calories:150 , Fat:4 g, Carbs:8 g, Protein:6 g, Sugars:2 g, Sodium:700 mg

604. Kelp salad

Preparation Time: 15 mins
Servings: 2

Ingredients:

- ½ c. chopped spring onions
- ¼ shredded white cabbage head
- 1 oz. boiled kelp
- 1 tbsp. olive oil
- 1 peeled and sliced cucumber
- 1 hard-boiled and wedged egg

Directions:

1. Prepare the ingredients and combine them in a salad bowl.
2. Dress with olive oil.

Nutrition:

Calories: 162, Fat:9.8 g, Carbs:23 g, Protein:3 g, Sugars:1 g, Sodium:761 mg

605. Chicken celery salad

Preparation Time: 10 mins
Servings: 2

Ingredients:

- ¼ c. chopped celery
- 2 tbsps. olive oil
- 3¼ c. skinless cubed chicken meat
- 2 tbsps. raisins
- 1 peeled, cored and cubed apple
- 2 tbsps. lemon juice

Directions:

1. Preheat a non-stick pan and cook the chicken cubes in olive oil until golden.
2. In a salad bowl combine all the ingredients and dress with olive oil and lemon juice.

Nutrition:

Calories: 345, Fat:16.5 g, Carbs:16.7 g, Protein:10.7 g, Sugars:0.5 g, Sodium:191 mg

606. Garlic Potato Salad

Preparation Time: 10 mins
Servings: 6

Ingredients:

- ¼ c. olive oil
- 3 minced garlic cloves
- 2 tsps. chopped fresh rosemary
- Freshly ground black pepper
- 6 medium potatoes
- 1 c. sliced scallions
- 2 tbsps. unflavored rice vinegar

Directions:

1. Put the potatoes into a pot and add enough water to cover by 1 inch. Place over high heat and bring to a boil. Boil until fork tender but still solid; depending upon size, roughly 20 minutes.
2. Once cooked, remove from heat and place under cold running water. Drain and set potatoes aside to cool. Once cool enough to handle, cut into bite-sized cubes.
3. Place cubed potatoes, garlic, and scallions into a mixing bowl and toss to combine.
4. Measure the olive oil, vinegar, and rosemary into a small mixing bowl. Add freshly ground black pepper and whisk well to combine.
5. Pour the dressing over the salad and stir gently to coat. Serve immediately, or cover and refrigerate until serving.

Nutrition:

Calories: 204, Fat:9 g, Carbs:28 g, Protein:2 g, Sugars:6 g, Sodium:195 mg

607. Spring salad

Preparation Time: 8 hours
Servings: 2

Ingredients:

- 1 bunch minced dill
- 7 oz. halved small radishes
- 3 halved cucumbers
- ½ c. water
- 3 tbsps. lemon juice
- ¼ c. presoaked skinless almonds
- 1 minced garlic clove
- 1 tsp. honey

Directions:

1. Soak the almonds in water overnight.
2. Using a blender mix the almonds with garlic, honey, lemon juice and water.
3. Arrange the cucumbers, radish and dill in a salad bowl and pour the almond-garlic dressing over the salad.

Nutrition:

Calories: 197, Fat:6.8 g, Carbs:4.4 g, Protein:2 g, Sugars:2 g, Sodium:15 mg

608. Appetizing Cucumber Salad

Preparation Time: 10 mins
Servings: 8

Ingredients:

- 1 peeled and minced garlic clove
- 1 tbsp. fresh lemon juice
- 2 peeled cucumber
- 2 tbsps. low-fat, low-sodium mayonnaise

- 1 tsp. mustard
- 1/3 c. roughly chopped fresh dill leaves
- ½ tsp. pepper
- ½ c. sour cream

Directions:
1. Slice cucumber into 3 equal lengths. Then slice lengthwise into quarters or smaller to create cucumber sticks. Drain in a colander and set aside.
2. In a medium bowl whisk well the remaining ingredients.
3. Add the drained cucumber into bowl of dressing and toss well to coat.
4. Serve and enjoy.

Nutrition:
Calories: 37.9, Fat:2.3 g, Carbs:3.3 g, Protein:1 g, Sugars:5 g, Sodium:246 mg

609. Tuna Caprese Salad

Preparation Time: 10 mins
Servings: 2

Ingredients:
- 2 thinly sliced Roma tomatoes
- 2 tsps. balsamic vinegar
- 2 oz. cubed fresh mozzarella part-skim
- 8 large fresh basil leaves
- 1 tsp. olive oil
- 6 oz. fresh tuna steak
- Pepper
- 4 tsps. divided extra virgin olive oil

Directions:
1. On medium high fire, place a large skillet and heat 1 teaspoon olive oil.
2. Once hot, pan fry tuna for 3 minutes per side. Transfer to a plate with paper towel and dab dry. Place in ref to cool for at least an hour.
3. To assemble, layer tomatoes and tuna on a plate.
4. Season with pepper. Sprinkle with basil and mozzarella,
5. Drizzle balsamic vinegar and olive oil before serving.

Nutrition:
Calories: 267, Fat:14.6 g, Carbs:5.3 g, Protein:29.0 g, Sugars:2 g, Sodium:760 mg

610. Cabbage and Carrot Salad

Preparation Time: 5 mins
Servings: 4

Ingredients:
- 2 grated carrots
- 1 tbsp. lime juice
- 2 chopped shallots
- 1 tbsp. red vinegar
- ¼ tsp. black pepper
- 1 tbsp. olive oil
- 1 shredded big red cabbage head

Directions:
1. In a bowl, mix the cabbage with the shallots and the other ingredients, toss and serve as a salad.

Nutrition:
Calories: 106, Fat:3.8 g, Carbs:18 g, Protein:3.3 g, Sugars:1 g, Sodium:44 mg

611. Warm Asparagus Salad with Oranges

Preparation Time: 5 mins
Servings: 4

Ingredients:
- 1 lb. peeled and sliced fresh asparagus
- 2 tbsps. tomato basil seasoning blend
- 2 tbsps. olive oil
- 1 peeled and sectioned fresh orange

Directions:
1. Heat a 9 inch sauté pan to medium heat. Add olive oil.
2. When hot, add and toss asparagus. Cook 1 minute, tossing every 30 seconds.
3. Remove from heat, and toss with tomato basil seasoning blend and orange sections.

Nutrition:
Calories: 87.5, Fat:4.1 g, Carbs:8.1 g, Protein:5.1 g, Sugars:11 g, Sodium:10 mg

612. Chicken in Orange Sauce

Preparation Time: 10 mins
Servings: 4

Ingredients:

- ½ c. flour
- ¼ tsp. pepper
- 4 boneless and skinless chicken breasts
- ¼ tsp. salt
- 1 ½ c. orange juice
- 4 tbsps. margarine

Directions:

1. Rinse and pat dry the chicken. Cut into bite size pieces.
2. Place the flour in a shallow bowl.
3. In a large skillet, heat the margarine.
4. Dip the pieces of chicken in flour, fry in the margarine 4 - 6 minutes on each side, until golden brown.
5. Pour the orange juice over the chicken. Simmer until the orange juice is reduced, approximately 15 minutes.

Nutrition:

Calories: 160, Fat:18 g, Carbs:62 g, Protein:22 g, Sugars:19 g, Sodium:430 mg

613. Pumpkin salad

Preparation Time: 15 mins
Servings: 2

Ingredients:

- Juice of ½ lemon
- 2 tbsps. pumpkin seeds
- 2 oz. peeled, cored and sliced apples
- 1 tbsp. honey
- 2 oz. peeled and sliced Canary melon
- 2 oz. peeled and grated pumpkin

Directions:

1. Coat the grated pumpkin with honey.
2. Arrange the pumpkin, melon, apples and pumpkin seeds in a salad bowl.
3. Sprinkle with lemon juice.

Nutrition:

Calories: 213, Fat:6.5 g, Carbs:13 g, Protein:5 g, Sugars:1 g, Sodium:381 mg

614. Sweet Jicama Salad

Preparation Time: 12 mins
Servings: 1 - 2

Ingredients:

- 1 small fennel bulb
- ¼ tsp. salt
- ¼ lb. Jicama
- 1/8 tsp. fresh ground pepper
- ½ thinly sliced red onion
- Juice of 1 small tangerine
- 1 tbsp. chopped fennel leaves

Directions:

1. Peel and slice the Jicama into ¼ inch pieces.
2. Stem and core the fennel bulb, slice into thin half-moons.
3. In a large bowl, add the sliced Jicama and fennel. Squeeze the tangerine over the fennel and Jicama. Season with salt.
4. Garnish with black pepper and chopped fennel leaves. Serve immediately.

Nutrition:

Calories: 99, Fat:17 g, Carbs:35 g, Protein:45 g, Sugars:2 g, Sodium:405 mg

615. Heart Healthy Chicken Salad

Preparation Time: 10 mins
Servings: 5

Ingredients:

- ½ tsp. onion powder
- 1 tbsp. lemon juice
- 3 ¼ c. cooked, cubed, and skinless chicken breast
- 1 chopped lettuce head
- 3 tbsps. low-fat mayonnaise
- ¼ c. chopped celery

Directions:

1. Except for chicken and lettuce, combine all ingredients in a bowl and whisk well.
2. Add chicken and toss well to coat.
3. Evenly divide chopped lettuce in 5 bowls and top evenly with chicken salad.
4. Enjoy!

Nutrition:

Calories: 164, Fat:4.9 g, Carbs:1.9 g, Protein:28.3 g, Sugars:7 g, Sodium:179 mg

616. Cashews and Blueberries Salad

Preparation Time: 10 mins
Servings: 2

Ingredients:

- ¼ c. blueberries
- 1 peeled and sliced banana
- ¼ c. raw cashews
- 1 tsp. cinnamon powder
- 1 tbsp. almond butter

Directions:

1. In a bowl, combine the banana with cashews, blueberries, almond butter and cinnamon, toss and serve each day.
2. Enjoy!

Nutrition:

Calories: 120, Fat:0.3 g, Carbs:7 g, Protein:5 g, Sugars:5 g, Sodium:262 mg

617. Radish Salad

Preparation Time: 5 mins
Servings: 4

Ingredients:

- 1 lb. cubed radishes
- 1 c. pitted and halved black olives
- 2 tbsps. balsamic vinegar
- 2 tbsps. olive oil
- 2 green onions
- 1 tsp. chili powder
- ¼ tsp. black pepper

Directions:

1. In a large salad bowl, combine radishes with the onions and the other ingredients, toss and serve as a side dish.

Nutrition:

Calories: 123, Fat:10.8 g, Carbs:7 g, Protein:1.3 g, Sugars:1.7 g, Sodium:168 mg

618. Tarragon Tomatoes

Preparation Time: 5 mins
Servings: 4

Ingredients:

- 1 lb. sliced tomatoes
- 2 tbsps. chopped tarragon
- ¼ tsp. black pepper
- 1 ½ tbsps. olive oil
- 1 tbsp. grated lime zest
- 1 tbsp. lime juice

Directions:

1. In a bowl, combine the tomatoes with the other ingredients, toss and serve as a side salad.

Nutrition:

Calories: 170, Fat:4 g, Carbs:11.8 g, Protein:6 g, Sugars:9 g, Sodium:430 mg

Snacks

619. Seeds Bowls

Preparation time: 10 minutes
Cooking time: 15 minutes
Servings: 4

Ingredients:

- ½ cup sunflower seeds
- ½ cup chia seeds
- ½ cup pine nuts
- ½ cup pumpkin seeds
- 1 tablespoon coconut oil, melted
- 1 teaspoon sweet paprika

Directions:

1. Spread the seeds on a baking sheet lined with parchment paper, add the oil and the paprika, toss and cook for 15 minutes at 400 degrees F.
2. Divide into bowls and serve.

Nutrition: calories 110, fat 1, fiber 5, carbs 7, protein 5

Snow Peas and Tomato Salsa

Preparation time: 10 minutes
Cooking time: 0 minutes
Servings: 4

Ingredients:

- 1 cup cherry tomatoes, halved
- 2 cups snow peas, steamed and cooled
- 1 tablespoon lemon juice
- 2 garlic cloves, minced
- 1 avocado, peeled, pitted and cubed
- 1 tablespoon olive oil
- 1 tablespoon cilantro, chopped
- A pinch of cayenne pepper

Directions:

1. In a bowl, mix the cherry tomatoes with the peas and the other ingredients, toss well, divide into smaller bowls and serve.

Nutrition: calories 120, fat 2, fiber 4, carbs 6, protein 6

Apple Chips

Preparation time: 10 minutes
Cooking time: 1 hour
Servings: 4

Ingredients:

- Cooking spray
- 2 apples, cored thinly sliced
- 1 tablespoon cinnamon powder
- A pinch of nutmeg, ground

Directions:

2. Arrange the apples on a lined baking sheet, add the other ingredients, toss and cook at 360 degrees F for 1 hour.
3. Divide into bowls and serve as a snack

Nutrition: calories 141, fat 2, fiber 2, carbs 7, protein 5

622. Dill Cucumber Dip

Preparation time: 10 minutes
Cooking time: 0 minutes
Servings: 4

Ingredients:

- 2 cups coconut cream
- 2 cucumbers, chopped
- 1 tablespoon dill, chopped
- 2 teaspoons thyme, dried
- 2 teaspoons parsley, dried
- 2 teaspoons chives, chopped
- A pinch of sea salt and black pepper

Directions:

1. In a blender, combine the cream with the cucumbers and the other ingredients, pulse, divide into bowls and serve cold.

Nutrition: calories 120, fat 3, fiber 5, carbs 5, protein 3

623. Beans Salsa

Preparation time: 15 minutes
Cooking time: 0 minutes

Servings: 6

Ingredients:

- 1 cup canned garbanzo beans, drained and rinsed
- 1 cup canned black beans, drained and rinsed
- ½ cup cherry tomatoes, cubed
- 1 cucumber, cubed
- 2 tablespoons lime juice
- 1 tablespoon olive oil
- 5 garlic cloves, minced
- ½ teaspoon cumin, ground
- A pinch of salt and black pepper

Directions:

1. In a bowl, combine the beans with the tomatoes, cucumber and the other ingredients, toss well and serve cold as a snack.

Nutrition: calories 170, fat 3, fiber 7, carbs 10, protein 8

624. Bell Peppers and Zucchinis Patties

Preparation time: 10 minutes
Cooking time: 10 minutes
Servings: 6

Ingredients:

- 1 tablespoon olive oil
- ½ cup cilantro, chopped
- 2 spring onions, chopped
- 1 red bell pepper, chopped
- 1 green bell pepper, chopped
- 1 egg
- ½ cup almond flour
- A pinch of salt and black pepper
- 2 garlic cloves, minced
- 3 zucchinis, grated

Directions:

1. In a bowl, combine the zucchinis with the bell peppers and the other ingredients except the oil, stir well and shape medium patties out of this mix.
2. Heat up a pan with the oil over medium heat, add the patties, cook for 5 minutes on each side, arrange on a platter and serve.

Nutrition: calories 120, fat 4, fiber 2, carbs 6, protein 6

625. Broccoli Bites

Preparation time: 10 minutes
Cooking time: 25 minutes
Servings: 4

Ingredients:

- 1 pound broccoli florets
- Cooking spray
- 2 eggs, whisked
- 1 teaspoon Italian seasoning
- A pinch of sea salt and black pepper
- 1 teaspoon smoked paprika
- 1 teaspoon cumin, ground

Directions:

1. In a bowl, mix the eggs with the Italian seasoning and the other ingredients except the broccoli and the cooking spray and whisk well.
2. Dip the broccoli florets in the eggs mix, arrange them on a baking sheet lined with parchment paper, grease them with cooking spray and bake at 380 degrees F for 25 minutes.
3. Divide the broccoli bites into bowls and serve.

Nutrition: calories 120, fat 6, fiber 2, carbs 6, protein 7

626. Balsamic Mushrooms Mix

Preparation time: 10 minutes
Cooking time: 25 minutes
Servings: 6

Ingredients:

- 2 pound brown mushroom caps
- 1 tablespoon olive oil
- A pinch of sea salt and black pepper
- 1 tablespoon balsamic vinegar
- 1 tablespoon chives, chopped
- 1 teaspoon sweet paprika

Directions:

1. Arrange mushroom caps on a baking sheet lined with parchment paper, add the oil, salt, pepper and the other ingredients, toss well and bake at 390 degrees F for 25 minutes.
2. Divide the mushroom caps in bowls and serve.

Nutrition: calories 120, fat 2, fiber 2, carbs 6, protein 5

627. Almond Artichoke Dip

Preparation time: 10 minutes
Cooking time: 35 minutes
Servings: 8

Ingredients:

- ½ cup almond milk
- 1 cup coconut cream
- 10 ounces canned artichoke hearts, drained
- 4 garlic cloves, minced
- A pinch of black pepper
- 1 tablespoon oregano, dried

Directions:

1. In a pan, combine the cream with the almond milk and the other ingredients, toss, bring to a simmer and cook over medium heat for 35 minutes.
2. Blend the mix using an immersion blender, divide into bowls and serve as a party dip.

Nutrition: calories 130, fat 5, fiber 4, carbs 6, protein 6

628. Balsamic Pineapple Bites

Preparation time: 10 minutes
Cooking time: 20 minutes
Servings: 6

Ingredients:

- 14 ounces canned pineapple, cubed
- ½ teaspoon ginger, grated
- 1 tablespoon balsamic vinegar
- ½ teaspoon rosemary, dried
- 1 tablespoon olive oil

Directions:

1. In a bowl, combine the pineapple bites with the ginger and the other ingredients, toss, divide into bowls and serve as a snack.

Nutrition: calories 54, fat 2.4, fiber 1, carbs 8.9, protein 0.4

629. Parsley Pearl Onions Mix

Preparation time: 10 minutes
Cooking time: 12 minutes
Servings: 4

Ingredients:

- 2 cups pearl onions, peeled
- Juice of 1 lime
- 1 tablespoon olive oil
- 1 tablespoon ginger, grated
- 1 teaspoon turmeric powder
- 1 small parsley bunch, chopped
- A pinch of salt and black pepper

Directions:

1. Heat up a pan with the oil over medium-high heat, add the pearl onions, lime juice and the other ingredients, toss and cook over medium heat for 12 minutes.
2. Divide the mix into bowls and serve as a snack.

Nutrition: calories 135, fat 2, fiber 4, carbs 9, protein 12

630. Clam Platter

Preparation time: 10 minutes
Cooking time: 12 minutes
Servings: 4

Ingredients:

- 1 pound clams, scrubbed
- 3 garlic cloves, minced
- 1 tablespoon olive oil
- 1 teaspoon ginger, grated
- 1 teaspoon chili powder
- A pinch of sweet paprika
- ½ cup chicken stock

Directions:

1. Heat up a pan with the oil over medium heat, add the garlic and the ginger and sauté for 2 minutes.
2. Add the clams and the other ingredients, toss, bring to a simmer and cook over medium heat for 10 minutes.
3. Arrange the clams on a platter and serve.

Nutrition: calories 93, fat 4, fiber 0.8, carbs 14, protein 1

631. Mustard Tuna Bites

Preparation time: 10 minutes
Cooking time: 12 minutes
Servings: 6

Ingredients:

- 1 pound tuna fillets, boneless and cut into cubes
- 2 teaspoons dill, chopped
- 2 tablespoons olive oil
- 1 teaspoon garlic powder
- Salt and black pepper to the taste
- 2 tablespoon chives, chopped
- 1 tablespoon mustard

Directions:

1. In a bowl, mix the tuna with the dill, oil and the other ingredients except the chives, toss well and arrange on a baking sheet lined with parchment paper.
2. Bake the tuna bites at 400 degrees F for 12 minutes, divide into small bowls, sprinkle the chives on top and serve.

Nutrition: calories 140, fat 2, fiber 5, carbs 7, protein 6

632. Kale Chips

Preparation time: 10 minutes
Cooking time: 15 minutes
Servings: 4

Ingredients:

- 2 tablespoons olive oil
- 1 pound kale leaves, pat dried
- 2 tablespoons garlic, minced
- 1 tablespoon lemon zest, grated
- Salt and black pepper to the taste

Directions:

1. Spread the kale leaves on a baking sheet lined with parchment paper, add the oil and the other ingredients, toss a bit and cook in the oven at 400 degrees F for 15 minutes.
2. Cool the kale chips down, divide into bowls and serve as a snack.

Nutrition: calories 149, fat 4, fiber 3, carbs 9, protein 6

633. Avocado Salsa

Preparation Time: 10 minutes
Servings: 4

Ingredients:

- 2 avocados, pitted, peeled and chopped.
- 1/2 tomato, chopped.
- 1 small red onion, chopped.
- 3 jalapeno pepper, chopped.
- 2 tablespoons cumin powder
- 2 tablespoons lime juice
- Salt and black pepper to the taste.

Directions:

1. In a bowl, mix onion with avocados, peppers, salt, black pepper, cumin, lime juice and tomato pieces and stir well.
2. Transfer this to a bowl and serve with toasted baguette slices as a keto appetizer.

Nutrition: Calories:- 120; Fat : 2; Fiber : 2; Carbs : 0.4; Protein : 4

634. Keto Marinated Eggs

Preparation Time: 2 hours 17 minutes
Servings: 4

Ingredients:

- 1/4 cup unsweetened rice vinegar
- 4 ounces cream cheese
- 6 eggs
- 2 garlic cloves, minced
- 1 teaspoon stevia
- 1 tablespoon chives, chopped.
- 1¼ cups water
- 2 tablespoons coconut aminos

- Salt and black pepper to the taste.

Directions:
1. Put the eggs in a pot, add water to cover, bring to a boil over medium heat; cover and cook for 7 minutes
2. Rinse eggs with cold water and leave them aside to cool down.
3. In a bowl, mix 1 cup water with coconut aminos, vinegar, stevia and garlic and whisk well.
4. Put the eggs in this mix, cover with a kitchen towel and leave them aside for 2 hours rotating from time to time
5. Peel eggs, cut in halves and put egg yolks in a bowl.
6. Add 1/4 cup water, cream cheese, salt, pepper and chives and stir well.
7. Stuff egg whites with this mix and serve them.

Nutrition: Calories:- 210; Fat : 3; Fiber : 1; Carbs : 3; Protein : 12

635. Keto Bread Sticks

Preparation Time: 25 minutes
Servings: 24

Ingredients:
- 2 cups mozzarella cheese, melted for 30 seconds in the microwave
- 1 teaspoon baking powder
- 1 teaspoon onion powder
- 1 egg
- 2 tablespoons Italian seasoning
- 3 tablespoons cream cheese, soft
- 1 tablespoon psyllium powder
- ¾ cup almond flour
- 3 ounces cheddar cheese, grated
- Salt and black pepper to the taste.

Directions:
1. In a bowl, mix psyllium powder with almond flour, baking powder, salt and pepper and whisk.
2. Add cream cheese, melted mozzarella and egg and stir using your hands until you obtain a dough.
3. Spread this on a baking sheet and cut into 24 sticks
4. Sprinkle onion powder and Italian seasoning over them.
5. Top with cheddar cheese, introduce in the oven at 350 degrees F and bake for 15 minutes
6. Serve them as a keto snack!

Nutrition: Calories:- 245; Fat : 12; Fiber : 5; Carbs : 3; Protein : 14

636. Special Keto Hummus

Preparation Time: 10 minutes
Servings: 5

Ingredients:
- 4 cups zucchinis, finely chopped.
- 1/4 cup olive oil
- 4 garlic cloves, minced
- ¾ cup tahini
- 1/2 cup lemon juice
- 1 tablespoon cumin, ground
- Salt and black pepper to the taste.

Directions:
1. In your blender, mix zucchinis with salt, pepper, oil, lemon juice, garlic, tahini and cumin and blend very well.
2. Transfer to a bowl and serve

Nutrition: Calories:- 80; Fat : 5; Fiber : 3; Carbs : 6; Protein : 7

637. Keto Sausage And Cheese Dip

Preparation Time: 2 hours 20 minutes
Servings: 28

Ingredients:
- 1 pound Italian sausage, ground
- 8 ounces cream cheese
- 15 ounces canned tomatoes mixed with habaneros
- 16 ounces sour cream
- 8 ounces pepper jack cheese, chopped.
- A pinch of salt and black pepper
- 1/4 cup green onions, chopped.

Directions:
1. Heat up a pan over medium heat; add

sausage; stir and cook until it browns
2. Add tomatoes mix; stir and cook for 4 minutes more
3. Add a pinch of salt, pepper and the green onions; stir and cook for 4 minutes
4. Spread pepper jack cheese on the bottom of your slow cooker.
5. Add cream cheese, sausage mix and sour cream, cover and cook on High for 2 hours
6. Uncover your slow cooker; stir dip, transfer to a bowl and serve

Nutrition: Calories:- 144; Fat : 12; Fiber : 1; Carbs : 3; Protein : 6

638. Chicken Egg Rolls

Preparation Time: 25 minutes
Servings: 12

Ingredients:

- 4 ounces blue cheese
- 2 cups chicken, cooked and finely chopped.
- 12 egg roll wrappers
- 1/2 cup tomato sauce
- 1/2 teaspoon erythritol
- 2 green onions, chopped.
- 2 celery stalks, finely chopped.
- Vegetable oil
- Salt and black pepper to the taste.

Directions:

1. In a bowl, mix chicken meat with blue cheese, salt, pepper, green onions, celery, tomato sauce and sweetener; stir well and keep in the fridge for 2 hours
2. Place egg wrappers on a working surface, divide chicken mix on them, roll and seal edges
3. Heat up a pan with vegetable oil over medium high heat; add egg rolls, cook until they are golden, flip and cook on the other side as well.
4. Arrange on a platter and serve them.

Nutrition: Calories:- 220; Fat : 7; Fiber : 2; Carbs : 6; Protein : 10

639. Easy Jalapeno Crisps

Preparation Time: 35 minutes
Servings: 20

Ingredients:

- 5 jalapenos, sliced
- 8 ounces parmesan cheese, grated
- 1/2 teaspoon onion powder
- 3 tablespoons olive oil
- Tabasco sauce for serving
- Salt and black pepper to the taste.

Directions:

1. In a bowl, mix jalapeno slices with salt, pepper, oil and onion powder, toss to coat and spread on a lined baking sheet.
2. Introduce in the oven at 450 degrees F and bake for 15 minutes
3. Take jalapeno slices out of the oven, leave them to cool down.
4. In a bowl, mix pepper slices with the cheese and press well.
5. Arrange all slices on an another lined baking sheet, introduce in the oven again and bake for 10 minutes more
6. Leave jalapenos to cool down, arrange on a plate and serve with Tabasco sauce on the side

Nutrition: Calories:- 50; Fat : 3; Fiber : 0.1; Carbs : 0.3; Protein : 2

640. Keto Crab Dip

Preparation Time: 40 minutes
Servings: 8

Ingredients:

- 8 bacon strips, sliced
- 12 ounces crab meat
- 1/2 cup mayonnaise
- 1/2 cup sour cream
- 4 garlic cloves, minced
- 4 green onions, minced
- 8 ounces cream cheese
- 2 poblano pepper, chopped.
- 2 tablespoons lemon juice
- 1/2 cup parmesan cheese+ 1/2 cup parmesan cheese, grated

- Salt and black pepper to the taste.

Directions:
1. Heat up a pan over medium high heat; add bacon, cook until it's crispy, transfer to paper towels, chop and leave aside to cool down.
2. In a bowl, mix sour cream with cream cheese and mayo and stir well.
3. Add 1/2 cup parmesan, poblano peppers, bacon, green onion, garlic and lemon juice and stir again.
4. Add crab meat, salt and pepper and stir gently.
5. Pour this into a heatproof baking dish, spread the rest of the parm, introduce in the oven and bake at 350 degrees F for 20 minutes
6. Serve your dip warm with cucumber stick.

Nutrition: Calories:- 200; Fat : 7; Fiber : 2; Carbs : 4; Protein : 6

641. Keto Chili Lime Chips

Preparation Time: 30 minutes
Servings: 4

Ingredients:
- 1 cup almond flour
- 1 egg
- 1½ teaspoons lime zest
- 1 teaspoon lime juice
- Salt and black pepper to the taste.

Directions:
1. In a bowl, mix almond flour with lime zest, lime juice and salt and stir.
2. Add egg and whisk well again.
3. Divide this into 4 parts, roll each into a ball and then spread well using a rolling pin.
4. Cut each into 6 triangles, place them all on a lined baking sheet, introduce in the oven at 350 degrees F and bake for 20 minutes

Nutrition: Calories:- 90; Fat : 1; Fiber : 1; Carbs : 0.6; Protein : 3

642. Zucchini Rolls

Preparation Time: 15 minutes
Servings: 24

Ingredients:
- 2 tablespoons olive oil
- 3 zucchinis, thinly sliced
- 24 basil leaves
- 2 tablespoons mint, chopped.
- 1/4 cup basil, chopped.
- 1 ⅓ cup ricotta cheese
- Tomato sauce for serving
- Salt and black pepper to the taste.

Directions:
1. Brush zucchini slices with the olive oil, season with salt and pepper on both sides, place them on preheated grill over medium heat; cook them for 2 minutes, flip and cook for another 2 minutes
2. Place zucchini slices on a plate and leave aside for now.
3. In a bowl, mix ricotta with chopped basil, mint, salt and pepper and stir well.
4. Spread this over zucchini slices, divide whole basil leaves as well, roll and serve as an appetizer with some tomato sauce on the side

Nutrition: Calories:- 40; Fat : 3; Fiber : 0.3; Carbs : 1; Protein : 2

643. Italian Style Meatballs

Preparation Time: 16 minutes
Servings: 16

Ingredients:
- 1 pound turkey meat, ground
- 1/4 cup almond flour
- 2 tablespoons olive oil
- 2 tablespoon basil, chopped.
- 1 egg
- 1/2 teaspoon garlic powder
- 2 tablespoons sun-dried tomatoes, chopped.
- 1/2 cup mozzarella cheese, shredded
- Salt and black pepper to the taste.

Directions:
1. In a bowl, mix turkey with salt, pepper,

egg, almond flour, garlic powder, sun-dried tomatoes, mozzarella and basil and stir well.
2. Shape 12 meatballs, heat up a pan with the oil over medium high heat; drop meatballs and cook them for 2 minutes on each side
3. Arrange on a platter and serve

Nutrition: Calories:- 80; Fat : 6; Fiber : 3; Carbs : 5; Protein : 7

644. Keto Mushrooms Appetizer

Preparation Time: 30 minutes
Servings: 5

Ingredients:
- 24 ounces white mushroom caps
- 1/4 cup mayo
- 1/4 cup sour cream
- 1/2 cup Mexican cheese, shredded
- 1 teaspoon garlic powder
- 1 small yellow onion, chopped.
- 1 teaspoon curry powder
- 4 ounces cream cheese, soft
- 1 cup shrimp, cooked, peeled, deveined and chopped.
- Salt and black pepper to the taste.

Directions:
1. In a bowl, mix mayo with garlic powder, onion, curry powder, cream cheese, sour cream, Mexican cheese, shrimp, salt and pepper to the taste. and whisk well.
2. Stuff mushrooms with this mix, place on a baking sheet and cook in the oven at 350 degrees F for 20 minutes
3. Arrange on a platter and serve

Nutrition: Calories:- 244; Fat : 20; Fiber : 3; Carbs : 7; Protein : 14

645. Keto Broccoli Sticks

Preparation Time: 30 minutes
Servings: 20

Ingredients:
- 2 cups broccoli florets
- 1/3 cup panko breadcrumbs
- A drizzle of olive oil
- 1 egg
- 1/3 cup Italian breadcrumbs
- 2 tablespoons parsley, chopped.
- 1/3 cup cheddar cheese, grated
- 1/4 cup yellow onion, chopped.
- Salt and black pepper to the taste.

Directions:
1. Heat up a pot with water over medium heat; add broccoli, steam for 1 minute, drain, chop and put into a bowl.
2. Add egg, cheddar cheese, panko and Italian bread crumbs, salt, pepper and parsley and stir everything well.
3. Shape sticks out of this mix using your hands and place them on a baking sheet which you've greased with some olive oil.
4. Introduce in the oven at 400 degrees F and bake for 20 minutes
5. Arrange on a platter and serve

Nutrition: Calories:- 100; Fat : 4; Fiber : 2; Carbs : 7; Protein : 7

646. Caviar Salad

Preparation Time: 6 minutes
Servings: 16

Ingredients:
- 4 ounces black caviar
- ¾ cup mayonnaise
- 4 ounces red caviar
- 8 eggs, hard-boiled, peeled and mashed with a fork
- 1 yellow onion, finely chopped.
- Some toast baguette slices for serving
- Salt and black pepper to the taste.

Directions:
1. In a bowl, mix mashed eggs with mayo, salt, pepper and onion and stir well.
2. Spread eggs salad on toasted baguette slices, and top each with caviar.

Nutrition: Calories:- 122; Fat : 8; Fiber : 1; Carbs : 4; Protein : 7

647. Tasty Bacon Delight

Preparation Time: 1 hour 35 minutes
Servings: 16

Ingredients:
- 16 bacon slices
- 1 tablespoon coconut oil
- 3 ounces dark chocolate
- 1/2 teaspoon cinnamon, ground
- 2 tablespoons erythritol
- 1 teaspoon maple extract

Directions:
1. In a bowl, mix cinnamon with erythritol and stir.
2. Arrange bacon slices on a lined baking sheet and sprinkle cinnamon mix over them.
3. Flip bacon slices and sprinkle cinnamon mix over them again.
4. Introduce in the oven at 275 degrees F and bake for 1 hour.
5. Heat up a pot with the oil over medium heat; add chocolate and stir until it melts
6. Add maple extract; stir, take off heat and leave aside to cool down a bit.
7. Take bacon strips out of the oven, leave them to cool down, dip each in chocolate mix, place them on a parchment paper and leave them to cool down completely. Serve cold.

Nutrition: Calories:- 150; Fat : 4; Fiber : 0.4; Carbs : 1. 1; Protein : 3

648. Delicious Corndogs

Preparation Time: 20 minutes
Servings: 4

Ingredients:
- 1 cup almond meal
- 1½ cups olive oil
- 2 tablespoons heavy cream
- 4 sausages
- 1 teaspoon baking powder
- 1 teaspoon Italian seasoning
- 1/2 teaspoon turmeric
- 2 eggs
- A pinch of cayenne pepper
- Salt and black pepper to the taste.

Directions:
1. In a bowl, mix almond meal with Italian seasoning, baking powder, turmeric, salt, pepper and cayenne and stir well.
2. In another bowl, mix eggs with heavy cream and whisk well.
3. Combine the 2 mixtures and stir well.
4. Dip sausages in this mix and place them on a plate
5. Heat up a pan with the oil over medium high heat; add sausages, cook for 2 minutes on each side and transfer to paper towels
6. Drain grease, arrange on a platter and serve

Nutrition: Calories:- 345; Fat : 33; Fiber : 4; Carbs : 5; Protein : 16

649. Keto Almond Butter Bars

Preparation Time: 2 hours 12 minutes
Servings: 12

Ingredients:
- ounces dark chocolate, chopped.
- 1 cup almond butter
- 2 tablespoons almond butter
- ¾ cup coconut, unsweetened and shredded
- ¾ cup almond butter
- ¾ cup stevia
- 2 tablespoons coconut oil

Directions:
1. In a bowl, mix almond flour with stevia and coconut and stir well.
2. Heat up a pan over medium-low heat; add 1 cup almond butter and the coconut oil and whisk well.
3. Add this to almond flour and stir well.
4. Transfer this to a baking dish and press well.
5. Heat up another pan with the chocolate stirring often.
6. Add the rest of the almond butter and whisk well again.
7. Pour this over almond mix and spread evenly.

8. Introduce in the fridge for 2 hours, cut into 12 bars and serve as a keto snack.

Nutrition: Calories:- 140; Fat : 2; Fiber : 1; Carbs : 5; Protein : 1

650. Easy Keto Zucchini Snack

Preparation Time: 25 minutes
Servings: 4

Ingredients:

- 1 cup mozzarella, shredded
- 1 zucchini, sliced
- 1/4 cup tomato sauce
- A pinch of cumin
- Cooking spray
- Salt and black pepper to the taste.

Directions:

1. Spray a cooking sheet with some oil and arrange zucchini slices
2. Spread tomato sauce all over zucchini slices, season with salt, pepper and cumin and sprinkle shredded mozzarella.
3. Introduce in the oven at 350 degrees F and bake for 15 minutes
4. Arrange on a platter and serve

Nutrition: Calories:- 140; Fat : 4; Fiber : 2; Carbs : 6; Protein : 4

651. Green Crackers

Preparation Time: 24 hours 10 minutes
Servings: 6

Ingredients:

- 2 cups flax seed, soaked overnight and drained
- 2 cups flax seed, ground
- 1 bunch basil, chopped.
- 4 bunches kale, chopped.
- 1/3 cup olive oil
- 1/2 bunch celery, chopped.
- 4 garlic cloves, minced

Directions:

1. In your food processor mix ground flaxseed with celery, kale, basil and garlic and blend well.
2. Add oil and soaked flaxseed and blend again.
3. Spread this on a tray, cut into medium crackers, introduce in your dehydrator and dry for 24 hours at 115 degrees F, turning them halfway.
4. Arrange them on a platter and serve

Nutrition: Calories:- 100; Fat : 1; Fiber : 2; Carbs : 1; Protein : 4

652. Beef Jerky Snack

Preparation Time: 10 hours
Servings: 6

Ingredients:

- 2 pounds beef round, sliced
- 24 ounces amber
- 2 tablespoons black peppercorns
- 2 tablespoons black pepper
- 2 cups soy sauce
- 1/2 cup Worcestershire sauce

Directions:

1. In a bowl, mix soy sauce with black peppercorns, black pepper and Worcestershire sauce and whisk well.
2. Add beef slices, toss to coat and leave aside in the fridge for 6 hours
3. Spread this on a rack, introduce in the oven at 370 degrees F and bake for 4 hours
4. Transfer to a bowl and serve

Nutrition: Calories:- 300; Fat : 12; Fiber : 4; Carbs : 3; Protein : 8

653. Spinach Garlic Dip

Preparation Time: 45 minutes
Servings: 6

Ingredients:

- 6 bacon slices
- 5 ounces spinach
- 1/2 cup sour cream
- 8 ounces cream cheese, soft
- 1 tablespoon garlic, minced
- 1½ tablespoons parsley, chopped.
- ounces parmesan, grated
- 1 tablespoon lemon juice

- Salt and black pepper to the taste.

Directions:
1. Heat up a pan over medium heat; add bacon, cook until it's crispy, transfer to paper towels, drain grease, crumble and leave aside in a bowl.
2. Heat up the same pan with the bacon grease over medium heat; add spinach; stir, cook for 2 minutes and transfer to a bowl.
3. In another bowl, mix cream cheese with garlic, salt, pepper, sour cream and parsley and stir well.
4. Add bacon and stir again.
5. Add lemon juice and spinach and stir everything.
6. Add parmesan and stir again.
7. Divide this into ramekins, introduce in the oven at 350 degrees f and bake for 25 minutes
8. Turn oven to broil and broil for 4 minutes more
9. Serve with crackers

Nutrition: Calories:- 345; Fat : 12; Fiber : 3; Carbs : 6; Protein : 11

654. Marinated Keto Kebabs

Preparation Time: 30 minutes
Servings: 6

Ingredients:
- 2 pounds sirloin steak, cut into medium cubes
- 1 red bell pepper, cut into chunks
- 1 green bell pepper, cut into chunks
- 1 orange bell pepper, cut into chunks
- 4 garlic cloves, minced
- 1/4 cup tamari sauce
- 1/4 cup lemon juice
- 1/2 cup olive oil
- 1 red onion, cut into chunks
- 2 tablespoons Dijon mustard
- 2½ tablespoons Worcestershire sauce
- Salt and black pepper to the taste.

Directions:
1. In a bowl, mix Worcestershire sauce with salt, pepper, garlic, mustard, tamari, lemon juice and oil and whisk very well.
2. Add beef, bell peppers and onion chunks to this mix, toss to coat and leave aside for a few minutes
3. Arrange bell pepper, meat cubes and onion chunks on skewers alternating colors, place them on your preheated grill over medium high heat; cook for 5 minutes on each side, transfer to a platter and serve as a summer keto appetizer.

Nutrition: Calories:- 246; Fat : 12; Fiber : 1; Carbs : 4; Protein : 26

655. Pesto And Cheese Terrine

Preparation Time: 30 minutes
Servings: 10

Ingredients:
- 1/2 cup heavy cream
- 1/4 cup pine nuts, toasted and chopped.
- 10 ounces goat cheese, crumbled
- 3 tablespoons basil pesto
- 5 sun-dried tomatoes, chopped.
- 1 tablespoons pine nuts, toasted and chopped.
- Salt and black pepper to the taste.

Directions:
1. In a bowl, mix goat cheese with the heavy cream, salt and pepper and stir using your mixer.
2. Spoon half of this mix into a lined bowl and spread.
3. Add pesto on top and also spread.
4. Add another layer of cheese, then add sun dried tomatoes and 1/4 cup pine nuts
5. Spread one last layer of cheese and top with 1 tablespoon pine nuts
6. Keep in the fridge for a while, turn upside down on a plate and serve

Nutrition: Calories:- 240; Fat : 12; Fiber : 3; Carbs : 5; Protein : 12

Desserts

656. Low Carb Chocolate Coconut Fat Bombs

Preparation time: 95 minutes
Servings: 11-12 balls

Ingredients

- 1 cup almond butter
- 1 tsp. vanilla extract (gluten free.
- 4 Tbsps. quality cocoa powder
- 1 tsp stevia powder extract
- 3-4 drops of peppermint essential oil (if desired.
- 1 cup coconut shreds
- 1 cup coconut milk

Direction

1. With a few inches of water in a sauce pan, place a glass bowl over it to create a double boiler.
2. Over medium heat, place all the ingredients except shredded coconut in a double boiler.
3. Combine the ingredients and stir while waiting for them to melt together.
4. Remove the bowl from the heat when all ingredients are well combined.
5. Place the bowl in the fridge for about 30 minutes or until it is hard enough to roll into balls.
6. Roll the contents into one-inch balls and roll them through the coconut shreds.
7. Place the balls on a plate and refrigerate for one hour.
8. Serve and enjoy.
9. Refrigerate if not serving immediately.

Nutrition: Calories 251, Carbs 12.8g, Total Fat 21.7g, Protein 2.8g

657. Crunchy Cherry Chocolate Confections

Preparation time: 20 minutes + freezing time
Servings: 30-36 candy cups

Ingredients

- 1 tablespoon cherry flavor
- 1 1/2 cups slivered almonds
- 4 oz. dark chocolate (85 % cocoa solids.
- 1/2 cup organic heavy cream
- 20 drops liquid stevia

Directions

1. Chop the chocolate into tiny pieces and set aside. Then, into small saucepan pour the cream and heat over very low heat until the cream is steaming hot. Don't let boil. Remove from heat.
2. Add the chopped chocolate to the steaming cream. Then, cover and let it stand for about 5 minutes.
3. Mix the cream and chocolate mixture with spoon after the 5 minutes until the mixture is thick and smooth.
4. Add the stevia and the cherry flavor and stir until well combined.
5. Add the slivered almonds and stir again until well combined.
6. Spoon the mixture into small foil or paper candy cups.
7. Let set at room temperature overnight, or in the fridge for a couple of hours.

Nutrition: Calories 72, Carbs 1.1g, Total Fat 1.8g, Protein 6.2g

658. Low Carb Keto Caramels

Preparation time: 15 minutes + refrigeration time
Servings: 10

Ingredients

- 1 cup butter
- 2 cups heavy whipping cream
- 6 tsps. stevia powder extract

Directions

1. In a small non-stick saucepan over medium low heat, melt the butter and let it cook until it is a light brown color.
2. Add the cream and stevia to the butter and continue to paddle for about 2 minutes or until it begins to feel sticky and the sauce has thickened.

3. Remove the pan from the heat and continue mixing until it has cooled slightly, to keep it from separating.
4. Pour into candy molds and refrigerate until it hardens, about 3-4 hours.

Nutrition: Calories 242, Carbs 1g, Total Fat 44g, Protein 1g

659. Coconut Chocolate Bars

Preparation time: 35 minutes+ refrigeration time

Servings: 10

Ingredients

- ⅓ cup coconut cream
- 4 tablespoons coconut oil
- 2 tablespoons unsweetened cocoa powder
- 1 cup unsweetened, shredded coconut
- 1 packet or ½ teaspoon of powdered Stevia
- 1 teaspoon vanilla extract

OPTION - instead of coconut oil for the coating

- 2 oz. cocoa butter

Directions

1. Combine shredded coconut with coconut cream, 1/2 of the vanilla extract and ½ packet of stevia and blend well with a spatula
2. On a small cookie sheet lined with parchment paper, place the shredded coconut mixture
3. Shape it into a flat rectangle about 4 inches by 6 inches and 1 inch thick. A kitchen wrap can help you accomplish this
4. Place in the freezer until frozen solid, about 2 hours
5. Remove from the freezer and cut into 5 bars
6. Preparing the chocolate coating:
7. In a small sauce pan, melt the coconut oil until liquefied
8. Add cocoa powder remaining stevia and vanilla extract to the coconut oil
9. Combine well on low heat until all ingredients are well blended, about 2 minutes, then let it cool to room temperature, but still liquid
10. Dip the bars in the cocoa mixture, and turn to all sides to coat evenly. It helps if the bars are frozen solid so they won't break.
11. Place bars back on the cookie sheet
12. When all bars are all coated put in the refrigerator to harden.
13. The bars can be kept in the fridge for harder consistency or at room temperature for softer.
14. Cacao will melt if kept at a temperature too high.

Nutrition: Calories 210, Carbs 4.8g, Total Fat 22g, Protein 1g

660. Keto Pumpkin Fudge

Preparation time: 2 hours
Servings: 25

Ingredients

- 1 teaspoon ground cinnamon
- ¼ teaspoon ground nutmeg
- 1 tablespoon coconut oil
- 1 ¾ cups coconut butter
- 1 cup pumpkin puree

Directions

1. Line your baking pan with aluminum foil and set aside.
2. Into a saucepan, spoon coconut butter and warm over low heat until coconut butter is melted.
3. Stir and remove from heat.
4. Add pumpkin and spices; stir. The mixture will be thick and almost grainy.
5. Add the coconut oil and vigorously stir to combine the ingredients and distribute the oil.
6. Into the prepared pan, spoon the mixture and spread evenly with the back of a spoon.
7. Place a piece of wax paper over the top of the fudge and use your hands to press the fudge mixture evenly into the pan.
8. Remove the wax paper and discard. Place fudge in the refrigerator for until cooled and firm. This takes about 1 to 2 hours.
9. Remove the fudge from the refrigerator

and carefully lift out the foil pan lining along with the fudge. Peel back the foil from the edges of the fudge.
10. Use a sharp knife to cut the large brick of fudge into 25 equal squares.
11. Store the fudge in a sealed container up to 1 week in the refrigerator.

Nutrition: Calories 109, Carbs 2.19g, Total Fat 10.6g, Protein 1.2g

661. Low-Carb, Keto Strawberry Fat Bombs

Preparation time: 2 hours
Servings: 15

Ingredients

- 1 cup strawberries chopped
- 3 tbsp. powdered erythritol
- 4 oz. cream cheese very soft
- 3 tbsp. butter very soft

Directions

1. Combine the butter and cream cheese in a bow. Using a fork, mash to combine.
2. Mash the strawberries in a separate bowl. Mix in the sweetener.
3. You can either try to incorporate the strawberries into the cream cheese mixture with a spatula, or place everything in a food processor and pulsing a few times.
4. Pipe the mixture into ice cube molds and freeze for at least 2 hours. Keep frozen.

Nutrition: Calories 49, Carbs 1g, Total Fat 4g, Protein 0g

662. Paleo Vegan Peppermint Patties

Preparation time: 5 minutes
Servings: 24 cups

Ingredients

- 1/2 cup coconut oil
- 1 serving liquid sweetener of choice
- 1/2 cup coconut butter, melted
- 2 tsps. peppermint extract
- ½ cup cocoa powder

Directions

1. With muffin liners and set aside, line a 24-count mini muffin tin.
2. Melt 1 cup of your chocolate chips and evenly distribute between the mini muffins tins, ensuring the sides are covered in the chocolate. Refrigerate.
3. Slightly melt your coconut butter until smooth and creamy if required. Add your peppermint extract and stir well.
4. Remove the firm chocolate shells and evenly distribute the coconut butter/mint mixture amongst them.
5. Melt the remaining half-cup of chocolate chips and cover the tops of the peppermint patties. Refrigerate until firm.

Nutrition: Calories 82, Carbs 2g, Total Fat 8g, Protein 2g

663. Keto Marshmallows

Preparation time: 2-3 hours
Servings: 36 cups

Ingredients

- 1/4 cup cold + 3/4 cup boiling water
- 1 heaping tbsp. coconut flour to coat the outsides of the marshmallows (12 g / 0.4 oz..
- pinch salt
- 3 large egg whites
- 4 tbsps. / 4 envelopes gelatin
- 1 tsp. cream of tartar (to stabilize the egg whites.
- 1/2 cup powdered Erythritol
- Topping
- 1 package dark chocolate, 85% coco solids or more (100 g / 3.5 oz..
- 3 tbsps. Unsweetened desiccated coconut (18 g / 0.6 oz..
- Coating Options
- ground or chopped nuts
- cinnamon
- raw cacao powder
- fruit powder (freeze-dried.

Directions

1. Line a pan with parchment paper and

sprinkle with a layer of coconut flour or any other coating
2. Into a pot, place a gelatin and add 1/4 cup of cold water. Tilt the pot to circulate the water. The gelatin will become firm in just a couple of minutes.
3. Separate the egg whites from the egg yolks. Cut the vanilla bean and scrape the seeds out (cut lengthwise.
4. Start beating the egg whites using an electric mixer, then slowly add the cream of tartar, powdered Erythritol, vanilla seeds and salt. Continue beating for a minute or two until it becomes thick and creates soft peaks
5. Add the remaining boiling water to the pot with the gelatin and stir until dissolved. Briefly boil over low heat if you still see some lumps and stir well until they go away.
6. Turn the mixer to medium and very slowly pour a steady stream of gelatin into the egg whites. Turn the mixer to high after pouring all the gelatin and continue beating until it becomes thick and creamy, about 3-5 minutes.
7. Turn off the mixer and quickly transfer the marshmallow cream into the pan lined with parchment paper and sprinkled with fine coconut flour.
8. Spread evenly all over the pan.
9. Sprinkle more coating (coconut flour on top and pat level.
10. Place in the fridge for 2-3 hours or overnight until the marshmallow cream is set. When done, remove the pan and peel the parchment paper off. Cut into cubes, 6 by 6 to create 36 marshmallows.
11. If you make plain marshmallows with no topping, place on a plate and cover with a towel for a few hours. Then, store them in an air-tight container to avoid drying.
12. If you are adding a topping, melt the chocolate in a water bath. Dip a lollypop stick into the chocolate.
13. Then, dip each marshmallow into the melted chocolate and keep turning until the chocolate stops dripping.
14. Store in an air-tight container to avoid the marshmallows from getting too dry.

Nutrition: Calories 22.3, Carbs 1.2g, Total Fat 1.4g, Protein .2g

664. White Chocolate Butter Pecan Fat Bombs

Preparation time: 20 minutes
Servings: 4 bombs

Ingredients

- 1/4 tsp. vanilla extract
- 1 pinch Stevia
- 1 pinch salt
- 1/2 cup chopped pecans
- 2 tbsps. coconut oil
- 2 tbsps. butter
- 2 oz. cocoa butter
- 2 tbsps. powdered erythritol

Directions

1. In a small pan, melt coconut oil, cocoa butter and butter together until melted.
2. If you don't have powdered erythritol, you can easily make it. Stir in 2 tablespoons of powdered erythritol into the butter mixture until mixed.
3. Add a pinch of salt to bring out the sweetness.
4. Add in an optional pinch of Stevia to counteract the cooling effects of erythritol.
5. Add in vanilla extract.
6. Add a few chopped pecans in some silicon cupcake molds. I added about 3-4 pecans total to each mold, but this can be altered. If you don't have pecans, walnuts and hazelnuts work well with white chocolate too!
7. Pour your white chocolate mix evenly into the molds over the nuts and place in freezer immediately.
8. Freeze for about 30 minutes.
9. Serve!

Nutrition: Calories 287, Carbs 0.5g, Total Fat 30g, Protein 0.5g

665. Keto Low Carb Gummy Bears

Preparation time: 40 minutes

Servings: 2

Ingredients

- 0.25 oz. packet of powdered unflavored gelatin Knox or similar
- ¼ - ⅓ cup of water see main text for quantities
- 0.3 oz. packet of sugar free Jello

Directions

1. To a small saucepan, add the Jello, and water, then place over a low heat, and cook until all the crystals have dissolved.
2. Remove from the heat and use the dropper to fill the cavities.
3. When all the cavities are complete, transfer the tray to the fridge until the bears are set, for around 30 minutes.
4. Pop them out of the mold and serve!

Nutrition: Calories 20, Carbs 0.01g, Total Fat 3g, Protein 3g

666. Keto Chocolate Chip Cookies

Preparation time: 50 minutes
Servings: 12 cookies

Ingredients

- 1/2 tsp. baking powder
- 1/4 tsp. Salt
- 1/2 tsp. xanthan gum (optional.
- 3/4 Cup Sugar Free Chocolate Chips
- 1 1/2 Cups Almond Flour
- 1/2 Cup Salted Butter
- 3/4 Cup Natvia (Or Erythritol.
- 1 tsp. Vanilla Extract
- 1 Egg

Direction

1. Preheat your oven to 180C (355 and melt the butter for 30 seconds. Don't make it hot.
2. Into a mixing bowl, place the butter and whisk with the natvia. Add the vanilla and egg, mix on low for another 15 seconds exactly.
3. Add the almond flour, xanthan gum, baking powder and salt. Mix until well combined.
4. Press the dough together and remove from the bowl. Mix the chocolate chips into the dough with your hands.
5. Roll the dough to Make 12 balls and place on a baking tray. Bake for 10 mins.
6. Let them cool, and serve.
7. Keep in an airtight container.

Nutrition: Calories 168, Carbs 2.3g, Total Fat 17.3g, Protein 4g

667. Bakery-Style' Salted Chocolate Chip Cookies

Preparation time: 50 minutes
Servings: 12 cookies

Ingredients

- 110-144 g golden erythritol to taste
- 1 teaspoon blackstrap molasses (optional.
- 1 teaspoon vanilla extract
- 1 egg
- 85-120 g Lily's Sweets dark chocolate bar broken up (or chips.
- 70 g pecans broken up
- flakey sea salt to garnish
- 120 g almond flour
- 16 g coconut flour
- 1 tablespoon konjac powder (i.e. glucomannan arrowroot powder, or more coconut flour
- 1 teaspoon kosher salt
- 1/2 teaspoon baking soda
- 1/2 teaspoon xanthan gum
- 150 g grass-fed unsalted butter at room temperature

Directions

1. In a medium bowl, put almond flour, coconut flour, konjac powder (or arrowroot/more coconut flour, salt, baking soda and xanthan gum. Mix until thoroughly combined and set aside.
2. In a large bowl, cream butter with an electric mixer until softened, 1-2 minutes.
3. Add in sweetener and molasses (optional, and continue to cream until light and fluffy (about 8 minutes.
4. Add in vanilla extract and egg, mixing

until just combined. The mixture will appear slightly 'broken' (i.e. not thoroughly smooth.
5. Add in half of your flour mixture with your mixer on low- mixing until just combined.
6. Mix in the rest.
7. Fold in chocolate and pecan bits. Cover with cling film and refrigerate for 1 hour.
8. Preheat oven to 350°F/180°C and line a baking tray with parchment paper
9. Divide cookie dough into 18 rounds for 3 1/2-inch cookies (or 12 for jumbo style!, and flatten them slightly.
10. Place cookie dough on the prepared baking tray. Bake for 9-10 minutes for smaller cookies and 12-13 minutes for the jumbo, flipping tray around 180° half way through.
11. Garnish with flakey sea salt and allow the cookies to cool completely on the trays
12. Store in an airtight container for three to four days.

Nutrition: Calories 149, Carbs 3g, Total Fat 13g, Protein 2.2g

668. Chocolate Chip Keto Cookie

Preparation time: 30 minutes
Servings: 20

Ingredients

- 3/4 cup erythritol
- 1/2 tsp. baking soda
- 1/4 tsp. cream of tartar
- 1/2 tsp. pink Himalayan salt
- 3 cups almond flour
- 3 oz. 100% cacao baking chocolate bar
- 1/3 cup coconut oil, room temperature
- 1/2 cup grass-fed butter, room temperature
- 2 eggs
- 1 tsp. vanilla extract

Directions

1. Preheat oven to 350 degrees and line two baking sheets with parchment paper
2. With a hand mixer, mix together coconut oil and butter in a medium bowl, using a hand mixer. Add eggs and vanilla extract once mixed and continue mixing with hand mixer.
3. Add erythritol, baking soda, cream of tartar, and salt in the same bowl. Mix using hand mixer until well-combined.
4. One cup at a time, add almond flour and mix together with hand mixer.
5. Microwave chocolate pieces in a bowl in 15 second increments until just barely soft.
6. Transfer chocolate to plastic baggie and carefully break pieces apart using a rolling pin or the bottom of a hard object.
7. Pour chocolate pieces into bowl of dough and fold in until combined.
8. Form dough into balls and lightly press down and place on prepared cookie sheets, allowing plenty of room in between cookies for dough to spread during baking process.
9. Bake cookies until edges are golden brown, about 20 minutes.
10. Remove from oven and allow to cool completely before serving.
11. Serve!

Nutrition: Calories 191, Carbs 11.5g, Total Fat 18g, Protein 4.3g

669. Peanut Butter Cookies

Preparation time: 20 minutes
Servings: 15

Ingredients

- 1/2 cup granular erythritol
- 1 large egg
- 1 cup peanut butter

Directions

1. Preheat your oven to 350°F
2. Place half a cup of granular erythritol into a Nutribullet and blend for a few seconds.
3. Combine the peanut butter, powdered erythritol and the egg and mix very well.
4. Roll the cookie dough into 1-inch balls and place on a parchment paper lined baking sheet. Press down with a fork twice to create the iconic peanut butter cookie pattern.

5. Bake in the oven for about until you see the cookie edges turn a darker brown, about 10-15 minutes
6. Let them cool on a wire rack and enjoy with a yummy glass of nut milk!

Nutrition: Calories 105, Carbs 4g, Total Fat 9g, Protein 2g

670. Low Carb Keto Cream Cheese Cookies

Preparation time: 25 minutes
Servings: 24

Ingredients

- 1 large Egg white
- 2 tsps. Vanilla extract
- 3 cup Almond flour
- 1/4 tsp. Sea salt
- 1/4 cup Butter (softened.
- 2 oz. Plain cream cheese (softened.
- 1/2 cup Erythritol

Directions

1. Preheat the oven to 350 degrees F (177 degrees C.
2. Line a large cookie sheet with parchment paper.
3. Use a hand mixer or stand mixer to beat together the butter using a hand mixer, cream cheese, and erythritol, until it's fluffy and light in color.
4. Beat in the vanilla extract, salt and egg white.
5. Beat in the almond flour, 1/2 cup (64 g at a time.
6. Use a medium cookie scoop (about 1 1/2 tbsps., 22 mL volume to scoop balls of the dough onto the prepared cookie sheet.
7. Flatten with your palm.
8. Bake for about 15 minutes, until the edges are lightly golden. Allow to cool completely in the pan before handling

Nutrition: Calories 106, Carbs 3g, Total Fat 9g, Protein 2g

671. Sugar-Free Paleo Pecan Snowball Cookies

Preparation time: 40 minutes
Servings: 24

Ingredients

- 1/2 cup stevia
- 1 tsp. vanilla extract
- 1/2 tsp. vanilla liquid stevia
- 1/4 tsp. salt
- extra confectioners to roll balls in
- 8 tbsps. Ghee 1 1/2 cup almond flour 150 grams
- 1 cup pecans 120 grams, chopped

Directions

1. Preheat oven to 350 degrees F.
2. Into a food processor, place all ingredients and process until batter forms a ball. Pulse if required.
3. Taste batter, adjust sweetener if needed.
4. Line a baking sheet with silpat or parchment.
5. Use a cookie scoop and make 24 mounds, then roll each mound in the palm of your hand.
6. Place in freezer for 20-30 minutes.
7. Place in oven until golden around edges, about 15 minutes.
8. Allow to cool slightly.
9. Once able to handle roll each in stevia.
10. Allow to cool completely before storing in an air tight container.

Nutrition: Calories 112, Carbs 2g, Total Fat 11g, Protein 1g

672. Chocolate Chip Cookies with Coconut Flour

Preparation time: 20 minutes
Servings: 9

Ingredients

- 2 eggs, large
- 3 tbsps. sugar free chocolate chips
- ½ tsp. organic blackstrap molasses
- ¼ tsp. vanilla extract
- ⅛ tsp. salt
- ¼ cup coconut flour
- ⅓ cup unsalted butter

- 3 tbsps. Stevia

Directions
1. Preheat oven to 350 deg F.
2. Mix together the dry ingredients of coconut flour, stevia, chocolate chips, and salt in a large bowl
3. Mix together the wet ingredients of unsalted butter, eggs, molasses, molasses, and vanilla extract in another medium bowl.
4. Slowly stir the wet ingredients into the dry ingredients.
5. Place the cookies on while measuring two tablespoons of batter using a cookie mat.
6. Bake in the oven until browned on the bottom, about 15 minutes.

Nutrition: Calories 111, Carbs 6g, Total Fat 10g, Protein 1g

673. Cinnamon Keto French Toast Cookies

Preparation time: 30 minutes
Servings: 12

Ingredients
- Rolling Cinnamon
- 2 tsp. Cinnamon Ground
- 2 tbsps. Erythritol
- Cookies
- 1/3 Cup Sugar Free Maple Syrup
- 1/2 tsp. xanthan gum
- 1/2 tsp. baking soda
- 1/2 tsp. Salt
- 1 tsp. Vanilla Extract
- 2 Cups Almond Flour
- 1/2 Cup Butter slightly melted
- 1/4 Cup Erythritol
- 1 Egg

Directions
1. Preheat your oven to 180C (355 F. Zap the butter to melt for 30 seconds, don't make it hot.
2. Place the butter into a mixing bowl and beat with the erythritol and sugar free maple syrup. Add the vanilla and egg and combine on low for another 15 seconds exactly.
3. Add the almond flour, xanthan gum, baking soda and salt and mix until well combined.
4. Place in the fridge for 20 mins to let the ingredients solidify slightly
5. Roll the dough to Make 12 balls, place the cinnamon and natvia onto a place and roll the biscuits around in the mixture
6. Place on a baking tray and bake for 10 mins.
7. Serve when cool. Refrigerate in an air-tight container

Nutrition: Calories 106, Carbs 2g, Total Fat 10g, Protein 2g

674. Gluten-free Flourless Chocolate Cookies

Preparation time: 22 minutes
Servings: 24

Ingredients
- ½ cup very dark chocolate chips 63%
- ½ cup chopped pecans
- 3-4 large egg whites
- 1 teaspoon vanilla extract
- 1 ½ cups Stevia
- 6 Tablespoons unsweetened cocoa powder
- ¼ teaspoon salt

Directions
1. Heat oven to 350 degrees.
2. Cover baking sheet in baking parchment and spray with cooking spray.
3. In a mixing bowl, mix stevia, cocoa, salt, chocolate chips, and pecans together.
4. Add vanilla with three egg whites and stir to moisten batter. If all the dry ingredients aren't moistened or it is too thick, add one more egg white. (It should be very soft / sticky, but not soupy..
5. Place rounded teaspoons of dough onto cookie sheet, 2"-3" apart as cookies will spread and thin while baking.
6. Bake for 11-12 minutes.
7. Allow cookies to set-up on the pan for 5-

8 minutes before removing to cooling rack.

Nutrition: Calories 30, Carbs 2.4g, Total Fat 2.4g, Protein 1g

675. Low Carb Shortbread Cookies Recipe

Preparation time: 22 minutes
Servings: 18

Ingredients

- 1/2 cup Erythritol
- 1 tsp. Vanilla extract
- 2 1/2 cups Almond flour
- 6 tbsps. Butter

Directions

1. Preheat the oven to 350 degrees F.
2. Line a cookie sheet with parchment paper.
3. Beat together the butter and erythritol using a hand mixer, until it's fluffy and light in color.
4. Beat in the vanilla extract. Beat in the almond flour, 1/2 cup at a time.
5. Expose rounded tablespoonful of the dough onto the prepared cookie sheet. Flatten each cookie to about 1/3" thick or to your liking. They will not spread or thin out during baking, so make them as thin as you want them when done.
6. Bake until the edges are golden, ABOUT 12-15 minutes.
7. Allow to cool completely in the pan before handling.

Nutrition: Calories 124, Carbs 3.3g, Total Fat 12g, Protein 3g

676. Coconut Mousse

Preparation Time: 10 mins
Servings: 12

Ingredients:

- 1 tsp. vanilla flavoring
- 1 tsp. coconut extract
- 1 c. toasted coconut
- 2 ¾ c. coconut milk
- 4 tsps. coconut sugar

Directions:

1. In a bowl, combine the coconut milk with the coconut extract, vanilla flavor, coconut and sugar, whisk well, divide into small cups and serve cold.
2. Enjoy!

Nutrition:

Calories: 152, Fat:5 g, Carbs:11 g, Protein:3 g, Sugars:0.1 g, Sodium:13 mg

677. Blueberry Cream

Preparation Time: 5 mins
Servings: 1

Ingredients:

- 1 tbsp. low-fat peanut butter
- 2 dates
- ¾ c. blueberries
- 1 peeled banana
- ¾ c. almond milk

Directions:

1. In a blender, combine the blueberries with peanut butter, milk, banana and dates, pulse well, divide into small cups and serve cold.
2. Enjoy!

Nutrition:

Calories: 120, Fat:3 g, Carbs:6 g, Protein:7 g, Sugars:2.5 g, Sodium:55 mg

678. Lemon Apple Mix

Preparation Time: 10 mins
Servings: 6

Ingredients:

- 4 tbsps. coconut sugar
- 2 tsps. vanilla flavoring
- 2 tsps. cinnamon powder
- 2 tsps. lemon juice
- 6 cored and chopped apples
- Directions:
- In a little pan, combine the apples with all

the sugar, vanilla, fresh lemon juice and cinnamon, toss, heat over medium heat, cook for 10-15 minutes, divide between small dessert plates and serve.
- Enjoy!

Nutrition:
Calories: 120, Fat:4 g, Carbs:8 g, Protein:5 g, Sugars:13 g, Sodium:175 mg

679. Minty Rhubarb

Preparation Time: 10 mins
Servings: 4

Ingredients:
- 1/3 c. water
- 2 lbs. roughly chopped rhubarb
- 1 tbsp. chopped mint
- 3 tbsps. coconut sugar

Directions:
1. Put the river inside a tiny pot, get hot over medium heat, add the sugar and whisk well.
2. Add rhubarb and mix, toss, cook for 10 minutes, divide into bowls and serve.
3. Enjoy!

Nutrition:
Calories: 160, Fat:2 g, Carbs:8 g, Protein:5 g, Sugars:15 g, Sodium:39 mg

680. Nigella Mango Sweet Mix

Preparation Time: 10 mins
Servings: 8

Ingredients:
1. 1 tsp. cinnamon powder
2. 1 ½ lbs. peeled and cubed mango
3. 3 tbsps. coconut sugar
4. ½ c. apple cider vinegar treatment
5. 1 tsp. nigella seeds

Directions:
1. In a tiny pot, combine the mango while using nigella seeds, sugar, vinegar and cinnamon, toss, bring using a simmer over medium heat, cook for 10 minutes, divide into bowls and serve.
2. Enjoy!

Nutrition:
Calories: 160, Fat:3 g, Carbs:8 g, Protein:3 g, Sugars:6 g, Sodium:147 mg

681. Blueberry Compote

Preparation Time: 10 mins
Servings: 6

Ingredients:
- 1 lb. blueberries
- 1 oz. orange juice
- 5 tbsps. coconut sugar

Directions:
1. In a pot, combine the sugar with all the orange juice and blueberries, toss, bring which has a boil over medium heat, cook for 15 minutes, divide into bowls and serve cold.
2. Enjoy!

Nutrition:
Calories: 120, Fat:2 g, Carbs:6 g, Protein:9 g, Sugars:3 g, Sodium:1 mg

682. Lentils and Dates Brownies

Preparation Time: 10 mins
Servings: 8

Ingredients:
- 1 peeled and chopped banana
- 2 tbsps. powered cocoa
- ½ tsp. baking soda
- 28 oz. no-salt-added, rinsed and drained canned lentils
- 1 tbsp. coconut sugar
- 4 tbsps. almond butter
- 12 dates

Directions:
1. Put lentils inside food processor, pulse, add dates, sugar, banana, baking soda, almond butter and cocoa powder, pulse well, pour right in to a lined pan, spread, bake inside oven at 3750F for quarter-hour, leave the amalgamation aside to cool down the down a little bit, cut into medium pieces and serve.
2. Enjoy!

Nutrition:

Calories: 202, Fat:4 g, Carbs:12 g, Protein:6 g, Sugars:8 g, Sodium:8 mg

683. Blueberry Curd

Preparation Time: 10 mins
Servings: 4

Ingredients:

- 12 oz. blueberries
- 3 tbsps. coconut sugar
- 2 eggs
- 2 tbsps. melted coconut oil
- 2 tbsps. fresh lemon juice

Directions:

1. Put the oil in a pot, get hot over medium heat, add freshly squeezed freshly squeezed lemon juice and coconut sugar and whisk well.
2. Add the blueberries plus the eggs, whisk well, cook for ten minutes, divide into small cups and serve cold.
3. Enjoy!

Nutrition:

Calories: 201, Fat:3 g, Carbs:6 g, Protein:3 g, Sugars:8 g, Sodium:10 mg

684. Almond Peach Mix

Preparation Time: 10 mins
Servings: 4

Ingredients:

- 2 c. rolled oats
- ½ c. chopped almonds
- 1 chopped peach
- 4 c. water
- 2 tbsps. flax meal
- 1 tsp. vanilla flavoring

Directions:

1. In a pan, combine water while using oats, vanilla flavoring, flax meal, almonds and peach, stir, give a simmer over medium heat, cook for 10 minutes, divide into bowls and serve.
2. Enjoy!

Nutrition:

Calories: 161, Fat:3 g, Carbs:7 g, Protein:5 g, Sugars:8.5 g, Sodium:17.5 mg

685. Coconut Cream

Preparation Time: 1 hour
Servings: 4

Ingredients:

- 1 tsp. cinnamon powder
- 5 tbsps. coconut sugar
- 2 c. coconut cream
- Zest of one grated lemon
- 3 whisked eggs

Directions:

1. In just a little pan, combine the cream with cinnamon, eggs, sugar and lemon zest. Whisk well
2. Simmer over medium heat for 10 minutes.
3. Divide into ramekins and inside fridge for an hour before serving.
4. Enjoy!

Nutrition:

Calories: 130, Fat:5 g, Carbs:8 g, Protein:6 g, Sugars:1.8 g, Sodium:0 mg

686. Cinnamon Apples

Preparation Time: 10 mins
Servings: 4

Ingredients:

- 1 tbsp. cinnamon powder
- 4 tbsps. raisins
- 4 cored big apples

Directions:

1. Stuff the apples while using the raisins, sprinkle the cinnamon, stick them inside a baking dish, introduce inside oven at 375 0F, bake for 20 minutes and serve cold.
2. Enjoy!

Nutrition:

Calories: 200, Fat:3 g, Carbs:8 g, Protein:5 g, Sugars:26 g, Sodium:120 mg

687. Green Tea Cream

Preparation Time: 1 hour | Servings: 6

Ingredients:

- 2 tbsps. green tea extract powder
- 3 tbsps. coconut sugar
- 14 oz. coconut milk
- 14 oz. coconut cream

Directions:

1. Put the milk in the very pan, add sugar and green tea herb powder, stir, give your simmer, cook for two minutes, remove heat, cool down, add coconut cream, whisk well, divide into small bowls whilst from the fridge for just two hours before serving.
2. Enjoy!

Nutrition:

Calories: 160, Fat:3 g, Carbs:7 g, Protein:6 g, Sugars:20 g, Sodium:45 mg

688. Coconut Figs

Preparation Time: 6 mins
Servings: 4

Ingredients:

- 12 halved figs
- 1 c. toasted and chopped almonds
- 2 tbsps. coconut butter
- ¼ c. coconut sugar

Directions:

1. Put butter inside the pot, get hot over medium heat, add sugar, whisk well, include almonds and figs, toss, cook for 5 minutes, divide into small cups and serve cold.
2. Enjoy!

Nutrition:

Calories: 150, Fat:4 g, Carbs:7 g, Protein:4 g, Sugars:12 g, Sodium:15 mg

689. Cocoa Banana Dessert Smoothie

Preparation Time: 5 mins
Servings: 2

Ingredients:

- ½ pitted, peeled and mashed big avocado
- 2 tsps. powered cocoa
- 2 peeled medium bananas
- ¾ c. almond milk

Directions:

1. In your blender, combine the bananas with the cocoa, avocado and milk, pulse well, divide into 2 glasses and serve.
2. Enjoy!

Nutrition:

Calories: 155, Fat:3 g, Carbs:6 g, Protein:5 g, Sugars:17 g, Sodium:66 mg

690. Chocolate Pomegranate Fudge

Preparation Time: 1 hour
Servings: 6

Ingredients:

- 1 tsp. vanilla flavoring
- 1 ½ c. chopped chocolate brown
- ½ c. coconut milk
- ½ c. pomegranate seeds
- ½ c. chopped almonds

Directions:

1. Put milk in a very pan, get hot over medium-low heat, add chocolate, stir well, cook for 5 minutes, remove heat, combine with all the vanilla flavoring, 50 % from the pomegranate seeds and 50 % of the almonds, stir well, spread on the lined baking sheet, sprinkle the rest using the almonds and pomegranate seeds, keep within the fridge for just two hours, cut and serve.
2. Enjoy!

Nutrition:

Calories: 148, Fat:3 g, Carbs:6 g, Protein:5 g, Sugars:3 g, Sodium:500 mg

691. Cheese Stuffed Apples

Preparation Time: 20-25 min.
Servings: 4

Ingredients:

- 1 tbsp. raisins
- 1 whisked egg
- 8 oz. cottage cheese
- 1 tsp. confectioners' sugar
- 2 tbsps. honey
- 4 cored apples

Directions:
1. Preheat the oven to 400 0F.
2. In a mixing bowl, thoroughly mix the egg, cheese, honey, and raisins.
3. Spoon some flesh from the core part of the apples and fill with the cheese mix.
4. Bake for 18-20 minutes; top with confectioner's sugar and serve.

Nutrition:
Calories: 194, Fat:5.2 g, Carbs:23.8 g, Protein:3.6 g, Sugars:7 g, Sodium: 280mg

692. Green Apple Bowls

Preparation Time: 10 mins
Servings: 3

Ingredients:
- 1 tbsp. coconut sugar
- ½ tsp. vanilla flavoring
- 1 c. halved strawberries
- 3 cored and cubed big green apples
- ½ tsp. cinnamon powder

Directions:
1. In a bowl, combine the apples with strawberries, sugar, cinnamon and vanilla, toss and serve.
2. Enjoy!

Nutrition:
Calories: 205, Fat: 1 g, Carbs:8 g, Protein:4 g, Sugars:95 g, Sodium:9 mg

693. Peach Dip

Preparation Time: 10 mins
Servings: 2

Ingredients:
- 1 c. chopped peaches
- ½ c. nonfat yogurt
- ¼ tsp. ground nutmeg
- ¼ tsp. cinnamon powder

Directions:
1. In a bowl, combine the yogurt while using the peaches, cinnamon and nutmeg, whisk, divide into small bowls and serve being a snack.
2. Enjoy!

Nutrition:
Calories: 165, Fat:2 g, Carbs:14 g, Protein:13 g, Sugars:2 g, Sodium:2 mg

694. Cashew Nut Cuppas

Preparation Time: 15 mins
Servings: 12

Ingredients:
- 15 g coconut cream
- 85 g maple syrup
- 30 g mini dark chocolate chips.
- 255 g unsalted cashew butter
- 5 g vanilla extract
- 70 g coconut oil

Directions:
1. Preheat oven to about 400 0F.
2. In a large bowl, add the cashew butter, coconut cream, coconut oil, vanilla and maple syrup, mix well.
3. Once the mixture is smooth, grease a cupcake pan, set with liners and set aside.
4. Carefully fold in the mini-chocolate chips, remember to always fold, or else you'll end up with runny chocolate which isn't' necessarily the worst thing in the world, but still, aesthetics right?
5. Pour into pan molds, and freeze.
6. Serve whenever the cups seem to have solidified, a couple hours in the deep is perfect!

Nutrition:
Calories: 163, Fat:11.9 g, Carbs:13 g, Protein:3 g, Sugars:1.7 g, Sodium:3.4 mg

695. Pecan Granola

Preparation Time: 5 mins

Servings: 10

Ingredients:

- 50 g maple syrup
- ½ g nutmeg
- 2 ½ g salt
- 1400 g raw pecans
- 2 ½ g cayenne pepper
- 5 g ground cinnamon

Directions:

1. Preheat oven to about 400 0F.
2. In a large bowl, mix the pecans maple syrup, and spices, and toss till perfectly coated.
3. Spread out nuts on a baking sheet and roast for about 10 minutes.
4. Cool for another 10 minutes, then store or serve.

Nutrition:

Calories: 174, Fat:100.8 g, Carbs:23 g, Protein:13 g, Sugars:7 g, Sodium:135 mg

696. Walnut Green Beans

Preparation Time: 15-20 mins
Servings: 2-3

Ingredients:

- 2 c. roughly cut green beans
- 1 tbsp. olive oil
- 3 minced garlic cloves
- ½ c. chopped walnuts

Directions:

1. In a cooking pot, add and boil the beans in salted water until tender.
2. In a saucepan, add the beans, garlic, oil, and walnuts; cook for about 5-7 minutes stirring constantly.
3. Serve warm.

Nutrition:

Calories: 130, Fat:7 g, Carbs:15 g, Protein:5 g, Sugars:0 g, Sodium:104 mg

697. Banana Sashimi

Preparation Time: 5 mins
Servings: 1

Ingredients:

- ¼ tsp. chia seeds
- 15 g almond butter
- 1 medium banana

Directions:

1. Peel banana and cover one side in the nut butter, while placing it face up.
2. Slice banana evenly into even 1-centimeter thick pieces.
3. Sprinkle on toppings and serve!

Nutrition:

Calories: 194, Fat:8 g, Carbs:30 g, Protein:5 g, Sugars:0 g, Sodium:43 mg

698. Maple Malt

Preparation Time: 10 mins
Servings: 2

Ingredients:

- 2 ½ g vanilla essence
- 45 g maple syrup
- 5 g cinnamon
- 30 g chocolate
- 45 g cocoa powder
- 340 g almond milk

Directions:

1. Literally just pour it all into a saucepan and boil till it thickens.

Nutrition:

Calories: 1180, Fat:85.8 g, Carbs:80 g, Protein:40 g, Sugars:13 g, Sodium:0 mg

699. Parmesan Roasted Chickpeas

Preparation Time: 10 mins
Servings: 12

Ingredients:

- 1 tsp. thyme
- 2 crushed and minced garlic cloves
- 4 c. cooked garbanzo beans
- ½ c. fresh grated parmesan cheese
- 2 tbsps. olive oil

Directions:

1. Preheat oven to 400°F.
2. Pat dry the garbanzo beans to remove as much moisture as possible.
3. Place the garbanzo beans in bowl and combine with olive oil, garlic, thyme, and Parmesan cheese.
4. Spread the beans out on a baking sheet and place in the oven.
5. Bake for approximately 1 hour, tossing once halfway through.
6. Remove from oven and let cool before enjoying.

Nutrition:
Calories: 134.1, Fat:4.4 g, Carbs:18.3 g, Protein:5.7 g, Sugars:1 g, Sodium:202 mg

700. Apricot Nibbles

Preparation Time: 10 mins
Servings: 4

Ingredients:

- 1 tbsp. chopped pecans
- 2 tbsps. goat cheese
- Honey
- 12 dried apricots
- 1 tsp. rosemary
- 2 tbsps. blue cheese

Directions:

1. In a bowl, combine the pecans, goat cheese, blue cheese, and rosemary. Mix well. If you desire a creamier texture, place in the blender and pulse until smooth.
2. Add a dollop to the top of each dried apricot.
3. Serve with drizzled honey, if desired.

Nutrition:
Calories: 13.6, Fat:5.0 g, Carbs:20.8 g, Protein:4.1 g, Sugars:24 g, Sodium:5 mg

701. All Dressed Crispy Potato Skins

Preparation Time: 10 mins
Servings: 2

Ingredients:

- Butter-flavored cooking spray
- 1/8 tsp. freshly ground black pepper
- 1 tbsp. minced fresh rosemary
- 2 medium russet potatoes

Directions:

1. Preheat the oven to 375 0F.
2. Wash the potatoes with fresh water.
3. Pierce the potatoes with a fork.
4. Bake the potatoes in an oven about 1 hour or until the skins are crisp.
5. Cut the hot potatoes in half and scoop out most of the flesh, leaving about 1/8 inch from the skin.
6. Use a butter-flavored cooking spray to spray the insides of each potato skin.
7. Press rosemary and pepper into the potato skin.
8. Bake the potato skins again for another 5 to 10 minutes.
9. Serve immediately.

Nutrition:
Calories: 92.3, Fat:3.8 g, Carbs:9.6 g, Protein:4.6 g, Sugars:3.4 g, Sodium:803 mg

702. Delightful Coconut Shrimp

Preparation Time: 10 mins
Servings: 3

Ingredients:

- ¼ c. coconut milk
- 2 tbsps. panko breadcrumbs
- 2 tbsps. sweetened coconut
- 6 peeled and deveined large shrimp
- ¼ tsp. kosher salt

Directions:

1. Preheat your oven to 375 0F. Spray a baking sheet lightly with cooking spray.
2. Add the panko, coconut, and salt to a blender and run until the mixture has an even consistency.
3. Transfer the mixture to a small bowl. Then, pour the coconut milk into a separate small bowl.
4. Dip your shrimps in the coconut milk and then in the panko mixture one by one and place on the coated baking sheet.
5. Spray the top of the shrimps lightly with

cooking spray. Bake the coated shrimps in the oven for about ten to fifteen minutes or until golden brown.

Nutrition:

Calories: 75, Fat:4 g, Carbs:4 g, Protein:5 g, Sugars:18 g, Sodium:450 mg

703. Creamy Peanuts with Apples

Preparation Time: 10 mins
Servings: 2

Ingredients:

- 4 oz. fat-free cream cheese
- 1 tbsp. diced peanuts
- ¼ c. orange juice
- 2 cored and sliced medium apples
- 1 tbsp. brown sugar
- ¾ tsp. vanilla

Directions:

1. Set your cream cheese on the counter for about five minutes to soften it.
2. Make the dip by mixing the cream cheese, vanilla, and brown sugar in a bowl. Add peanuts and mix until combined.
3. Add the sliced apples in a separate bowl and drizzle with orange juice to stop the apples from turning brown.
4. Serve the apples with the dip and enjoy!

Nutrition:

Calories: 110, Fat:2 g, Carbs:18 g, Protein:5 g, Sugars:3 g, Sodium:140 mg

21-days meal plan

DAY	BREAKFAST	MAINS	DESSERT
1	Breakfast Granola	Lime Chicken Soup	Low Carb Chocolate Coconut Fat Bombs
2	Green Smoothie	Spinach Soup	Crunchy Cherry Chocolate Confections
3	Muffins Breakfast	Hot Turkey Meatballs	Low Carb Keto Caramels
4	Special Burrito	Cauliflower Soup	Coconut Chocolate Bars
5	Coconut and Almonds Granola	Tarragon Cod with Olives	Keto Pumpkin Fudge
6	Red Breakfast Smoothie	Kale Soup	Low-Carb, Keto Strawberry Fat Bombs
7	Tomato and Eggs Breakfast	Salmon with Balsamic Fennel	Paleo Vegan Peppermint Patties
8	Plantain Pancakes	Carrot Soup	Keto Marshmallows
9	Strawberry and Kiwi Breakfast Smoothie	Leeks Cream Soup	White Chocolate Butter Pecan Fat Bombs
10	Eggs and Artichokes	Blue Cheese Chicken Wedges	Keto Low Carb Gummy Bears
11	Beef Burrito	Lasagna Spaghetti Squash	Coconut Mousse
12	Spinach Frittata	Mashed Garlic Turnips	Low Carb Shortbread Cookies Recipe
13	Blueberry Smoothie	Green Beans Soup	Gluten-free Flourless Chocolate Cookies
14	Nuts Porridge	Chicken Chili	Cinnamon Keto French Toast Cookies
15	Breakfast Waffles	Turmeric Cauliflower and Cod Stew	Sugar-Free Paleo Pecan Snowball Cookies
16	Maple Nut Porridge	Smoked Salmon Salad	Chocolate Chip Cookies with Coconut Flour
17	Squash Blossom Frittata	Turmeric Broccoli and Leeks Stew	Low Carb Keto Cream Cheese Cookies
18	Pork Skillet	Shrimp with Zucchini	Chocolate Chip Keto Cookie
19	Sweet Potato Breakfast	Salmon and Green Beans	Blueberry Cream
20	Turkey Breakfast Sandwich	Chicken Stew	Peanut Butter Cookies
21	Eggplant French Toast	Beans and Salmon Pan	Bakery-Style' Salted Chocolate Chip Cookies

Conclusion

You do not need to stay hungry all the time to lose weight. This is the most common mistake committed by people who start a low carb diet. In the Ketogenic diet, you do not have to be scared of fats. Carbohydrates and fats are two major sources of energy for our body. If you are snatching carbs from your body, you need to give it an ample supply of fats. Low fats and low carbs equal to starvation, and we do not want that, do we? Starvation results in cravings and fatigue. That is why, people who starve give up easily on their diet plans. The better solution is to consume natural fat till the time you are satisfied.

All the best!!

Made in the USA
Columbia, SC
27 January 2020